Hypertensive Disease in
PREGNANCY

Hypertensive Disease in
PREGNANCY

Editors

Sabaratnam Arulkumaran MD PhD DSc FRCS FRCOG
Professor Emeritus of Obstetrics and Gynecology
St George's University of London
Cranmer Terrace
London, United Kingdom

Sanjay A Gupte MD DGO FICOG FRCOG (Honoris Causa) LLB
Consultant Obstetrician and Gynecologist
Director, Gupte Hospital and Center for Research in Reproduction
Pune, Maharashtra, India

Evita Fernandez FRCOG
Consultant Obstetrician and Managing Director
Fernandez Hospital Pvt Ltd
Hyderabad, Andhra Pradesh, India

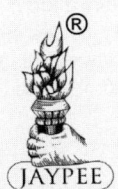

JAYPEE

JAYPEE BROTHERS MEDICAL PUBLISHERS (P) LTD

New Delhi • London • Philadelphia • Panama

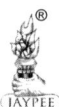

Jaypee Brothers Medical Publishers (P) Ltd

Headquarters

Jaypee Brothers Medical Publishers (P) Ltd
4838/24, Ansari Road, Daryaganj
New Delhi 110 002, India
Phone: +91-11-43574357
Fax: +91-11-43574314
Email: jaypee@jaypeebrothers.com

Overseas Offices

J.P. Medical Ltd
83, Victoria Street, London
SW1H 0HW (UK)
Phone: +44-2031708910
Fax: +02-03-0086180
Email: info@jpmedpub.com

Jaypee-Highlights.
Medical Publishers Inc
City of Knowledge, Bld. 237
Clayton, Panama City, Panama
Phone: +507-301-0496
Fax: +507-301-0499
Email: cservice@jphmedical.com

Jaypee Medical Inc.
The Bourse
111 South Independence Mall East
Suite 835, Philadelphia, PA 19106, USA
Phone: + 267-519-9789
Email: jpmed.us@gmail.com

Jaypee Brothers
Medical Publishers (P) Ltd
17/1-B Babar Road, Block-B
Shaymali, Mohammadpur
Dhaka-1207, Bangladesh
Mobile: +08801912003485
Email: jaypeedhaka@gmail.com

Jaypee Brothers
Medical Publishers (P) Ltd
Shorakhute, Kathmandu
Nepal
Phone: +00977-9841528578
Email: jaypee.nepal@gmail.com

Website: www.jaypeebrothers.com
Website: www.jaypeedigital.com

Inquiries for bulk sales may be solicited at: jaypee@jaypeebrothers.com

This book has been published in good faith that the contents provided by the contributors contained herein are original, and is intended for educational purposes only. While every effort is made to ensure accuracy of information, the publisher and the editors specifically disclaim any damage, liability, or loss incurred, directly or indirectly, from the use or application of any of the contents of this work. If not specifically stated, all figures and tables are courtesy of the editors. Where appropriate, the readers should consult with a specialist or contact the manufacturer of the drug or device.

Hypertensive Disease in Pregnancy

First Edition: 2014

ISBN 978-93-5090-951-5

Printed at: Rajkamal Electric Press, Plot No. 2, Phase-IV, Kundli, Haryana.

Contributors

Anthony Addei MBChb FRCA
Consultant Obstetric Anesthetist
St George's Healthcare, NHS Trust
London, United Kingdom

Gita Arjun FACOG
Obstetrician and Gynecologist
Director, EV Kalyani Medical
Foundation Pvt Ltd
Chennai, Tamil Nadu, India

Nishkantha Arulkumaran MBBS
MRCP
Specialist Registrar in Critical Care
and Nephrology, Wellcome Trust
Research Fellow University College
London, United Kingdom

Sabaratnam Arulkumaran MD
PhD DSc FRCS FRCOG
Professor Emeritus of
Obstetrics and Gynecology
St George's University of London
Cranmer Terrace
London, United Kingdom

Michael A Belfort MD PhD
Professor of Obstetrics and
Gynecology
Chairman of the Department of
Obstetrics and Gynecology
Baylor College of Medicine
Houston, Texas, USA

Nirmala Chandrasekaran MRCOG
Clinical Fellow
Fetal Medicine Unit
St George's Hospital
NHS Trust, London, United Kingdom

Rana Choudhary DNB (Obs & Gyne)
DGO FCPS DFP MNAMS
Project Research Officer
Department of Clinical Research
National Institute for Research in
Reproductive Health (NIRRH)
Indian Council of Medical
Research (ICMR)
Parel, Mumbai, Maharashtra, India

Jarita Deb DGO MD (Obs/Gyn)
Research Consultant
Divakars Speciality Hospital
Bengaluru, Karnataka, India

Hema Divakar DGO MD (Obs/Gyn)
Consultant Obstetrician and
Gynecologist
Divakars Speciality Hospital
Bengaluru, Karnataka, India

Evita Fernandez FRCOG
Consultant Obstetrician and
Managing Director
Fernandez Hospital Pvt Ltd
Hyderabad, Andhra Pradesh, India

Sirisha Rao Gundabattula MD
Consultant Gynecologist
Fernandez Hospital Pvt. Ltd.
Hyderabad, Andhra Pradesh, India

Sanjay A Gupte MD DGO FICOG
FRCOG (Honoris Causa) LLB
Consultant Obstetrician and
Gynecologist
Director, Gupte Hospital and Center
for Research in Reproduction
Pune, Maharashtra, India

Boon H Lim MBBS FRCOG
FRANZCOG
Associate Professor and Director
Department of Obstetrics and
Gynecology
Royal Hobart Hospital
Hobart, Tasmania, Australia

Gorakh G Mandrupkar MBBS
DGO FCPS
Incharge, High Risk Pregnancy Unit
Prakash Memorial Clinic
Islampur, Maharashtra, India

Isaac T Manyonda BSc PhD
MRCOG FICOG (Hon)
Professor and Consultant
Department of Obstetrics and
Gynecology
St George's Hospital
NHS Trust, London, United Kingdom

Hiten D Mistry BSc (Hons) PhD
Division of Women's Health
Women's Health Academic Center
KHP King's College
London School of Medicine
North Wing
St Thomas' Hospital
Westminster, London
United Kingdom

Suchitra N Pandit MD FRCOG
DNB DFP FICOG B Pharma MNAMS
Senior Consultant
Obstetrics and Gynecology
Kokilaben Dhirubhai
Ambani Hospital and
Research Center
Mumbai Maharashtra, India
President, Mumbai Society of OBS/GYN
President Elect FOGSI 2014
Fellow of Executive Council
West Zone RCOG, India

Fiona Broughton Pipkin MA
DPhil FRCOG ad eundem
Emeritus Professor of
Perinatal Physiology
Department of Obstetrics and
Gynecology
Maternity Unit, City Hospital
Nottingham, United Kingdom

Lavanya Rai MD DGO
Professor and Head
Department of Obstetrics and
Gynecology
Kasturba Medical College
Manipal, Bengaluru
Karnataka, India

PK Shah MD FCPS FICOG FICMU
DGO DEP
Professor
Department of Obstetrics and
Gynecology
Seth GS Medical College and
King Edward VII
Memorial Hospital
Mumbai, Maharashtra, India

Vikram Sinai Talaulikar MD MRCOG

Clinical Research Fellow
Department of Obstetrics and
Gynecology
Clinical Sciences Jenner 1
St George's University of
London, Cranmer Terrace
London, United Kingdom

Parikshit D Tank MD DNB FCPS
DGO DFP MNAMS MICOG MRCOG
Consultant, Ashwini Maternity and
Surgical Hospital
Center for Endoscopy and
Assisted Reproduction
Honorary Clinical Associate
Nowrosjee Wadia Maternity Hospital
Mumbai, Maharashtra, India

Basky Thilaganathan MD FRCOG

Professor and Director
Fetal Medicine Unit
St George's Hospital
NHS Trust, London
United Kingdom

Alex C Vidaeff MD MPH

Professor
Division of Maternal-Fetal Medicine
Department of Obstetrics and
Gynecology, Baylor College of
Medicine, Texas Children's Hospital
Pavillion for Women
Maine Street
Suite F 1020 Houston
Texas, USA

Girija Wagh MD FICOG
Dip Endoscopy
Professor and Head
Obstetrics and Gynecology
Bharati Vidyapeeth University
Medical College
Pune, Maharashtra, India
Consultant, Girija
Hospital and Meera Hospital
Pune, Maharashtra, India

Adele Zito B Med Sci MBBS (Hons)
Specialist Registrar
Department of Obstetrics and
Gynecology
Royal Hobart Hospital
Hobart, Tasmania, Australia

Preface

Out of the eight the Millennium Development Goals, the fifth goal had an ambitious target of reducing the maternal mortality of 540,000 per year in the 1990s by 75% by the year 2015. The 2010 estimates suggest that the mortality has reduced to 280,000 per year, i.e. less than the target but substantial reduction. Hypertensive disorders in pregnancy is the second highest direct cause of maternal deaths globally. Maternal death is the tip of the iceberg—for every death, twenty mothers suffer morbidity. The perinatal wastage due to preterm birth, intrauterine growth restriction, stillbirths and early neonatal deaths are far greater in magnitude than the maternal problems.

Although hypertensive disease in pregnancy is common, it carries major morbidity and mortality in the mother and the offspring. Very few texts are available to cover the entire spectrum of this bizarre illness. Hence, seventeen chapters are dedicated to this enigmatic condition. Chapter 1 deals with the classification with a practical approach useful to the clinician. Chapter 2 provides information on the etiology and the pathophysiology that is essential to understand the nature of the illness. Biochemical and biophysical prediction, maternal vascular differences and possible prevention strategies are discussed in Chapters 3, 4 and 5. If it cannot be prevented, it need to be treated and is discussed in Chapter 6 followed by fetal (Chapter 7) and maternal assessment (Chapter 8). Medical disorders can give rise to hypertension and may mimic or complicate pregnancy-induced hypertension. The different conditions that can give rise to hypertension are discussed in Chapter 9. Complications that lead to severe morbidity could be typical like the HELLP syndrome (Chapter 10) or atypical (Chapter 11) and are discussed in detail. Timing and mode of delivery need to consider several factors and similar consideration is essential for analgesia and anesthesia and is tackled in Chapters 12 and 13.

Management of second and third stage poses special problems in hypertensive disease and are described in Chapter 14 followed by care of the critically ill hypertensive mother (Chapter 15). Mothers who have hypertensive disease in pregnancy may develop hypertension after the delivery and slowly progress to become candidates with cardiac and hypertensive cerebrovascular complications. Regular follow-up should be arranged and any hypertension and its complications properly treated. This important aspect is discussed in Chapter 16. Despite good knowledge and facilities, still we loose mothers. Confidential inquiries into maternal deaths identify two-thirds of the deaths to have had substandard care and teach us very valuable lessons. These are provided in Chapter 17. These chapters should provide the comprehensive knowledge needed by a health care professional to provide the best of care for a pregnant mother with hypertension.

This book may not be perfect and may have inadvertent mistakes or points of confusion or contention. The editors would be grateful if the readers could contact any of the editors or publishers so that we can correct factual errors and clarify any misunderstanding.

Sabaratnam Arulkumaran
Sanjay A Gupte
Evita Fernandez

Acknowledgments

The editors are privileged to have internationally renowned experts to contribute chapters to this comprehensive book. We are most grateful to them. Our publishers M/s Jaypee Brothers Medical Publishers (P) Ltd, New Delhi, India, deserve a special mention for their patience and hard work. To our families we are indebted for the time away from them. Our gratitude to all our patients, as we learn from the experiences of providing the care and interacting with colleagues.

Contents

xviii

1 Classification and Diagnosis of Hypertensive Disorders of Pregnancy: A Practical Approach

Sanjay A Gupte, Girija Wagh

■ INTRODUCTION

The very first step of effective treatment of hypertensive disorders in pregnancy (HTNP) is diagnosis and classification. The literature is rife with several definitions of HTNP for the purpose of research as well as clinical management. In the current context we need to identify the most practical and acceptable definition to aid quick and correct diagnosis. This has to be followed up with the classification of the disorder to identify the systemic involvement, prognosticate the outcome and plan prompt interventions.

Many classifications have been promoted by different groups of experts or representative bodies.[1-5] These have led to confusion and difficulties in interpretation. The availability of investigative modalities to identify mothers at risk, fetal compromise and laboratory evaluations for multisystemic involvement were not available when the older classification systems were proposed.[6,7] The recent classifications are better for clinical usage and a superior reflection of associated pathophysiology.

■ DEFINITION OF HYPERTENSION DURING PREGNANCY

Hypertension during pregnancy is defined as systolic blood pressure (SBP) greater than or equal to 140 mm Hg or diastolic blood pressure (DBP) greater than or equal to 90 mm Hg with the patient sitting quietly (10 minutes), by a mercury sphygmomanometer with the right arm cuff at the heart level. The 5th Korotkoff (K5) sound is used to mark the DBP. Where K5 is absent, 4th Korotkoff sound

should be accepted.[8] The reading of 140/90 mm Hg is included in the definition because above these levels both the adverse fetal outcome and perinatal mortality was seen to rise.[9]

The correct diagnosis and classification of HTNP is essential for proper management of the mother and the baby. The classification proposed by the International Society for the Study of Hypertension in Pregnancy (ISSHP)[10] is easy to use in clinical settings (Table 1.1).[11,12] It is also self-explanatory and practical.

Gestational Hypertension

Gestational hypertension is characterized by mild to moderate elevation of blood pressure after 20 weeks of gestation without proteinuria. Occasionally, severe hypertension may be encountered to begin with which later may manifest other signs and symptoms of preeclampsia. The cause of gestational hypertension is unclear. However, it appears to identify women destined to develop essential hypertension in later life similar to the correlation of gestational diabetes to the subsequent development of type 2 diabetes mellitus.[13,14] Blood pressure returns to normal during the immediate puerperium. Thus, the diagnosis of gestational hypertension is always retrospective. Such women may present as hypertensive in all or most of their subsequent pregnancies.[15]

Preeclampsia

Hypertension after 20 weeks of pregnancy with proteinuria is defined as preeclampsia, a condition which is a serious disorder with a broad clinical

Table 1.1: The ISSHP classification of hypertension in pregnancy[11,12]

Gestational hypertension	• Hypertension that:
	  – develops beyond 20 weeks of gestation
	  – returns to normal within 42nd postpartum day and
	  – is not associated with any other features of preeclampsia
		6–7% of pregnancies

Preeclampsia/eclampsia	• Hypertension presenting beyond 20 weeks of gestation with > 300 mg protein in a 24 hour urine collection or 1+ (0.3 g/L) on urine dipstick. • Eclampsia is the occurrence of seizures in a pregnant woman with preeclampsia	5–7% of pregnancies
Chronic hypertension	• Blood pressure—140/90 mm Hg • Present before pregnancy, before the 20th week of gestation, or persisting beyond the 42nd post-partum day	1–5% of pregnancies
Preeclampsia superim-posed on chronic hyperten-sion	• The onset of features diagnostic of preeclampsia in a woman with chronic hypertension beyond 20 weeks of gestation	20–25% of chronic hyper-tension pregnancies

Source: Report of the National High Blood Pressure Education Program Working Group on High Blood Pressure in Pregnancy. Am J Obstet Gynecol. 2000;183(1):S1-S22.
European Society of Gynecology (ESG), Association for European Paediatric Cardiology (AEPC), German Society for Gender Medicine (DGesGM), et al. ESC guidelines on the management of cardiovascular disease during pregnancy: the Task Force on the Management of Cardiovascular Diseases during Pregnancy of the European Society of Cardiology (ESC). Eur Heart J. 2011;32(24):3147-97.

spectrum. Preeclampsia is a multisystemic disorder primarily characterized by new onset hypertension and proteinuria in pregnancy. Proteinuria is defined as an excretion of 300 mg/24 hour, a urine protein/creatinine ratio of 0.3, or a qualitative 1+ dipstick reading.

Preeclampsia is a pregnancy-specific condition characterized by placental dysfunction and a maternal response featuring systemic inflammation with activation of the endothelium and coagulation. This multifactorial disease presents as a syndrome of symptoms and signs with associated hematological and biochemical abnormalities. Most consider hypertension and proteinuria to be the hallmarks of preeclampsia, but the clinical manifestation of this syndrome is heterogeneous. Some women develop severe maternal disease requiring intensive care, whereas others remain asymptomatic with mild hypertension and proteinuria. The condition is also associated with adverse neonatal outcomes. Experience shows that the hostile (immunological) response to the pregnancy by the maternal body is an ongoing process which is usually contained by

the protective mechanisms of the body. But there appears to be a "turning point" when suddenly this process of protection is overwhelmed and the cascade of preeclampsia syndrome ensues.

It is also recommended that preeclampsia may be diagnosed when hypertension rises after 20 weeks and is associated with any of the following complications like renal (significant proteinuria, serum or plasma creatinine > 90 µmol/L, oliguria), hepatic (raised serum transaminases, severe epigastric or right upper quadrant pain), hematological [thrombocytopenia, hemolysis, disseminated intravascular coagulation (DIC)] or neurologic involvement (eclampsia, hyperreflexia).[16]

Atypical Preeclampsia

Hypertension and proteinuria before 20 weeks (e.g in gestational trophoblastic disease), pre-eclampsia with hypertension but without proteinuria or preeclampsia with proteinuria without hypertension when associated with above mentioned systemic involvement is designated at atypical preeclampsia. Preeclampsia arising first time after 48 hours of delivery can also be included in this definition.[17] This is an important entity for diagnosis and management of certain unusual cases. This has been elaborated in Chapter 11 by Prof Alex Vidaeff.

Eclampsia is defined as the development of grand mal seizures in a woman with preeclampsia. It is the most severe and life-threatening manifestation, with an estimated incidence of 4–5 cases per 10,000 live births.[18] Eclampsia usually is preceded by a history of preeclampsia but rarely may arise in a woman with minimally increased blood pressure and no proteinuria. There is significant risk of cardiorespiratory arrest during or after the seizure. Seventy-two percent of eclamptic seizures occur in the antepartum period, 9% are intrapartum and 28% occur in the postpartum period. Late postpartum seizures, arising more than 48 hours after delivery, are increasingly documented.[19] The FOGSI-ICOG (Federation of Obstetrics and Gynaecological Societies of India- Indian College of Obstetrics and Gynaecology) National Eclampsia Registry (NER) reveals eclampsia prevalence among registry patients as 1.9%. This is out of the 111,725 deliveries analyzed and reported by the 175 reporting centers. Interestingly out of all the eclampsia reported in the NER 76.78% were antepartum, 9.5% were intrapartum and 13.72% were postpartum.

Gestational Hypertension and Preeclampsia

Gestational hypertension and preeclampsia are separate disease processes with different mechanisms. Nulliparity is a strong preeclampsia risk factor while it is not so for gestational hypertension. Preeclampsia is associated with specific histologic changes in the placenta and kidneys and also increase in antiangiogenic peptides which is not so in gestational hypertension. The total circulating volume is lower in women with preeclampsia compared to women with gestational hypertension.[20]

Chronic Hypertension

It is defined as hypertension that presents before pregnancy or within the first 20 weeks of gestation.[21]

About 1–5% pregnancies are associated but the incidence may be underestimated.[10] Women classified as chronic hypertension have essential hypertension (90%), mostly mild in intensity to begin with and their pregnancies are many a times uncomplicated though some variables may occur with grave outcomes.[22] Advanced maternal age, obesity ($> 30 \, kg/m^2$), heredity, race and diabetes are identified risk factors. They are at an increased risk for the development of superimposed preeclampsia and abruptio placentae.[23] Less commonly (10%), chronic hypertension is secondary to specific causes such as underlying kidney disease, collagen vascular diseases (systemic lupus erythematosus, scleroderma and periarteritis nodosa), endocrine disorders (diabetes mellitus, pheochromocytoma, thyrotoxicosis, hyperaldosteronism, Cushing's disease) or other vascular diseases (coarctation of the aorta, renal artery stenosis). Women with such secondary chronic hypertension may have grave obstetric outcomes.[24,25] Pheochromocytoma, although rare, may present for the first time during pregnancy and is especially fatal when unsuspected, but if diagnosed it can be managed to a successful outcome, either surgically or pharmacologically, depending on the gestational period.[26,27] Chronic hypertension may be masked by physiological hemodynamic changes in pregnancy, in particular the second trimester reduction in arterial blood pressure, secondary to increasing vasodilatation. Women presenting with hypertension in the first half of pregnancy should be evaluated keeping in mind the above mentioned causes.

Preeclampsia Superimposed on Chronic Hypertension

The onset of features diagnostic of preeclampsia in a woman with chronic hypertension beyond 20 weeks of gestation is classified as superimposed preeclampsia. This may include new onset of proteinuria, thrombocytopenia ($< 100,000/\mu L$) or any other systemic involvement of preeclampsia. Pre-existing hypertension is a strong risk factor for development of eclampsia.

Paradox

In spite of such elaborate classification it is tempting to say that there is no need to classify hypertensive disorders in clinical practice. Presence of rising blood pressure should alert the clinician to seek evidence for the development of preeclampsia and associated abnormalities of fetal growth and/or maternal renal, cerebral, hepatic or coagulation functions which may necessitate specific interventions. This is more so in low resource countries like India where traditional health workers in remote areas can be provided with modified blood pressure apparatuses with which they may be able to detect only systolic blood pressures (SBP) as the risk factor for early referral and further management.

CLINICAL CLASSIFICATION OF PREECLAMPSIA

Classification as early onset preeclampsia and late onset preeclampsia is clinically useful (Table 1.2). Appearance of preeclampsia before 34 weeks is called as early onset preeclampsia. Early preeclampsia is associated with greater morbidity[28] (four-fold increased risk of stillbirth in a subsequent pregnancy, higher recurrence risk in subsequent pregnancy than when the disorder presents later). In this context, suggestions are made to subdivide preeclampsia into two groups by time of onset because of differences in prognosis and management.[29] This distinction is held important as there is a suspicion that these two are separate entities with distinct predisposing factors.

The early onset disease may be associated with the underlying genetic or environmental factors leading to abnormal placentation. The late onset disease may be the result of obesity, diabetes, cardiovascular abnormalities or multifetal pregnancy.

SEVERITY CLASSIFICATION OF PREECLAMPSIA

Preeclampsia is a syndrome with a significant potential for fetal and maternal morbidity and mortality. These specific risks not only depend upon the gestational age at the time of disease onset and/or presence of comorbidities, but also on the severity of the condition. Severe preeclampsia is characterized by advent of coagulation or liver function abnormalities, occurs commonly in nulliparous usually after 20 weeks of gestation, and most frequently near term. Several classifications for disease severity in preeclampsia are proposed. These are based on the severity of hypertension, timing of delivery and pregnancy outcome. The National Institute for Health and Clinical Excellence (NICE, UK) classification of severity is based on blood pressure measurement (Table 1.3). American College of Obstetricians and Gynecologists (ACOG) classifies severity based on blood pressure measurement as well as the presence of signs of systemic involvement (Table 1.4).

HELLP SYNDROME

HELLP is a severe form of preeclampsia which includes hemolysis (abnormal blood smear, LDH > 600 IU, elevated indirect bilirubin), elevated

Table 1.2: Clinical classification of preeclampsia	
Early Onset Pre-eclampsia (Before 34 Weeks)	Late Onset Preeclampsia (After 34 Weeks)
• A fetal disorder that is typically associated with placental dysfunction	• Maternal disorder due to underlying maternal constitutional factors
• Reduction in placental volume	• Normal or larger placental volume
• Intrauterine growth restriction	• Normal fetal growth
• Abnormal uterine and umbilical artery Doppler evaluation	• Normal uterine and umbilical artery Doppler evaluation
• Low birthweight	• Normal birthweight
• Adverse maternal and neonatal outcomes	• More favorable maternal and neonatal outcomes

Table 1.3: Severity classification NICE UK based on blood pressure measurement	
NICE Severity Classification	Blood Pressure
• Mild	• 140–149 mm Hg systolic and/or 90–99 mm Hg diastolic
• Moderate	• 150–159 mm Hg systolic and/or 100–109 mm Hg diastolic
• Severe	• ≥ 160 mm Hg systolic and/or ≥ 110 mm Hg diastolic

Table 1.4: ACOG severity classification—blood pressure along with signs and systemic involvement	
• Mild to Moderate	• Blood Pressure (BP) is 140–159 mm Hg Systolic and/or 90–109 mm Hg Diastolic
• Severe (any two if present)	• BP is ≥ 160 mm Hg systolic and/or ≥ 110 mm Hg diastolic (on two occasions at least 6 hours apart, while the patient is on bed rest) • Proteinuria of ≥ 5 g/24 hours or ≥ 3+ (on two random urine samples, collected at least 4 hours apart). • Oliguria < 500 mL/24 hours • Cerebral or visual disturbances • Pulmonary edema or cyanosis • Epigastric or right upper quadrant pain • Impaired liver function • Thrombocytopenia

Table 1.5: HELLP syndrome classified on the basis of platelet count	
Class of HELLP	*Platelet count*
I	• < 50,000 per mm^3 (50 × 10^9 per L)
II	• 50,000 to < 100,000 per mm^3 (50–100 × 10^9 per L)
III	• 100,000–150,000 per mm^3 (100–150 × 10^9 per L)

hepatic enzymes (transaminases > 70 IU) and thrombocytopenia (platelets < 100,000/mL).[26] This complex syndrome occurs in approximately 10% of patients with preeclampsia and is associated with significant perinatal morbidity and mortality.[30] Common presenting complaints are right upper quadrant or epigastric pain, nausea and vomiting which may indicate hepatocellular injury such as subcapsular hematomas.[26] None of these symptoms may be present and only nonspecific symptoms such as malaise could be present.[30] The clinical features are similar to hemolytic uremic syndrome (HUS) and thrombotic thrombocytopenic purpura (TTP).[31] The clinical evaluation of preeclampsia patient should include a vigilance to detect HELLP syndrome. The maternal complications like acute renal failure, hemorrhage and neonatal complications like acute respiratory failure, hypoxic damage due to placental abruption, low birth weight, sudden neonatal death, are associated.[26,30]

Classification of HELLP

HELLP syndrome is classified either based on the number of abnormalities viz: (1) hemolysis, (2) thrombocytopenia and (3) elevated liver enzymes or by the range of the platelet count. In the first classification (Tennessee classification) based on the number of the three abnormalities patients are categorized as having partial HELLP syndrome with one or two abnormalities or full HELLP syndrome with all the three abnormalities. Women with full HELLP syndrome are at a higher risk for complications, including DIC, than women with the partial syndrome. Consequently, patients with the full syndrome should be considered for delivery within 48 hours, whereas those with partial HELLP syndrome may be candidates for temporizing.[32]

Alternatively, HELLP syndrome can be classified on the basis of platelet count as given in Table 1.5. This is the Mississippi or the Martin classification of HELLP.[33] Patients with class I HELLP syndrome are at higher risk for maternal morbidity and mortality than patients with class II or III HELLP syndrome. The utility of specific classifications as prognostic tools were compared and it was concluded that both models classified patients according to different criteria but were correlated with mortality. The two models seem to be complimentary. Development of an aggregate classification could refine the models.[34]

DIAGNOSIS OF HYPERTENSION IN PREGNANCY

Abnormal blood pressure reading is the first clue for the diagnosis of HTNP. Every pregnancy should be considered as a potentially dangerous one for the appearance of preeclampsia and appropriate laboratory tests should be performed. Women with the following features should be more closely evaluated and monitored:[31] first pregnancy, older maternal age, previous preeclampsia, duration of 10 years or more since last baby, body mass index greater than or equal to 35 kg/m², family history of hypertension, patient who herself is low birth weight, DBP greater than or equal to 80 mm Hg at booking, proteinuria (≥ +1 on more than one occasion and ≥ 0.3 g/24 hours), multiple pregnancy, underlying medical condition (pre-existing hypertension, diabetes, renal disease, presence of antiphospholipid antibodies, other thrombophilias, and autoimmune disease and infertility).

Hypertension in pregnancy always cannot be diagnosed definitively. Taking this into account both the ACOG[8] and the National High Blood Pressure Education Program (NHBPEP) Working Group (2000)[11] recommend more frequent prenatal visits even if preeclampsia is only suspected. Traditionally these visits increase in frequency toward the third trimester and this is of help in early detection of HTNP. Abnormal blood pressure reading can act as a starting point for investigations and warn the clinician to better plan the antenatal care. Blood pressure recorded as 140/90 mm Hg or more anytime during pregnancy needs evaluation and classification which would need laboratory investigations to help correctly segregate this diagnosis.

Existing chronic hypertension may be masked in early pregnancy because of the initial decrease in pressure. When the hypertension reappears later in the gestation, it may be misdiagnosed as a gestation-specific disorder. The absence of normal midpregnancy decrease in the DBP has been reported to be an early sign to be associated with hypertension.[35] In the past an increase of 15 mm Hg diastolic and 30 mm Hg systolic, respectively, even if the final value of 140/90 mm Hg was absent was also included in the definition. However, data demonstrating similar outcomes irrespective of the magnitude of rise when values remain less than 140/90 mm Hg, have led consensus groups to delete this latter definition. Nevertheless, the NHBPEP consensus report[11] stressed that patients with blood pressure readings below the 140/90 mm Hg cutoff who have experienced a 30 or 15 mm Hg rise in systolic and diastolic levels, respectively, be watched closely.

Proteinuria

Proteinuria is defined as the presence of 300 mg/L or more protein in a 24 hour urine specimen. This finding many times correlates with a finding of +1 or greater on the uristick measurements. The dipstick value of 1+ has many false-positive and false-negative results and is the least useful.[11,36] A diluted (< 1,010 specific gravity) or concentrated (> 1,030 specific gravity) urine or an alkaline specimen (pH > 8) may produce false results when tested with the reagent strips. Accurately, timed urine collections are difficult to obtain during pregnancy, and theoretically a urine creatinine/protein ratio eliminates such errors. Absence of proteins on dipstick needs further evaluation either by 24 hour urinary proteins or micro albuminuria. Like hypertension, proteinuria too is a poor predictor of either maternal (eclampsia, placental abruption) or fetal (still birth, neonatal or infant death or neonatal intensive care unit admission) complications.[37] Data from the Preeclampsia Integrated Estimate of Risk (PIERS)[38] study supports this observation.[39] NICE guideline recommends that once proteinuria is detected repeat measurements are not necessary and should not be used to guide clinical interventions.[40]

Weight Gain and Edema

Rapid weight gain and appearance of edema were considered the harbingers of preeclampsia in the past. Severe generalized edema or sudden weight gain in pregnancy may still prove to be significant early warning signs in the hands of the traditional health workers in remote areas in low resource settings.

■ SYMPTOMS

Preeclampsia is a strange condition which does not have any specific signs or symptoms of its own. Many vague signs and symptoms are associated. These can vary from something as basic as headache, nausea and vomiting to more ominous right upper quadrant or epigastric pain, chest pain or dyspnea and visual disturbances. Most of these symptoms are nonspecific and common in pregnancy and use of these for clinical diagnosis and severity assessment are controversial. Some workers found visual disturbances and epigastric pain to be associated with adverse maternal complications[41] while others found nausea and vomiting in the presence of HELLP syndrome like picture to be better associated[42] PIERS database found chest pain and dyspnea as predictors of adverse maternal outcomes but poor correlation was observed.[43] Thus, evidence suggests that symptoms are of limited value in risk assessment and should not guide clinical management.

■ LABORATORY EVALUATION

Women with chronic hypertension most likely have essential hypertension and baseline workup should be undertaken. Secondary causes too should be considered and appropriate relevant workup can be commenced. Women with suspected preeclampsia should undergo evaluation for end organ involvement and also to enable differential diagnoses. Hemoglobin may be higher due to hemoconcentration in the absence of microangiopathic anemia. Exaggerated neutrophilia may give rise to raised white blood cell and differential counts. Lower platelet counts aid in diagnosing and classifying HELLP. Peripheral smear showing microangiopathy with red blood cell fragments is characteristic of preeclampsia. Liver enzymes, aspartate aminotransferase; alanine aminotransferase are raised and are signs of liver involvement. Glucose levels are found to be low in acute fatty liver of pregnancy (AFLP). Renal function is assessed by serum creatinine and serum uric acid estimation. Increased breakdown of purines in the ischemic placenta leading to overproduction of uric acid may explain increased serum uric acid levels in preeclampsia. Tests for coagulation, such as activated partial thromboplastin time, international normalized ratio (INR), are recommended in the presence of thrombocytopenia or placental abruption. The validity of these tests either alone or in combination for prediction of adverse outcomes and the critical values for intervention has not been established.[44]

Initial laboratory test recommended by most of the guidelines for surveillance of severity are platelet count (< 100,000/mL), elevated creatinine (> 0.9 IU) raised liver enzymes, raised lactate dehydrogenase (LDH) (> 600). The SOMANZ[45] strongly recommend delivery in view of these parameters. Platelet counts less than 100,000/mL

have been found to be associated with adverse maternal and perinatal outcome,[46,47] while PIERS[38] database showed the utility of this level of platelets to be borderline in predicting adverse maternal outcomes, such an association with adverse fetal outcome is not evaluated. Likewise creatinine levels, uric acid levels, liver enzymes and LDH levels have been identified as risk factors and diagnostic parameters but cannot be used to predict adverse outcomes accurately.[48]

Hemodynamic Investigations

Preeclampsia is characterized by abnormal placentation. Uterine artery Doppler velocimetry may be useful in hypertensive pregnant women to support a placental origin for the hypertension, proteinuria and/or adverse conditions.[49] Umbilical artery Doppler velocimetry too may be useful. Absent or reversed end-diastolic flow in the umbilical artery would be more consistent with placental dysfunction than with decreased biological growth potential, incorrect dates, or aneuploidy as a cause of fetal growth restriction.

■ DIFFERENTIAL DIAGNOSIS

Wrong diagnosis is possible in preeclampsia patients especially with liver involvement, epigastric and right upper quadrant pain. Other diagnoses include hepatitis, gallbladder disease, peptic ulcer, gastroenteritis, pyelonephritis, nephrolithiasis, Reye's syndrome, AFLP, TTP and HUS.

Likewise in case of seizures a differential diagnosis of epilepsy, intracranial hemorrhage and thrombosis, rupture of cerebral aneurysm, meningitis, encephalitis, cerebral tumors, cerebral malaria should be borne in mind. Having said so it should be a ground rule that any convulsion in the later part of pregnancy should be considered as eclampsia unless proved otherwise.

■ CHALLENGES IN THE LOW RESOURCE SETTINGS

Low resource settings have altogether different challenges. The first issue is that the actual prevalence of the disease is unknown in most of the low and middle income countries. Low utilization and availability of the antenatal care is identified as a single deficiency contributing towards adverse obstetric outcomes. There also is a marked divide of health care access between the rural and urban population and the often observed delays are in triage, transport and treatment. Adoption of the standards of practice can be difficult in these settings due to lack of facility and resources. In such situations task shifting to the community level workers is important so that early detection of the disease can be undertaken based on risk assessment, signs and symptoms. The basic model consisting of increasing awareness amongst the community about the disease, and training community health workers in identifying the basic signs and symptoms and variables like maternal weight gain SBP, dipstick proteinuria can be adopted for early diagnosis.[29]

CONCLUSION

Hypertension in pregnancy is a major cause of maternal mortality and morbidity worldwide. Classification and early diagnosis is a challenge and prediction of adverse outcomes is a further challenge. Many international guidelines are in place for classification and assessment of the HTNP and therefore we have presented a practical guideline which is clinically useful. Some important points to remember have been listed in Box 1.1.

Box 1.1: Important points

- Existing classification systems and the one proposed by ISSHP is of value but has limitations due to its inability to predict adverse outcomes.
- Severity criteria as a single entity and in combination have limitations. The clinician should understand and take appropriate decisions with a complete overview.
- Standardization of antenatal interventions and surveillance for women with HTNP has shown improved outcomes and this therefore needs to be stressed.
- If we truly have to make a difference to the appalling maternal mortality and morbidity, clinical classification is more important for management.
- We have to find simpler ways of early detection for low resource settings that will bring about early referral to the community health worker to facilitate further treatment.

REFERENCES

1. Brown MA, Hague WM, Higgins J, et al. The detection, investigation and management of hypertension in pregnancy: full consensus statement. Aust N Z J Obstet Gynaecol. 2000;40(2):139-55.
2. Davey DA, MacGillivray I. The classification and definition of the hypertensive disorders of pregnancy. Am J Obstet Gynecol. 1988;158(4):892-8.
3. Helewa ME, Burrows RF, Smith J, et al. Report of the Canadian Hypertension Society Consensus Conference: 1. Definitions, evaluation and classification of hypertensive disorders in pregnancy. CMAJ. 1997;157(6):715-25.
4. Hughes EC (Ed). Obstetric–Gynecologic Terminology. Philadelphia: Davis; 1972. pp. 422-3.
5. Redman CW, Jefferies M. Revised definition of preeclampsia. Lancet. 1988;1(8589):809-12.
6. Chappell L, Poulton L, Halligan A, et al. Lack of consistency in research papers over the definition of pre-eclampsia. Br J Obstet Gynaecol. 1999; 106(9):983-5.
7. Harlow FH, Brown MA. The diversity of diagnoses of preeclampsia. Hypertens Pregnancy. 2001;20(1): 57-67.
8. ACOG Committee on Practice Bulletins—Obstetrics. ACOG practice bulletin. Diagnosis and management of preeclampsia and eclampsia. Number 33, January 2002. Obstet Gynecol. 2002;99(1):159-67.
9. MacGillivray I. Pre-eclampsia. The hypertensive diseases of pregnancy. London: WB Saunders; 1983. pp. 174-90.
10. Brown MA, Lindheimer MD, de Swiet M, et al. The classification and diagnosis of the hypertensive disorders of pregnancy: statement from the International Society for the Study of Hypertension in Pregnancy (ISSHP). Hypertens Pregnancy. 2001;20(1):9-14.
11. Report of the National High Blood Pressure Education Program Working Group on High Blood Pressure in Pregnancy. Am J Obstet Gynecol. 2000;183(1): S1-S22.
12. European Society of Gynecology (ESG), Association for European Paediatric Cardiology (AEPC), German Society for Gender Medicine (DGesGM), et al. ESC guidelines on the management of cardiovascular disease during pregnancy: the Task Force on the Management of Cardiovascular Diseases during Pregnancy of the European Society of Cardiology (ESC). Eur Heart J. 2011;32(24):3147-97.
13. Fisher KA, Luger A, Spargo BH, et al. Hypertension in pregnancy: clinical-pathological correlations and remote prognosis. Medicine (Baltimore). 1981; 60(4):267-76.

14. Villar J, Carroli G, Wojdyla D, et al. Preeclampsia, gestational hypertension and intrauterine growth restriction, related or independent conditions? Am J Obstet Gynecol. 2006;194(4):921-31.

15. Lindheimer MD, Taler SJ, Cunningham FG. Hypertension in Pregnancy. J Am Soc Hypertens. 2008;2(6):484-94.

16. South Australian Perinatal Practice Guidelines Workgroup. Hypertensive disorders in pregnancy. South Australian Perinatal Practice Guidelines workgroup at: cywhs.perinatalprotocol@health. sa.gov.au,2008.

17. Sibai BM, Stella CL. Diagnosis and management of atypical preeclampsia-eclampsia. Am J Obstet Gynecol. 2009;200(5):481.el-7.

18. Douglas KA, Redman CW. Eclampsia in the United Kingdom. BMJ. 1994;309(6966):1395-400.

19. Hirshfeld-Cytron J, Lam C, Karumanchi SA, et al. Late postpartum eclampsia: examples and review. Obstet Gynecol Surv. 2006;61(7):471-80.

20. Silver HM, Seebeck M, Carlson R. Comparison of total blood volume in normal, preeclamptic, and nonproteinuric gestational hypertensive pregnancy by simultaneous measurement of red blood cell and plasma volumes. Am J Obstet Gynecol. 1998; 179(1):87-93.

21. Roberts CL, Bell JC, Ford JB, et al. The accuracy of reporting of the hypertensive disorders of pregnancy in population health data. Hypertens Pregnancy. 2008;27(3):285-97.

22. Sibai BM, Abdella TN, Anderson GD. Pregnancy outcome in 211 patients with mild chronic hypertension. Obstet Gynecol. 1983;61(5):571-6.

23. Cunningham FG, MacDonald PC, Gant NF. Hypertensive disorders in pregnancy. In: Cunningham FG, MacDonald PC, Gant NF (Eds). Williams Obstetrics, 18th edition. Norwalk, CT: Appleton & Lange; 1989. pp. 653-94.

24. Lindheimer MD, Katz AI. Hypertension in pregnancy. N Engl J Med. 1985;313(11):675-80.

25. National High Blood Pressure Education Program Working Group report on high blood pressure during pregnancy. Am J Obstet Gynecol. 1990;163(5 Pt 1): 1691-712.

26. August P, Lindheimer M. Chronic hypertension and pregnancy. In: Lindheimer MD, Roberts JM, Cunningham FG (Eds). Chesley's Hypertensive Disorders in Pregnancy, 2nd edition. Stamford, CT: Appleton & Lange; 1999. pp. 605-33.

27. Dugas G, Fuller J, Singh S, et al. Pheochromocytoma and pregnancy: a case report and review of anesthetic management. Can J Anaesth. 2004;51(2):134-8.

28. Mbah AK, Alio AP, Marty PJ, et al. Pre-eclampsia in the first pregnancy and subsequent risk of stillbirth in black and white gravidas. Eur J Obstet Gynecol Reprod Biol. 2010;149(2):165-9.

29. von Dadelszen P, Magee LA, Roberts JM. Sub-classification of preeclampsia. Hypertens Pregnancy. 2003;22(2):143-8.

30. Hepburn IS, Schade RR. Pregnancy-associated liver disorders. Dig Dis Sci. 2008;53(9):2334-58.

31. Kaplan N, Victor R. Hypertension with pregnancy and the pill. In: Kaplan N, Victor R (Eds). Kaplan's Clinical Hypertension. Philadelphia: Lippincott Williams and Wilkins; 2010. pp. 410-29.

32. Audibert F, Friedman SA, Frangieh AY, et al. Clinical utility of strict diagnostic criteria for the HELLP (hemolysis, elevated liver enzymes, and low platelets) syndrome. Am J Obstet Gynecol. 1996; 175(2):460-4.

33. Martin JN, Blake PG, Lowry SL, et al. Pregnancy complicated by preeclampsia-eclampsia with the syndrome of hemolysis, elevated liver enzymes, and low platelet count: how rapid is postpartum recovery? Obstet Gynecol. 1990;76(5 pt 1):737-41.

34. R Souissi, Z Haddad, W Trabelsi, et al. HELLP syndrome: utility of specific classifications as prognostic tools. Critical Care. 2007,11(Suppl 2):383.

35. Silva LM, Steegers EA, Burdorf A, et al. No midpregnancy fall in diastolic blood pressure in women with a low educational level: the Generation R Study. Hypertension. 2008;52(4):645-51.

36. Shennan AH, Waugh J. The measurement of blood pressure and proteinuria in pregnancy. In: Critchly H, MacLean A, Poston L, Walker J (Eds). Pre-eclampsia. London, England: RCOG Press; 2003. pp. 305-24.

37. Thangaratinam S, Coomarasamy A, O'Mahony F, et al. Estimation of proteinuria as a predictor of complications of pre-eclampsia: a systematic review. BMC Med. 2009;7:10.

38. Laskin S, Payne B, Hutcheon J, et al. PIERS Study Group. The role of platelet counts in the assessment on in patient women with preeclampsia. Hypertens Pregnancy. 2010;1:57.

39. Payne B, Magee LA, Côté AM, et al. PIERS proteinuria: relationship with adverse maternal and perinatal outcome. J Obstet Gynaecol Can. 2011; 33(6):588-97.

40. National Institute of Health and Clinical Excellence. Hypertension in Pregnancy: The management of hypertensive disorders during pregnancy (clinical guideline 107). August 2010.

41. Cavkaytar S, Ugurlu EN, Karaer A, et al. Are clinical symptoms more predictive than laboratory parameters for adverse maternal outcome in HELLP syndrome? Acta Obstet Gynecol Scand. 2007; 86(6):648-51.

42. Martin JN, May WL, Magann EF, et al. Early risk assessment of severe preeclampsia; admission battery of symptoms and laboratory tests to predict likelihood of subsequent significant maternal morbidity. Am J Obstet Gynecol. 1999;180(6 Pt 1):1407-14.

43. Menzies J, von Dadelszen P, PIERS Study Group. The PIERS (Preeclampsia Integrated Estimate of Risk) models: univariable and cluster analyses. Hypertens Pregnancy. 2008;27:620-20.

44. The official voice of reproductive health care in Canada. J Obstet Gynaecol Can. 2008;30(3).

45. Lowe SA, Brown MA, Dekker GA, et al. Gudelines for the management of hypertensive disorders of pregnancy 2008. Aust N Z J Obstet Gynaecol. 2009;49(3):242-6.

46. Menzies J, Magee LA, Macnab YC, et al. Current CHS and NHBPEP criteria for severe preeclampsia do not uniformly predict adverse maternal or perinatal outcomes. Hypertens Preg. nancy. 2007;26(4): 447-62.

47. Romero R, Mazor M, Lockwood CJ, et al. Clinical significance, prevalence, and natural history of thrombocytopenia in pregnancy-induced hypertension. Am J Perinatol. 1989;6(1):32-8.

48. Brown MA, Buddle ML. Hypertension in pregnancy: maternal and fetal outcomes according to laboratory and clinical features. Med J Aust. 1996;165(7): 360-5.

49. Alkazaleh F, Chaddha V, Viero S, et al. Second-trimester prediction of severe placental complications in women with combined elevations in alpha-fetoprotein and human chorionic gonadotrophin. Am J Obstet Gynecol. 2006;194(3):821-7.

2 Etiology and Pathophysiology of Hypertensive Diseases

Hiten D Mistry, Fiona Broughton Pipkin

◼ INTRODUCTION

Hypertension is the most frequent medical complication occurring during pregnancy and this hypertension which develops de novo in pregnancy appears to be unique to man. Early animal models showed in several species that hypertension can be induced in pregnancy by banding the uterine arteries;[1,2] however, this presupposes a mechanical cause, and imposes its own conditions on the pregnancy. Other techniques which can induce hypertension ± proteinuria during pregnancy have been used, prominent among them are the knockout of possible candidate genes and dietary manipulation, mainly in rodents. However, implantation and placentation in rodents differ in a number of important respects from that in humans, and the fact that a considerable variety of maneuvers can induce preeclampsia like symptoms suggests that those symptoms are indicative of a vulnerable vascular endothelium in late pregnancy, such that any perturbation is potentially damaging. It is thus not clear whether these mechanisms are actually those inducing hypertensive disorders in pregnancy, therefore the main focus of this chapter will be on human pregnancies.

◼ PLACENTATION

The placenta is central, not only to a successful normal pregnancy, but also in the development of the hypertensive diseases of pregnancy. This section therefore briefly summarizes normal placental development, to allow better understanding of the disease process. The placenta is a unique organ, produced outside the embryo, connected by a cord of vessels and formed as a result of various degrees of interactions between fetal and maternal tissues within the pregnant uterus. The trophectoderm begins to differentiate from the blastocyst even before the inner cell mass, which will form the fetus. The placenta fulfills a variety of functions, which are completed by several different organs in adult life. Unlike the relatively stable mature adult organs, the placenta is programmed to complete very different functions during development. Thus, the placenta can be described as a constantly evolving organ. Its major role is the homeostasis of a protected environment for the undisturbed growth and development of the embryo/fetus.[3,4] With a balanced equilibrium between placental supply and fetal demand, the genetic growth potential is the major determinant for fetal growth. However, this balance varies throughout pregnancy due to a disproportional increase in fetal demand relative to placental supply.

During gestation, placental and fetal growth follows similar patterns in different mammalian species. Fetal growth is represented as sigmoidal, with a slow increase during early gestation followed by accelerated growth toward term which, in humans, decreases again after 36–37 weeks' gestation. In comparison, placental growth initially exceeds growth of the fetus and slowly increases during mid-gestation, but not to the same extent (Fig. 2.1).[3,5] In fact, placental growth almost stops by 35–36 weeks even in normal pregnancies, and this is reflected in the "placental ratio" (placental weight/birth weight), which is reduced after this time as fetal growth still continues.[6]

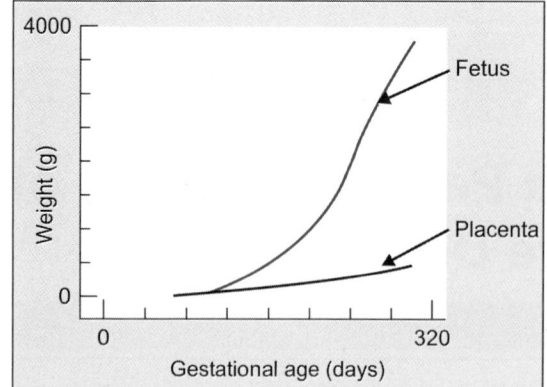

Fig. 2.1: Weight curves of placenta and fetus in humans (*Source*: Owens JA, Robinson JS. The effect of experimental manipulation of placental growth and development. New York: John Wiley; 1988)[7]

Implantation is usually completed by the second week after conception, during which time the embryoblast undergoes various morphological changes to produce the embryonic disk. Trophoblast differentiation is essential for correct implantation and continued trophoblast invasion of the uterus. During this period, extraembryonic structures, such as the amniotic cavity, amnion, yolk sac, connecting stalk and chorionic sac, are also formed.[8] These trophoblasts provide three main cell types in the human placenta:

1. The syncytiotrophoblasts, the main endocrine component of the placenta which forms the epithelial covering of the villous tree
2. The villous cytotrophoblasts, which proliferate throughout pregnancy and fuse to generate syncytiotrophoblasts
3. The extravillous trophoblasts, the cells which invade the maternal endometrium.[9] These extravillous trophoblasts are initially found in the central area of the placenta, within and around the spiral arteries; they gradually extend laterally, reaching the periphery of the placenta by around mid-gestation.

During implantation, erosive syncytiotrophoblasts invade endometrial connective tissues, which support the endometrial capillaries and glands. At this stage the blastocyst slowly embeds itself in the endometrium.[8] As a result, endometrial cells undergo apoptosis as the syncytiotrophoblast cells displace them in the central part of the implantation site.

Data collected from both human and murine systems have highlighted the importance of achieving implantation during the period of optimal uterine receptivity.[10,11] Delays in implantation induce restricted fetal and placental growth, abnormal uterine spacing of embryos in polytocous species and increased risk of early pregnancy loss.[8,12] Endovascular trophoblast invasion in humans has been reported to occur in two waves, which are required for a successful pregnancy.[13-15] The primary invasion occurs into the decidual segments of the spiral arteries at 8–10 weeks of gestation;[15-17] these spiral arteries in the placental bed are muscular arteries of between 200–300 μm diameter.[18] The secondary invasion takes place later at about 16–18 weeks gestation into the myometrial segments.[19] In normal pregnancy the transformation of spiral arteries into uteroplacental arteries is completed around mid-gestation,[17,20] although the mechanisms that control trophoblast invasion of the uterus are poorly understood.[18] The main purpose of these vascular changes is to optimize the distribution of maternal blood into a low-resistance uterine vascular network (Figs 2.2A and B). It is known that by term the uteroplacental circulation carries approximately 600 mL of maternal blood per minute.[21]

In the first trimester, placental tissues thrive in low oxygen concentrations, but the oxygen tension rises sharply when full maternal intervillous connectivity is established (10–12 weeks). This "hypoxia/reperfusion" state is accompanied by rapid degeneration of the syncytium. Although the capacity of trophoblast tissues to synthesize reactive oxygen species (ROS) such as superoxide (O_2^-) is three times higher in the first trimester than in the last, the total cellular antioxidant capacity is also twice as high. This "hypoxic" state appears to be necessary for normal placental development.[22] At present, delivery of the placenta is the only "cure" for preeclampsia, indicating the central role of the placenta in pathogenesis.

HYPERTENSIVE DISORDERS OF PREGNANCY

Hypertension during pregnancy occurs overall in 10–15% of all pregnancies[23,24] and can be broadly categorized into three groups: (1) chronic

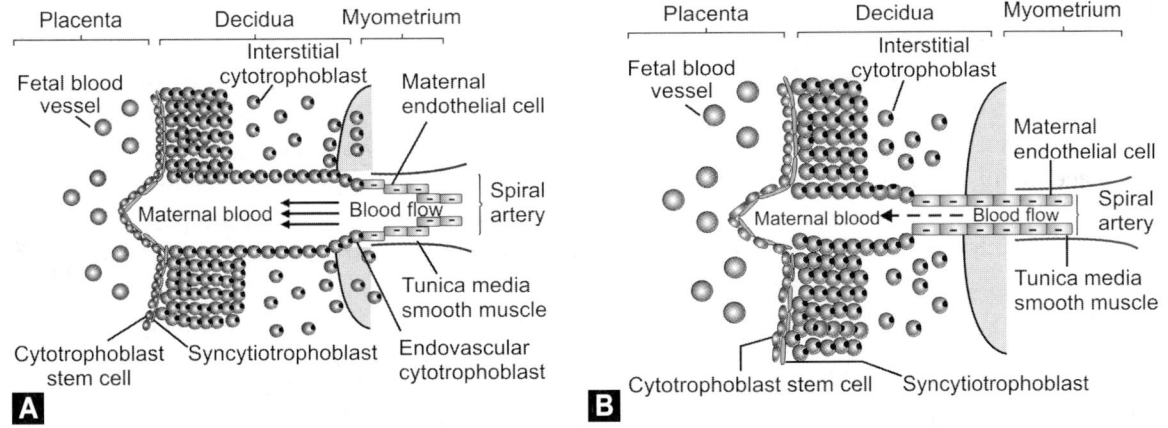

Figs 2.2A and B: Exchange of oxygen, nutrients, and waste products between the fetus and the mother depends on adequate placental perfusion by maternal vessels. (A) In normal placental development, invasive interstitial cytotrophoblasts of fetal origin invade the maternal spiral arteries, transforming them from small-caliber resistance vessels to high-caliber capacitance vessels capable of providing placental perfusion adequate to sustain the growing fetus; (B) In preeclampsia, the interstitial cytotrophoblasts fail to adopt an invasive endothelial phenotype. Instead, invasion of the spiral arteries is shallow and they remain small-caliber, resistance vessels

hypertension, (2) nonproteinuric hypertension [commonly called gestational hypertension (GH)] and preeclampsia[25,26] (See Chapter 1 for detailed definitions and general background). An important, but often overlooked point regarding the definitions is that in populations residing in warmer climates where vasodilation is normal, waiting for the blood pressure to reach more than 140/90 before taking any action is inappropriate as by the time blood pressure in such women reaches this level, they will already be in a serious condition. GH occurs in about 10–12% of first pregnancies, preeclampsia in approximately 2–5% (1 in 50 incident rate in the UK population).[27-29] Although the overwhelming majority of these will have successful pregnancy outcomes, the condition gives rise to severe multisystem complications including cerebral hemorrhage, hepatic and renal dysfunction and respiratory compromise. Hypertensive syndromes are also associated with perinatal morbidity and mortality, mainly from intrauterine growth restriction (IUGR) due to uteroplacental insufficiency and complications related to prematurity.[30] Even mild hypertension is associated with greater risk for prematurity and newborns who are small for gestational age.[31] While eclampsia is associated with hypertension in pregnancy, the rates are very low in the UK and no delivery unit sees more than

1 case a year due to improved antenatal care and the use of prophylactic treatments such as magnesium sulfate;[32] furthermore it has been reported that 11% of women who developed eclampsia had no hypertension or proteinuria;[33] therefore eclampsia will not be covered here.

Chronic Hypertension

Underlying hypertension is present in about 5% of pregnancies.[24] Unless accompanied by the development of superimposed preeclampsia, which has been reported to occur in up to 20% of such women,[34] its etiology is outside the scope of this chapter. However, women with pre-existing hypertension should receive prepregnancy care including determining the severity and cause of the hypertension and use of potentially teratogenic medications such as the angiotensin converting enzyme (ACE) inhibitors and angiotensin receptor blockers (three times the risk of congenital abnormality.[35] All women should be informed of the increased risks during pregnancy and should receive low-dose aspirin in pregnancy. Antihypertensives such as methyldopa, labetalol, nifedipine and hydralazine are the most commonly used, which have shown to have no association with congenital abnormalities.[24]

One of the main issue is that it is difficult to distinguish superimposed preeclampsia from worsening chronic hypertension, with the new onset of proteinuria being the only suitable differentiating factor. As mentioned above, in addition to superimposed preeclampsia, the perinatal mortality is also increased due to uteroplacental insufficiency leading to IUGR and death, although independent risk associated with uncomplicated chronic hypertension are less clear as most studies have focused on the development of superimposed preeclampsia.

Gestational Hypertension

Gestational hypertension is relatively common and it is noted that a substantial number of these women later develop proteinuria and are thus reclassified as preeclamptics. The National Institute for Health and Clinical Excellence (NICE) clinical guidelines states that aspirin prophylaxis and routine hospital admission is not required if the blood pressure is controlled.[24] It is also imperative that women with GH are followed up with a postnatal visit where their blood pressure is checked. At present, the mechanisms responsible for the pathogenesis of GH which does not progress to preeclampsia have yet to be elucidated. However, a number of the factors predisposing to GH and preeclampsia (Box 2.1) are also those which predispose to nonpregnant hypertension, and mild, late onset, GH may simply be identifying women at risk of future cardiovascular disease.

◼ PREECLAMPSIA

Preeclampsia is one of the leading causes of maternal and perinatal mortality and morbidity in the Western world.[28,36-38] Together with other hypertensive disorders of pregnancy it is responsible for approximately 60,000 deaths each year and thus remains one of the most frequently-cited causes of maternal death in the developed world.[27,39-41] Preeclampsia is the most frequent cause of elective premature delivery, accounting for 15% of all premature births and approximately one in five very low birth weight infants (< 15,000 g).[42] Since size at birth is related to future health, preeclampsia may have lifetime consequences in terms of greater predisposition to adult cardiovascular and renal diseases.[43-45] Preeclampsia is much more than hypertension and proteinuria; it is a syndrome affecting virtually every organ system. Preeclampsia is now regarded as being of two types: (1) early onset preeclampsia, which tends to develop before 34 weeks' gestation and (2) late onset preeclampsia, which develops at or after 34 weeks' gestation.[46] Early onset preeclampsia is typically associated with placental dysfunction, reduced placental volume, IUGR, abnormal uterine and umbilical artery Doppler evaluation, multiorgan dysfunction, perinatal death and adverse maternal and neonatal outcomes. Late onset preeclampsia is thought to arise from an underlying maternal constitutional disorder, it is more often associated with a normal placenta and Doppler evaluation, normal birth weight and more favorable maternal and fetal outcomes.[46] It is beyond the scope of this review to provide information on all the possible mechanisms which have been linked with preeclampsia, thus only the areas which have received the greatest research focus are considered below.

Risk Factors for Preeclampsia

Over the past 60 years, there have been many attempts to screen the antenatal population for preeclampsia, with over 100 potential biochemical, biophysical or epidemiological candidate tests. Despite the lack of a single universal test to apply, it is still possible to advise women regarding their potential risk of preeclampsia simply from their clinical history, as emphasized in the current NICE guidelines for routine antenatal care.[47] Box 2.1 outlines risk factors that should be identified at booking as risk factors for preeclampsia. As can be seen, some of these factors can be understood in relation to a maternal predisposition to cardiovascular disease. Furthermore, many are modifiable, which might lead to a reduction in risk either prior to or between pregnancies. The relative risk for some of these factors ranges from 1.55 for raised BMI at booking to 9.72 for antiphospholipid syndrome;[48] this suggests that the majority of these women who are at high risk will still not develop preeclampsia, whilst a considerable number of cases will still arise de novo in the "low-risk" population.

Box 2.1: Basic risk factors to identify women at increased risk of preeclampsia[35]

- High risk factors (any single)
  - Hypertensive diseases in a previous pregnancy
  - Chronic kidney disease
  - Autoimmune disease (e.g. lupus erythematosus or antiphospholipid syndrome)
  - Type 1 or type 2 diabetes
  - Chronic hypertension
- Moderate risk factors (two or more of these)
  - Primiparity
  - Age 40 years or older
  - New paternity
  - Pregnancy interval of 10 years or more
  - Elevated body mass index (BMI > 35 kg/m² at first visit)
  - Family history of preeclampsia
  - Multiple pregnancy
  - African American ethnicity

In what follows, it should always be remembered that what is observed in established disease may be a consequence, rather than a cause. The diagnostic criteria themselves relate to late features of a disease invisibly initiated at implantation.

The Cardiovascular System and Preeclampsia

In a normal pregnancy, the heart rate rises very early in the first trimester and is the initial driver of the increased cardiac output; stroke volume rises soon afterwards. There is substantial vasodilatation from the first trimester, allowing the increase in plasma volume. This vasodilatation is hormonally-driven, for example, by the substantial rise in synthesis of circulating prostacyclin (PGI$_2$) and locally synthesized nitric oxide (NO), and a fall in pressor response to angiotensin II (ANG II), and is not due to a withdrawal of sympathetic tone. Figure 2.3 summarizes some of the mechanisms which have been implicated in this vasodilatation.

There is a consequent well-documented small fall in systolic blood pressure during the first half of pregnancy, reaching a nadir at 16–20 weeks, followed by a small rise as pregnancy progresses.[50] Diastolic blood pressure also falls during the first half of pregnancy, reaching its lowest level at

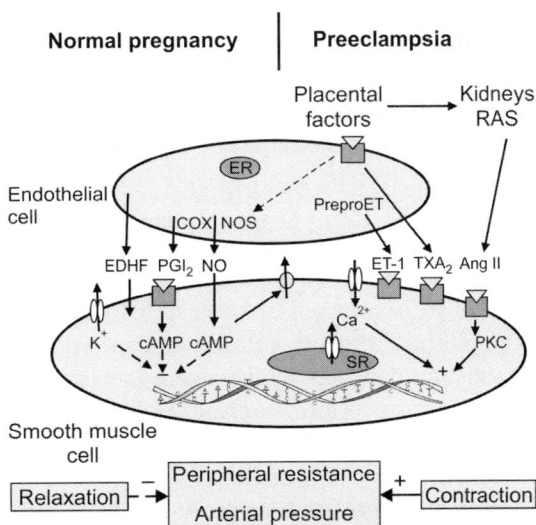

Fig. 2.3: Summary of the vascular changes during normal pregnancy and preeclampsia

Note: During normal pregnancy there is an increase in the activity of eNOS and cyclo-oxygenase (COX) and increased production of NO, PGI$_2$, and endothelium-derived hyperpolarizing factor (EDHF). NO increases cGMP and PGI$_2$ increases cAMP in smooth muscle, which decrease intracellular Ca²⁺ and the myofilament sensitivity to Ca²⁺. Also, EDHF opens K⁺ channels in smooth muscle, leading to membrane hyperpolarization. This leads to smooth muscle relaxation and decreased peripheral resistance and arterial pressure. In preeclampsia there is increased release of placental cytokines that inhibit the production of NO and thereby decrease smooth muscle relaxation. Cytokines also stimulate the release of endothelially-derived vasoactive hormones such as endothelin (ET-1) and could activate the renin-angiotensin system (RAS) in the kidney leading to increased ANG II. ET-1, thromboxane (TXA$_2$), and ANG II stimulate specific receptors in smooth muscle leading to increased intracellular Ca²⁺, protein kinase C (PKC) activity, smooth muscle contraction, and increased peripheral resistance and arterial pressure. (ER: Endoplasmic reticulum; SR: Sarcoplasmic reticulum)

(Source: Khalil RA, Granger JP. Vascular mechanisms of increased arterial pressure in preeclampsia: lessons from animal models. Am J Physiol Regul Integr Comp Physiol. 2002;283(1):R29-45)[50]

20 weeks gestation.[51] Thereafter, there is a progressive increase and by 38 weeks, diastolic blood pressure is significantly higher than preconception values.[51-53] Overall, the mean arterial pressure decreases approximately 10 mm Hg, reaching a nadir at 16–20 weeks gestation, with a slow rise toward nonpregnant values from 30 weeks.[54] These topics are reviewed in Khalil and Granger, 2002.[50]

The pathophysiological changes associated with preeclampsia suggest a strongly vasoconstricted maternal circulation, with reduced circulating volume, leading to decreased systemic organ perfusion.[55,56] This is thought to be due to increased sensitivity to pressor agents producing further increases in vascular tone.[57,58] In established preeclampsia, unlike normal pregnancy, cardiac output is reduced,[59,60] which has been suggested to be due to decreases in both heart rate and stroke volume.[61] Plasma volume is also reduced in established disease[62] while severe increases in vascular resistance and arterial pressure occur, enhanced by vasopressor agents, such as ANG II, or changes in receptor density/function and reduction of renal plasma flow (RPF).[63] This increased vascular reactivity to vasoconstrictors during preeclampsia could be due to decreased endothelium-dependent mechanisms of vascular relaxation and/or enhanced mechanisms of vascular smooth muscle contraction.[49] For example, whereas in normal pregnancy, the pressor response to ANG II falls from very early in gestation, women who go on to develop preeclampsia begin to show an increase toward nonpregnant responsiveness to ANG II from 10 weeks to 22 weeks of gestation;[57] those women also have raised platelet ANG II binding site density.[64]

Renal Function and Preeclampsia

In a normal pregnancy, glomerular filtration rate (GFR) rises by 40–50% and RPF by up to 80% by the end of the first trimester, both being maintained during the second trimester and beginning to fall in the third—RPF falling faster. Plasma concentrations of many analytes therefore fall in parallel. The rise in GFR would normally cause a loss of 5,000–10,000 mEq sodium daily. However, there are mitigating factors resulting in maintenance of sodium homeostasis such as increased tubular reabsorption,[65] and increases in mineralocorticoid-like compounds, mainly aldosterone[66] under the influence of the activated renin-angiotensin-aldosterone system (RAAS).

Both renal blood flow and GFR decrease in preeclampsia, although absolute values may remain above the nonpregnant range.[67-69] This reduction in GFR could be due to a decrease in the ultrafiltration coefficient (Kf) and/or reduced renal blood flow,

which are the most likely mechanisms.[67,68] Reduced GFR leads to decreased filtered load of uric acid, and plasma volume contraction contributes to increased proximal tubular reabsorption of uric acid coupled to sodium; increased serum uric acid levels (markers of renal function) in preeclampsia are common clinical findings.[69,70] Another characteristic of preeclampsia is abnormal glomerular morphology.[71-73] The glomerulus is diffusely enlarged and structural changes include hypertrophy of the cytoplasmic organelles in endothelial and occasionally mesangial cells, particularly the lysosomes, which undergo marked enlargement termed "glomerular capillary endotheliosis".[71,74]

Placentation and Preeclampsia

All cases of preeclampsia appear to be accompanied by the placental pathology described below, but apparently identical pathology can also occur in the absence of preeclampsia, although such pregnancies are usually accompanied by IUGR. The inadequate uteroplacental circulation leads to placental hypoxia, oxidative stress and in the most severe cases infarction.[75,76] It is important to make this kind of distinction, as it implies that some women and/or their fetuses can mount a defense against inadequate placentation, while others cannot.[77,78] Placentae from pregnant women with preeclampsia tend to be, on average, smaller than those from patients with uncomplicated pregnancies, but with an increased placental/fetal weight ratio.[79] In preeclampsia, there is reduced blood flow into the intervillous space with an increase in vascular resistance and characteristic "notch" apparent within the Doppler waveform; these have been demonstrated by uteroplacental Doppler blood flow studies from as early as the second trimester, before any clinical signs become apparent.[80] At present the causes of increased vessel stiffness are unknown, but is likely to be hormonally driven (Fig. 2.3) although further investigations are required to elucidate this.

Significantly, one of the most frequent findings in preeclampsia is a decreased or absent second wave of trophoblast invasion of maternal spiral arteries compared to normal pregnancies.[78,81] In a typical case of preeclampsia, the invasive interstitial trophoblasts fail to continue their journey into the spiral arteries as they only invade the endometrium, implying the absence of the second wave of endovascular trophoblast invasion (Figs 2.2A and B).[82] Placental bed biopsies from preeclamptic pregnancies revealed the presence of nonconverted spiral arteries, which remain muscular and narrow, thus resulting in placental hypoxia due to reduced maternal blood flow to the intervillous spaces with the secretion of vasoactive substances that might lead to maternal hypertension.[16,83]

Khong et al. detected intraluminal endovascular trophoblasts in placental bed spiral arteries in the third trimester, in patients with preeclampsia.[84] In normal pregnancy intraluminal endovascular trophoblasts are not found beyond the second trimester. Thus, presence of these endovascular trophoblast cells later in pregnancy in preeclampsia may represent a delayed response in an attempt to transform the maternal vasculature (described above) in order to achieve an adequate blood flow to the fetal-placental unit.[85,86] Clustering of interstitial trophoblasts has also been reported around nonconverted spiral arteries within the third trimester in pathological pregnancy,[83] and this may also represent a delayed response by the trophoblast to initiate spiral artery remodeling. This initial failure of trophoblast invasion, however caused, would be of relatively little biological significance when the fetus is small. However, later in gestation when there is rapid fetal growth (Fig. 2.1), its demands could begin to outstrip the ability of the uteroplacental circulation to deliver nutrients and excrete waste products. This puts strain on poor placentae, which manifests as clinical preeclampsia with ischemia to the placenta and kidney, and possible activation of the placental RAAS by analogy with the ischemic kidney.[87] An intrinsic placental angiotensin-generating system has been well documented based on the presence of major RAAS components including renin, angiotensinogen, ACE, and ANG II as well as its receptor subtypes.[88,89] A functioning placental RAAS appears necessary for an uncomplicated pregnancy.[90]

Oxidative Stress and Preeclampsia

Oxidative stress, defined as an imbalance between pro-oxidants and antioxidant capacity, has been implicated in suboptimal reproductive performance from the earliest stages of development through to labor and delivery.[91] ROS are substances with one or more unpaired electrons; because of this ROS are highly reactive, interacting with lipids, proteins or DNA leading to oxidation and cellular malfunction which may initiate pathological processes. The most commonly produced ROS in mammals is O_2^-. Depletion of antioxidant capacity, whether through low abundance of nonenzymatic (e.g. vitamins C, E, glutathione) or enzymatic [e.g. superoxide dismutase (SOD)], glutathione peroxidases [(GPxs), catalase] antioxidants renders the cell vulnerable to oxidative attack, even under physiological situations where redox status is maintained through careful balance of a low level of synthesis of ROS and the pathways of cellular defense.[92]

Preeclampsia is now commonly regarded as being a state of oxidative stress, thought to arise from a biochemical imbalance which occurs either from excessive generation of free radical formation and/or inadequate antioxidant capacity.[79,93-95] This point has been implicated from a wide range of studies in both the mother and the placenta;[29,79,96] oxidative stress is well documented in the placenta of women with established preeclampsia.[97-102] The reduced placental perfusion characteristic of preeclampsia and the resultant hypoxia, together with intermittent reperfusion, is hypothesized to provoke ROS synthesis in the placenta.[103] Furthermore, ROS synthesis is likely to increase with the degree of maternal spiral artery malfunction,[104] and proposed to activate a cascade of pathways leading to cytokine release, prostaglandin synthesis, increased expression of antiangiogenic factors [e.g. soluble fms-like tyrosine kinase-1 (sFlt-1)] and activation of apoptotic pathways. Changes in some circulating markers of oxidative stress precede the development of clinical symptoms,[105-107] indicating a primary phenomenon of chronic oxidative stress.[20] Moreover, oxidative stress in the placenta leads to an overload of debris by stimulating apoptosis and/or necrosis.[75]

Abnormally high O_2^- synthesis rates have been noted in placental tissue from women with preeclampsia.[108,109] The increases in placental ROS in preeclampsia have been suggested to be due to increased mitochondrial generation.[93]

Placental mitochondrial numbers have also been shown to be increased in preeclamptic placentae and these were also abnormal in appearance,[110] potentially due to oxidative damage indicated by increased lipid peroxidation markers.[111] Burton and Jauniaux have suggested the vessels may retain some of their vasoreactivity when incomplete trophoblast invasion occurs, leading to intermittent perfusion of the intervillous space and placental oxidative stress, thus predisposing the mother to preeclampsia.[76] Additionally, if the unplugging of the vessels is premature, this will result in overwhelming placental oxidative stress and pregnancy failure (Fig. 2.4).[76]

In addition to the placental oxidative stress, maternal oxidative stress has also been implicated in preeclampsia, with studies reporting reduced levels of antioxidants, reduced antioxidant enzymes and increases in products of oxidation.[79,96,112] The oxidative stress seen in the mother may also be observed in the babies.[79] Tastekin et al. found SOD levels to be increased in infants born to preeclamptic pregnancies compared to control infants,[113] indicating that the fetus may have some capacity to mount a defense against a state of oxidative stress.

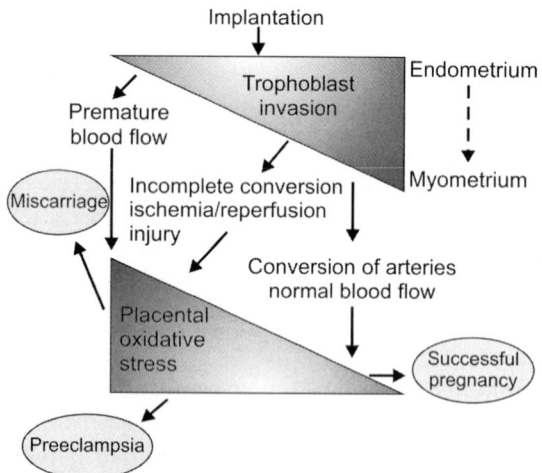

Fig. 2.4: Schematic representation of the relationship between the extent of trophoblast invasion, placental oxidative stress and pregnancy outcomes
(*Source*: Burton GJ, Jauniaux E. Placental oxidative stress: from miscarriage to preeclampsia. J Soc Gynecol Investig. 2004;11(6):342-52).

Antioxidant Supplementation in Preeclampsia

The recognition of oxidative stress in the placenta and the maternal circulation has prompted several supplementation trials of known risk factors of preeclampsia. An initial small randomized control trial of 283 women showed supplementation of 1 g vitamin C and 400 IU of vitamin E daily, from 16 weeks' gestation until delivery resulting in a reduction of markers of lipid peroxidation, in association with elevated plasma vitamin C and vitamin E concentrations.[107] However, the most recent meta-analysis of ten trials (6,533 women) published in 2008 of antioxidant supplementation (including vitamin C and E but also other supplements such as lycopene) showed no difference in the relative risk (RR) of preeclampsia (RR, 0.73; 95% CI, 0.51–1.06), preterm birth (before 37 weeks) (RR, 1.10; 95% CI, 0.99–1.22), small for gestational age infants (RR, 0.83; 95% CI, 0.62–1.11) or any baby death (RR, 1.12; 95% CI, 0.81–1.53).[114] Two subsequently published, recent multicenter, double-blinded randomized trials of a combination of vitamin C and E[115,116] also found supplementation did not reduce the rate of preeclampsia or gestational hypertension and like the vitamins in preeclampsia trial in 2006[117] increased the risk of fetal loss or perinatal death and preterm prelabor rupture of membranes. These disappointing results may relate to the use of isolated vitamins, without the cofactors found in complex vitamin sources such as fruit and vegetables. Further investigations are required as the concentrations of these vitamins remain significantly reduced in women with preeclampsia, but in the absence of further evidence, routine supplementation with isolated higher dose vitamins C and E is not recommended as they can be potentially dangerous in high concentrations.

Recent studies have now recognized associations between the essential antioxidant micronutrient selenium and preeclampsia, which may suggest a different approach from preventing oxidative stress.[79,118,119] Several selenoproteins particularly the GPxs play an important role in cellular antioxidant defense by reducing lipid hydroperoxides to their corresponding unreactive alcohols and reducing free hydrogen peroxide to water.[118,120] Numerous reports have now observed reduced maternal and fetal blood selenium concentrations and GPx activities, with increased thiobarbituric acid reactive substances (marker for lipid peroxidation), as well as decreased placental activities of the GPxs in women with preeclampsia.[79,96,121] Therefore, selenium supplementation offers another potential strategy for preventing preeclampsia, particularly in geographical regions with low soil selenium content.

Endothelial Dysfunction and Preeclampsia

Roberts et al. first formulated the concept of endothelial cell involvement in the pathogenesis of preeclampsia.[56] This hypothesis has received increased credence recently; this is due to the ubiquitous nature and diverse functions of the vascular endothelium which could account for clinical manifestations of the disease process.[56,94,122,123] At present, several lines of evidence suggest that impaired trophoblast invasion and hence reduced placental perfusion

may lead to the release of factor(s) that bring about widespread endothelial cell activation in susceptible women, leading to the multisystem dysfunction that characterizes preeclampsia (Fig. 2.5).[63] The nature of this factor or factors is unclear, but due to the fact that their effect diminishes rapidly after delivery, it is likely that they may be released from the placenta.[124] In addition, Roberts and Hubel supplemented this hypothesis by constructing a hypothetical two-stage model for the progression of preeclampsia.[125] This model proposes that a combination of several factors, including the endothelium, results in the final outcome of preeclampsia and this has now been updated to include other potential contributing factors (Fig. 2.5).[126] The major problem with preeclampsia diagnosis is that clinically, the disease is not seen until mid-gestation and not until the third trimester in the majority of women, but the abnormalities of implantation have occurred many weeks earlier. Thus, the identification of potential biomarkers of endothelial dysfunction that are able to predict preeclampsia could prove very useful in prevention and/or treatment.

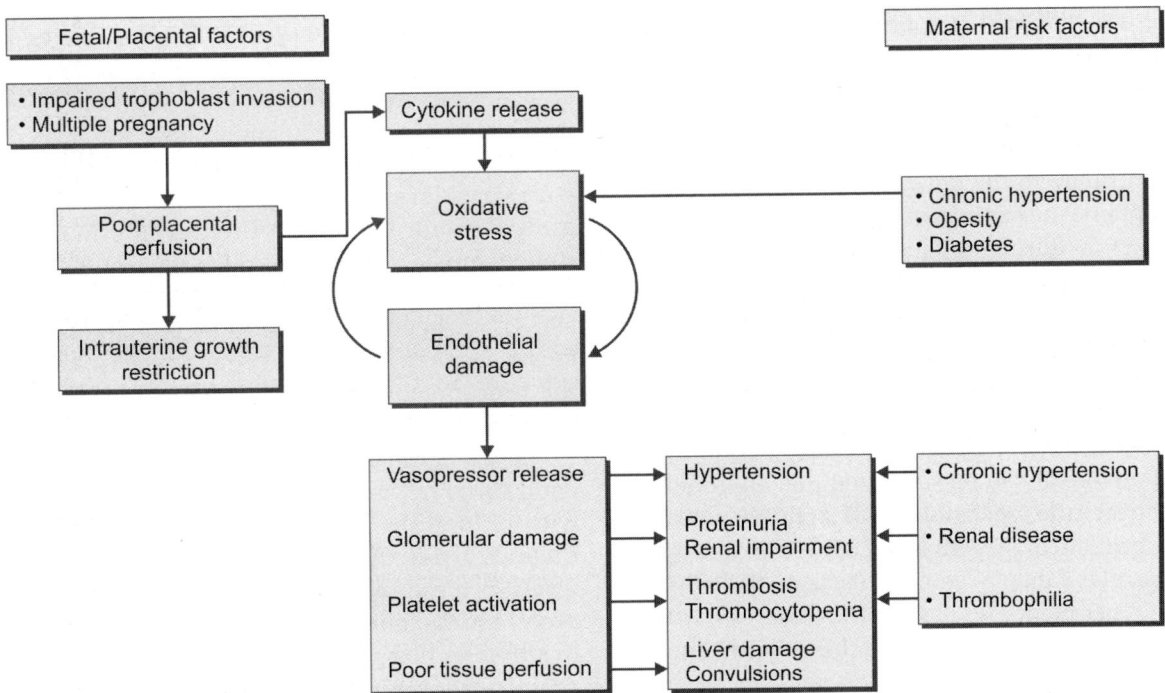

Fig. 2.5: Suggested pathophysiological mechanisms in preeclampsia. The diagram illustrates numerous factors that could potentially contribute to the final outcome of preeclampsia

(*Source*: Chappell S, Morgan L. Searching for genetic clues to the causes of preeclampsia. Clin Sci (Lond). 2006; 110(4):443-58).

20

Markers for Endothelial Dysfunction in Preeclampsia

In all cases, a change in any substance might be a cause or an effect. As noted above, observed differences found late in pregnancy are likely to be secondary; those which have been studied prospectively and found to be altered well before diagnostic symptoms present are much stronger candidates and this must be considered when looking at any of the observed changes seen in preeclampsia.

Endothelial Vasoactive Hormones

The increased vascular reactivity to vasoconstrictors during preeclampsia could be due to decreased endothelium-dependent mechanisms of vascular relaxation and/or enhanced mechanisms of vascular smooth muscle contractions.[49] PGI_2, which is synthesized in the vascular endothelium, may play a role in endothelial dysfunction. Urinary excretion of $PGF_{1\alpha}$ (the main metabolite of PGI_2) is raised several-fold by the end of the first trimester in pregnancies which remain normotensive, but in women who go on to develop severe preeclampsia, the excretion of $PGF_{1\alpha}$ is lower than in normal pregnant women during early (first trimester) as well as later pregnancy, indicating diminished renal PGI_2 synthesis in preeclampsia.[127-129] This decreased production of PGI_2, which could functionally contribute to the development of preeclampsia, supports the concept of abnormal endothelial cell function during this disease.[129-132] An eicosanoid which has opposing effects to PGI_2 is thromboxane (TXA_2), which is released by platelets and is a potent vasoconstrictor and platelet aggregating agent.[63] Placentae taken from preeclamptic pregnancies have been shown to synthesize more TXA_2 and less PGI_2 than those from normal pregnancies.[132] Therefore, it can be suggested that an imbalance between the prostanoids, PGI_2 and TXA_2 is likely to contribute to the enhanced platelet reactivity and vascular damage seen in preeclampsia.[49,133]

The potent vasodilator nitric oxide (NO) was first identified as a factor within the endothelium that mediated vascular relaxation and is synthesized by nitric oxide synthase (NOS).[134,135] NO exerts its vasodilator effect on vascular smooth muscle through the second messenger cyclic guanyl monophosphate (cGMP). NO has been implicated

in preeclampsia, however, there is currently no consensus as to whether they are higher or lower, mainly due to methodologic difficulties.[136]

Concentrations of circulating ACE fall in the first half of pregnancy of normotensive pregnancy, and then rise significantly over the third trimesters toward nonpregnant levels. In preeclampsia, these levels remain low in the third trimester, which may relate to the generalized endothelial dysfunction of preeclampsia.[137] In addition, angiotensin receptors, are increased (unlike normal pregnancies).[63] It has been suggested that a deficiency of PGI_2 may result in the increased ANG II sensitivity seen in preeclampsia,[138] furthermore, the increased pressor response may also be due to the increased production of endothelin-1 by activated endothelial cells.[139-141] Vessels from women with preeclampsia have been shown in vitro to have a significantly impaired response to acetylcholine suggesting altered endothelial responses in blood vessels.[142] Furthermore, in vivo evidence has shown impaired endothelial function associated with preeclampsia.[143,144]

Growth Factors and Preeclampsia

The placenta is a very highly vascularized organ; factors which affect vasculogenesis and angiogenesis might thus be expected to modify its development. Recent studies have implicated altered expression of growth factors associated with vascular angiogenesis, such as placental growth factor (PlGF), in the development of preeclampsia.[122,145,146] The receptor of vascular endothelial growth factor (VEGF) and PlGF, sFlt-1, has been suggested to be the circulating factor secreted by the placenta associated with the widespread endothelial dysfunction seen in preeclampsia.[147,148]

Levels of the growth factor sFlt-1 and soluble endoglin (sEng) are also increased in preeclampsia, with reductions in free circulating VEGF and PlGF.[149-153] Furthermore, the changes in the levels of these markers precede clinically overt preeclampsia, and disappears with resolution of the disease; this provides evidence for a possible causal relationship between endothelial cell injury and preeclampsia.[123,154] Serum levels of sFlt-1 have been reported to be increased and levels of free PlGF decreased in women with preeclampsia compared to normal pregnancy.[147,148] In addition, hypoxia, via the transcriptional protein complex, hypoxia-inducible factor-1 (HIF-1) upregulates VEGF.[155] HIF-1 has been found to be elevated in preeclampsia because its degradation pathway is inhibited,[156] which could also account for the increase in VEGF. Moreover, these changes in HIF-1 and VEGF further suggest that hypoxia is an important factor in preeclampsia pregnancies and ties in with the observed reduction in branching angiogenesis and impedance.[157]

Immunology and Preeclampsia

Immune maladaptation has also been postulated to be involved in the pathogenesis of preeclampsia,[158-160] although at present, disagreements about the exact involvement of immunology in preeclampsia exist. Aspects of the immune mechanism during pregnancy may be important contributing factors.[161] During pregnancy both the maternal and fetal immune systems should recognize the presence of each other's allogeneic cells. During invasion of the extravillous trophoblast into the maternal decidua, there is infiltration by the abundant natural killer (NK) cells together with other macrophages and a few CD3+ T cells. They secrete both prostaglandin E$_2$ (PGE$_2$) and TXA$_2$, and the balance tips to TXA$_2$ in hypoxic conditions. Decidual NK cells can recruit trophoblast cells through the secretion of chemokines and could induce vascular growth through their expression of angiogenic stimulants. They release various chemokines, and proangiogenic factors including VEGF and PlGF which both favor vascular growth in the decidua. Interactions between killer immunoglobulin-like receptors (KIR) on NK cell membranes and their appropriate ligands on target cells result in the production of positive or negative signals, which regulate NK cell function. Thus, the extremely polymorphic maternal KIR in the mother and the polymorphic human leukocyte antigen (HLA)-C in the fetus make up a potentially very variable receptor-ligand system, some combinations of which could predispose to preeclampsia by inhibiting trophoblast invasion.

These trophoblasts are allogeneic cells, however they express no HLA class II but do express three class I molecules, HLA-G, HLA-E and HLA-C. The classical major histocompatibility complex (MHC)

molecules, HLA-A and B, which are the dominant ligands used by T cells, are never expressed.[162] There have been reports that aberrant HLA-G expression is seen in preeclampsia placental tissue[163] and specifically extravillous cytotrophoblast cells.[164] Due to the unique expression pattern at the fetal-maternal interface, it has been hypothesized that it may play a critical role in maternal immune tolerance to the fetus.[163] Other studies have found that women with preeclampsia have autoantibodies capable of activating the angiotensin AT1 receptor, which are rarely seen in normal pregnancies.[165,166] This suggests that preeclampsia may actually be an autoimmune disease in which pathophysiological symptoms results from autoantibody-induced angiotensin receptor activation, possibly leading to increased plasminogen activator inhibitor-1 (PAI-1) production and shallow trophoblast invasion.[167]

Inflammatory Responses, Cytokines and Preeclampsia

It has been seen that all components of the inflammatory network appear to be engaged in preeclampsia, accounting for the diversity of the pathology presented in end-stage preeclamptic patients. Thus, the differences in the inflammatory response between normal and preeclamptic pregnancies are of intensity and not quality.[168] It is thought that the placental syncytium renews itself by shedding apoptotic debris into the maternal circulation, which imposes an increasing, but normal systemic inflammatory burden as the placenta grows. It has been suggested that oxidative stress stimulates syncytiotrophoblast apoptosis as it does in other tissues.[169,170] This could cause increases in shedding of syncytiotrophoblast microparticles, which has been observed in higher amounts in early onset preeclampsia.[171] Together, this debris could then activate an enhanced systemic inflammatory response including endothelial activation.[75,172]

Paternal Contribution

As mentioned in the genetics section below, there is also likely to be a paternal influence in the progression of preeclampsia; exposure to paternal antigens protects against the disease.[173] Anecdotally, severe preeclampsia has been reported in a woman who previously had an uncomplicated twin pregnancy; the two pregnancies were with separate fathers.[174] Immunological studies of the women and the two fathers demonstrated greater histoincompatibility between the mother and the second father;[174] this has been subsequently backed up by a further study.[175] Another two studies found that among women with no history of preeclampsia, a new father increased the risk of preeclampsia by 30%.[28,176] A potential explanation for this is that a mother with a non-preeclamptic first pregnancy may develop a tolerance to the paternal antigen to which she is exposed to during pregnancy. Changing the father will expose the mother to new paternal antigens to which she may not be tolerant. Thus, changing the father, for a woman with no history of preeclampsia, may increase her risk to the same level that she would have had as a primipara.[173]

Genetics and Preeclampsia

It has been recognized for many years that preeclampsia has a familial component, and the identification of susceptibility genes is one of a number of strategies designed to elucidate the underlying pathogenetic mechanisms.[41,126,177] Clustering of cases of preeclampsia within families has been recognized since the 19th century, suggesting a genetic component to the disorder.[178] Numerous studies from the USA, Scotland, Iceland, Scandinavia and Australia have been conducted, which recorded a two to five fold increase in risk to first-degree relatives of women with preeclampsia.[28,179-181] Many different models have been put forward, including maternal recessive or maternal dominant with partial penetrance;[179] it has also been noted that factors which modify the penetrance of maternal genes could include fetal genetic effects.[126]

It has also been postulated that a susceptibility gene, which is paternally imprinted could be involved; only the maternally inherited allele is active.[182] Thus, inheritance of a mutated copy of the gene from a heterozygous mother would effectively result in loss of gene activity in the fetus.[179] In addition, further paternal contribution has been suggested; this has already been discussed above in the immunology section. It has been shown that only 1.3% of women who had not had preeclampsia

in their first pregnancy developed preeclampsia in their second pregnancy.[28] This risk was doubled if they had a new partner who had previously fathered a preeclampsia pregnancy;[28,41] this is consistent with an effect of paternal genes acting via the fetus.

At present, the emphasis in genetic research into preeclampsia is focusing on linkage studies of large pedigrees. This strategy has been possible by new technologies developed in association with the Human Genome Project, which allows dense mapping of the entire human genome with highly polymorphic genetic markers.[183] There are two main approaches to this: the first approach to focus the search for linkage on genes with biologically plausible roles in the causation of preeclampsia, "the candidate gene" approach, although the number of potential candidates is large. The second approach makes no assumption as to which genes may be involved and the whole genome is searched systematically [genome wide association studies (GWAS)].[177]

Overall, a genetic component seems highly likely to be involved in the pathological changes in preeclampsia, which has been confirmed by epidemiological studies. Several candidate genes have been studied that fall into groups based on their proposed pathological mechanism, including endothelial function, oxidative stress.[177] However, although progress has been made in this field, much more work is required and it is highly unlikely that a single gene will be identified as the sole risk factor for preeclampsia, due to its multifactorial nature. A greater chance may be through numerous interactions between single nucleotide polymorphisms (SNPs) either alone or in combination with predisposing environmental factors. This area has highlighted that further collaboration is required between different research groups with the pooling of pedigree data to enable us to make significant progress in this area.[184]

■ CONCLUSION

There are two major difficulties for a clinician with a background in internal medicine in differentiating between hypertension during, as distinct from outside, pregnancy. Firstly, the time course of the disease process is greatly accelerated, with the consequences of hypertension being manifest in days or weeks rather than years. Secondly, there are two patients involved and although it is the mother who has the high blood pressure, it is often the fetus who is at most risk.[185] Therefore, hypertension during pregnancy highlights the need for interdisciplinary cooperation, in research and management. One of the major difficulties of research in this area is that there is poor agreement between investigators about diagnosing the various forms of hypertension during pregnancy. Although several attempts have been made over the past few decades, no classification system has so far been devised which suits both researcher and clinician. Furthermore, there are also considerable international differences in diagnostic criteria.

Preeclampsia and gestational hypertension continue to be relatively common and affect virtually all maternal organ systems. Although preeclampsia appears to be much less commonly complicated by eclampsia than it was in the past, the frequency of preeclampsia appears to be increasing.[32] Poor placental perfusion, frequently secondary to abnormal implantation, appears as the initiating factor. Placental and cardiovascular markers may provide tools for diagnosing and predicting preeclampsia however, there are still some very basic questions that remain unanswered. Among these are: Is preeclampsia one or many diseases? Can we accurately predict those women who will develop preeclampsia using a single set of parameters? If diagnosed early enough, can we even attempt to prevent it? If we know what caused it, could we at least treat it more rationally?

The plaques in the Chicago Lying-in Hospital reserved for the person who discovers the cause and/or cure for preeclampsia (Fig. 2.6) remains blank and may not be filled by a single person due to the multifactorial nature of preeclampsia. Data obtained from numerous studies highlights the enigma which is preeclampsia; it illustrates how the whole picture grows ever more complex as more data evolves, presumably because of the inter-individual variability. Further good quality research is still required in order to progress in our quest to conquer this syndrome.

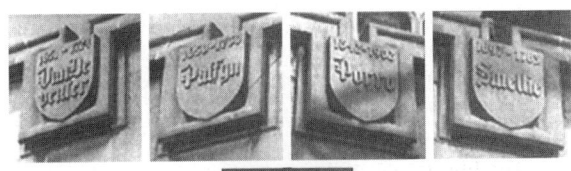

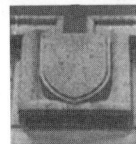

Fig. 2.6: Placards from the Chicago Lying-in Hospital honoring the famous physicians who made major contributions to the field of Obstetrics and Gynecology. This includes the empty plaque which is reserved for the individual who discovers the cause and/or cure of preeclampsia

(*Source*: Adapted from Lindheimer MD, Roberts JM, Cunningham FG, et al. In: Lindheimer MD, Roberts JM, Cunningham FG (Eds). Chesley's Hypertensive Disorders in Pregnancy. New York: Elsevier Academic Press; 2009).

23

■ ACKNOWLEDGMENTS

We are grateful to Dr Marta Ribeiro Hentschke for producing the figure (Figures 2.2A and B) demonstrating remodeling of the spiral arteries in normal and preeclamptic conditions.

■ REFERENCES

1. McCarthy FP, Kingdom JC, Kenny LC, et al. Animal models of preeclampsia; uses and limitations. Placenta. 2011;32(6):413-9.
2. Phippard AF, Horvath JS. Hypertension during pregnancy. In: Rubin PC (Ed). Handbook of Hypertension. Amsterdam: Elsevier; 1988. pp. 168-85.
3. Schneider H. Ontogenic changes in the nutritive function of the placenta. Placenta. 1996;17(1):15-26.
4. Huppertz B, Peeters LL. Vascular biology in implantation and placentation. Angiogenesis. 2005;8(2):157-67.
5. Salafia CM, Zhang J, Miller RK, et al. Placental growth patterns affect birth weight for given placental weight. Birth Defects Res A Clin Mol Teratol. 2007:79(4);281-8.
6. Perry IJ, Beevers DG, Whincup PH, et al. Predictors of ratio of placental weight to fetal weight in multiethnic community. BMJ. 1995;310(6977): 436-9.
7. Owens JA, Robinson JS. The effect of experimental manipulation of placental growth and development. New York: John Wiley; 1988.

8. Red-Horse K, Zhou Y, Genbacev O, et al. Trophoblast differentiation during embryo implantation and formation of the maternal-fetal interface. J Clin Invest. 2004;114(6):744-54.

9. Kaufmann P, Burton G. In: Knobil E, Neill J (Eds). The Physiology of Reproduction. New York: Raven Press, Ltd.; 1994.

10. Song H, Lim H, Paria BC, et al. Cytosolic phospholipase A2alpha is crucial [correction of A2alpha deficiency is crucial] for 'on-time' embryo implantation that directs subsequent development. Development. 2002;129(12):2879-89.

11. Psychoyos A. Uterine receptivity for nidation. Ann N Y Acad Sci. 1986;476:36-42.

12. Wilcox AJ, Baird DD, Weinberg CR. Time of implantation of the conceptus and loss of pregnancy. N Engl J Med. 1999;340(23):1796-9.

13. Pijnenborg R, Bland JM, Robertson WB, et al. Uteroplacental arterial changes related to interstitial trophoblast migration in early human pregnancy. Placenta. 1983;4(4):397-413.

14. Pijnenborg R, Robertson WB, Brosens I. The arterial migration of trophoblast in the uterus of the golden hamster, Mesocricetus auratus. J Reprod Fertil. 1974;40(2):269-80.

15. Robertson WB, Khong TY, Brosens I, et al. The placental bed biopsy: review from three European centers. Am J Obstet Gynecol. 1986;155(2):401-12.

16. Pijnenborg R. The placental bed. Hypertens Pregnancy. 1996;15:7-23.

17. Pijnenborg R, Dixon G, Robertson WB, et al. Trophoblastic invasion of human decidua from 8 to 18 weeks of pregnancy. Placenta. 1980;1(1):3-19.

18. Lyall F. Development of the utero-placental circulation: the role of carbon monoxide and nitric oxide in trophoblast invasion and spiral artery transformation. Microsc Res Tech. 2003;60(4):402-11.

19. Lyall F, Bulmer JN, Duffie E, et al. Human trophoblast invasion and spiral artery transformation: the role of PECAM-1 in normal pregnancy, preeclampsia, and fetal growth restriction. Am J Pathol. 2001;158(5):1713-21.

20. Jauniaux E, Poston L, Burton GJ. Placental-related diseases of pregnancy: Involvement of oxidative stress and implications in human evolution. Hum Reprod Update. 2006;12(6):747-55.

21. Ramsey EM, Donner NW. Placental Vasculature and Circulation. Stuttgart, Germany: Georg Thieme; 1980.

22. Raijmakers MT, Burton GJ, Jauniaux E, et al. Placental NAD(P)H oxidase mediated superoxide generation in early pregnancy. Placenta. 2006;27 (2-3):158-63.

23. National High Blood Pressure Education Program Working Group Report on High Blood Pressure in Pregnancy. Am J Obstet Gynecol. 1990;163(5 Pt 1):1691-712.

24. National Institute for Health and Clinical Excellence: Hypertension in pregnancy. The management of hypertensive disorders during pregnancy. NICE Clinical Guideline 107. Last modified January 2011 guidance.nice.org.uk/cg107.

25. Davey DA, MacGillivray I. The classification and definition of the hypertensive disorders of pregnancy. Am J Obstet Gynecol. 1988;158(4):892-8.

26. Higgins JR, de Swiet M. Blood-pressure measurement and classification in pregnancy. Lancet. 2001;357(9250):131-5.

27. Dekker G, Sibai B. Primary, secondary, and tertiary prevention of pre-eclampsia. Lancet. 2001; 357(9251):209-15.

28. Lie RT, Rasmussen S, Brunborg H, et al. Fetal and maternal contributions to risk of pre-eclampsia: population based study. BMJ. 1998;316(7141): 1343-7.

29. Hubel CA. Oxidative stress in the pathogenesis of preeclampsia. Proc Soc Exp Biol Med. 1999; 222(3):222-35.

30. Barra S, Cachulo Mdo C, Providência R, et al. Hypertension in pregnancy: the current state of the art. Rev Port Cardiol. 2012.

31. Ferrazzani S, Luciano R, Garofalo S, et al. Neonatal outcome in hypertensive disorders of pregnancy. Early Hum Dev. 2011;87(6):445-9.

32. Wallis AB, Saftlas AF, Hsia J, et al. Secular trends in the rates of preeclampsia, eclampsia, and gestational hypertension, United States, 1987-2004. Am J Hypertens. 2008;21(5):521-6.

33. Douglas KA, Redman CW. Eclampsia in the United Kingdom. BMJ. 1994;309(6966):1395-400.

34. Sibai B, Dekker G, Kupferminc M. Pre-eclampsia. Lancet. 2005;365(9461):785-99.

35. Waugh JJ, Smith MC. In: Edmonds DK (Ed). Dewhurst's Textbook of Obstetrics & Gynaecology. Oxford: John Wiley & Sons Ltd; 2012. pp. 101-10.

36. Cotter AM, Martin CM, O'leary JJ, et al. Increased fetal DNA in the maternal circulation in early pregnancy is associated with an increased risk of preeclampsia. Am J Obstet Gynecol. 2004;191(2):515-20.

37. Roberts JM. In: Creasy RK, Resnik R (Eds). Maternal Fetal Medicine: Principles and Practice. Philadelphia: W.B. Saunders; 1994.

38. Xiong X, Fraser WD. Impact of pregnancy-induced hypertension on birthweight by gestational age. Paediatr Perinat Epidemiol. 2004;18(3):186-91.

39. Geographic variation in the incidence of hypertension in pregnancy. World Health Organization International Collaborative Study of Hypertensive Disorders of Pregnancy. Am J Obstet Gynecol. 1988;158(1):80-3.

40. Roberts JM. Preeclampsia: what we know and what we do not know. Semin Perinatol. 2000;24(1):24-8.

41. Broughton Pipkin F. Risk factors for preeclampsia. N Engl J Med. 2001;344(12):925-6.

42. Jain A, Fleming P. Project 27/28. An enquiry into the quality of care and its effect on the survival of babies born at 27-28 weeks. Arch Dis Child Fetal Neonatal Ed. 2004;89(1):F14-6.

43. Barker D. Mothers, Babies and Disease in Later Life. London: BMJ Publishing Group; 1994.

44. Irgens HU, Reisaeter L, Irgens LM, et al. Long term mortality of mothers and fathers after pre-eclampsia: population based cohort study. BMJ. 2001;323(7323):1213-7.

45. Staff AC, Dechend R, Pijnenborg R. Learning from the placenta: acute atherosis and vascular remodeling in preeclampsia-novel aspects for atherosclerosis and future cardiovascular health. Hypertension. 2010;56(6);1026-34.

46. Raymond D, Peterson E. A critical review of early-onset and late-onset preeclampsia. Obstet Gynecol Surv. 2011;66(8):497-506.

47. National Institute for Health and Clinical Excellence: Hypertension in pregnancy. The management of hypertensive disorders during pregnancy. NICE Clinical Guideline 107. Last modified January 2011 guidance.nice.org.uk/cg107.

48. Duckitt K, Harrington D. Risk factors for pre-eclampsia at antenatal booking: systematic review of controlled studies. BMJ. 2005;330(7491):565.

49. Broughton Pipkin F. In: Edmonds DK (Ed). Dewhurst's textbook of Obstetrics and Gynaecology. Oxford: Blackwell Publishing; 2012.

50. Khalil RA, Granger JP. Vascular mechanisms of increased arterial pressure in preeclampsia: lessons from animal models. Am J Physiol Regul Integr Comp Physiol. 2002;283(1):R29-45.

51. Robson SC, Hunter S, Boys RJ, et al. Serial study of factors influencing changes in cardiac output during human pregnancy. Am J Physiol. 1989;256(4 Pt 2):H1060-5.

52. Duvekot JJ, Peeters LL. Maternal cardiovascular hemodynamic adaptation to pregnancy. Obstet Gynecol Surv. 1994;49(12 Suppl):S1-14.

53. MacGillivray I, Rose GA, Rowe B. Blood pressure survey in pregnancy. Clin Sci. 1969;37(2):395-407.

54. August P, Lenz T, Ales KL, et al. Longitudinal study of the renin-angiotensin-aldosterone system in hypertensive pregnant women: deviations related to the development of superimposed preeclampsia. Am J Obstet Gynecol. 1990;163(5 Pt 1):1612-21.

55. Brown MA. The physiology of pre-eclampsia. Clin Exp Pharmacol Physiol. 1995;22(11):781-91.

56. Roberts JM, Taylor RN, Musci TJ, et al. Preeclampsia: an endothelial cell disorder. Am J Obstet Gynecol. 1989;161(5):1200-4.

57. Gant NF, Daley GL, Chand S, et al. A study of angiotensin II pressor response throughout primigravid pregnancy. J Clin Invest. 1973;52(11): 2682-9.

58. Kyle PM, Buckley D, Kissane J, et al. The angiotensin sensitivity test and low-dose aspirin are ineffective methods to predict and prevent hypertensive disorders in nulliparous pregnancy. Am J Obstet Gynecol. 1995;173(3 Pt 1):865-72.

59. Visser W, Wallenburg HC. Central hemodynamic observations in untreated preeclamptic patients. Hypertension. 1991;17(6 Pt 2):1072-7.

60. Mabie WC, Ratts TE, Sibai BM. The central hemodynamics of severe preeclampsia. Am J Obstet Gynecol. 1989;161(6 Pt 1):1443-8.

61. Duvekot JJ, Cheriex EC, Pieters FA, et al. San Antonio: Society for Gynecological Investigations; 1992.

62. Gallery ED, Brown MA. Volume homeostasis in normal and hypertensive human pregnancy. Baillieres Clin Obstet Gynaecol. 1987;1(4):835-51.

63. Lyall F, Greer IA. The vascular endothelium in normal pregnancy and pre-eclampsia. Rev Reprod. 1996;1(2):107-16.

64. Broughton Pipkin F, Rubin PC. Pre-eclampsia—the 'disease of theories'. Br Med Bull. 1994;50(2):381-96.

65. Baylis C. Glomerular filtration and volume regulation in gravid animal models. Baillieres Clin Obstet Gynaecol. 1987;1(4):789-813.

66. Brown MA, Sinosich MJ, Saunders DM, et al. Potassium regulation and progesterone-aldosterone interrelationships in human pregnancy: a prospective study. Am J Obstet Gynecol. 1986; 155(2):349-53.

67. Lafayette RA, Druzin M, Sibley R, et al. Nature of glomerular dysfunction in pre-eclampsia. Kidney Int. 1998;54(4):1240-9.

68. Moran P, Lindheimer MD, Davison JM. The renal response to preeclampsia. Semin Nephrol. 2004;24(6):588-95.

69. Jeyabalan A, Conrad KP. Renal function during normal pregnancy and preeclampsia. Front Biosci. 2007;12:2425-37.

70. Powers RW, Bodnar LM, Ness RB, et al. Uric acid concentrations in early pregnancy among preeclamptic women with gestational hyperuricemia at delivery. Am J Obstet Gynecol. 2006;194(1):160.

71. Gaber LW, Spargo BH, Lindheimer MD. Renal pathology in pre-eclampsia. Baillieres Clin Obstet Gynaecol. 1994;8(2):443-68.

72. Kincaid-Smith P. The renal lesion of preeclampsia revisited. Am J Kidney Dis. 1991;17(2):144-8.

73. Sheehan HL. Renal morphology in preeclampsia. Kidney Int. 1980;18(2):241-52.

74. Stillman IE, Karumanchi SA. The glomerular injury of preeclampsia. J Am Soc Nephrol. 2007;18(8): 2281-4.

75. Redman CW, Sargent IL. Placental debris, oxidative stress and pre-eclampsia. Placenta. 2000;21(7):597-602.

76. Burton GJ, Jauniaux E. Placental oxidative stress: from miscarriage to preeclampsia. J Soc Gynecol Investig. 2004;11(6):342-52.

77. Brosens I, Dixon HG, Robertson WB. Fetal growth retardation and the arteries of the placental bed. Br J Obstet Gynaecol. 1977;84(9):656-63.

78. Brosens IA, Robertson WB, Dixon HG. The role of the spiral arteries in the pathogenesis of preeclampsia. Obstet Gynecol Annu. 1972;1:177-91.

79. Mistry HD, Wilson V, Ramsay MM, et al. Reduced selenium concentrations and glutathione peroxidase activity in preeclamptic pregnancies. Hypertension. 2008;52(5):881-8.

80. Bewley S, Cooper D, Campbell S. Doppler investigation of uteroplacental blood flow resistance in the second trimester: a screening study for pre-eclampsia and intrauterine growth retardation. Br J Obstet Gynaecol. 1991;98(9):871-9.

81. Meekins JW, Pijnenborg R, Hanssens M, et al. A study of placental bed spiral arteries and trophoblast invasion in normal and severe pre-eclamptic pregnancies. Br J Obstet Gynaecol. 1994; 101(8):669-74.

82. Redline RW, Patterson P. Pre-eclampsia is associated with an excess of proliferative immature intermediate trophoblast. Hum Pathol. 1995;26(6):594-600.

83. Pijnenborg R, Anthony J, Davey DA, et al. Placental bed spiral arteries in the hypertensive disorders of pregnancy. Br J Obstet Gynaecol. 1991;98(7):648-55.

84. Khong TY, De Wolf F, Robertson WB, et al. Inadequate maternal vascular response to placentation in pregnancies complicated by pre-eclampsia and by small-for-gestational age infants. Br J Obstet Gynaecol. 1986;93(10):1049-59.

85. Kliman HJ. Trophoblast of the human placenta. In: Knobil E, Neil J (Eds): Encyclcopedia of Reproduction. Elsevier 1998.

86. Lim KH, Zhou Y, Janatpour M, et al. Human cyto-trophoblast differentiation/invasion is abnormal in pre-eclampsia. Am J Pathol. 1997;151(6):1809-18.

87. Broughton Pipkin F. Hypertension in pregnancy: a physiological response to a pathological Problem? Dev Pharmol Ther. 1989;13(2-4):184-9.

88. Cooper AC, Robinson G, Vinson GP, et al. The localization and expression of the renin-angiotensin system in the human placenta throughout pregnancy. Placenta. 1999;20(5-6):467-74.

89. Williams PJ, Mistry HD, Innes BA, et al. Expression of AT1R, AT2R and AT4R and their roles in extravillous trophoblast invasion in the human. Placenta. 2010;31(5):448-55.

90. Irani RA, Xia Y. Renin angiotensin signaling in normal pregnancy and preeclampsia. Semin Nephrol. 2011;31(1):47-58.

91. Poston L, Igosheva N, Mistry HD, et al. Role of oxidative stress and antioxidant supplementation in pregnancy disorders. Am J Clin Nutr. 2011;94 (6 Suppl):1980S-1985S.

92. Forman HJ, Maiorino M, Ursini F. Signaling functions of reactive oxygen species. Biochemistry. 2010;49(5):835-42.

93. Poston L, Raijmakers MT. Trophoblast oxidative stress, antioxidants and pregnancy outcome—a review. Placenta. 2004;25 Suppl A:S72-8.

94. Zeeman GG, Dekker GA, van Geijn HP, et al. Endothelial function in normal and pre-eclamptic pregnancy: a hypothesis. Eur J Obstet Gynecol Reprod Biol. 1992;43(2):113-22.

95. Poston L. In: Critchley H, MacLean A, Poston L, Walker J (Eds). Pre-eclampsia. London: RCOG Press; 2004.

96. Mistry HD, Kurlak LO, Williams PJ, et al. Differential expression and distribution of placental glutathione peroxidases 1, 3 and 4 in normal and preeclamptic pregnancy. Placenta. 2010;31(5):401-8.

97. Chamy VM, Lepe J, Catalán A, et al. Oxidative stress is closely related to clinical severity of pre-eclampsia. Biol Res. 2006;39(2):229-36.

98. Hubel CA, Roberts JM, Taylor RN, et al. Lipid peroxidation in pregnancy: new perspectives on preeclampsia. Am J Obstet Gynecol. 1989; 161(4):1025-34.

99. Staff AC, Ranheim T, Khoury J, et al. Increased contents of phospholipids, cholesterol, and lipid peroxides in decidua basalis in women with preeclampsia. Am J Obstet Gynecol. 1999;180(3 Pt 1):587-92.

100. Walsh SW. Maternal-placental interactions of oxidative stress and antioxidants in preeclampsia. Semin Reprod Endocrinol. 1998;16(1):93-104.

101. Raijmakers MT, Roes EM, Poston L, et al. The transient increase of oxidative stress during normal pregnancy is higher and persists after delivery in women with pre-eclampsia. Eur J Obstet Gynecol Reprod Biol. 2008;138(1):39-44.

102. Bowen RS, Moodley J, Dutton MF, et al. Oxidative stress in pre-eclampsia. Acta Obstet Gynecol Scand. 2001;80(8):719-25.

103. Burton GJ, Yung HW, Cindrova-Davies T, et al. Placental endoplasmic reticulum stress and oxidative stress in the pathophysiology of unexplained intrauterine growth restriction and early onset preeclampsia. Placenta. 2009;30 Suppl A:S43-8.

104. Burton GJ, Jauniaux E. Oxidative stress. Best Pract Res Clin Obstet Gynaecol. 2011;25(3):287-99.

105. Wang YP, Walsh SW, Guo JD, et al. The imbalance between thromboxane and prostacyclin in

preeclampsia is associated with an imbalance between lipid peroxides and vitamin E in maternal blood. Am J Obstet Gynecol. 1991;165(6 Pt 1):1695-700.

106. Mikhail MS, Anyaegbunam A, Garfinkel D, et al. Preeclampsia and antioxidant nutrients: decreased plasma levels of reduced ascorbic acid, alpha-tocopherol, and beta-carotene in women with preeclampsia. Am J Obstet Gynecol. 1994;171(1):150-7.

107. Chappell LC, Seed PT, Briley A, et al. A longitudinal study of biochemical variables in women at risk of preeclampsia. Am J Obstet Gynecol. 2002;187(1):127-36.

108. Wang Y, Walsh SW. Increased superoxide generation is associated with decreased superoxide dismutase activity and mRNA expression in placental trophoblast cells in pre-eclampsia. Placenta. 2001;22(2-3):206-12.

109. Sikkema JM, van Rijn BB, Franx A, et al. Placental superoxide is increased in pre-eclampsia. Placenta. 2001;22(4):304-8.

110. Jones CJ, Fox H. An ultrastructural and ultra-histochemical study of the human placenta in maternal pre-eclampsia. Placenta. 1980;1(1):61-76.

111. Wang Y, Walsh SW. Placental mitochondria as a source of oxidative stress in pre-eclampsia. Placenta. 1998;19(8):581-6.

112. Holmes VA, McCance DR. Could antioxidant supplementation prevent pre-eclampsia? Proc Nutr Soc. 2005;64(4):491-501.

113. Tastekin A, Ors R, Demircan B, et al. Oxidative stress in infants born to preeclamptic mothers. Pediatr Int. 2005;47(6):658-62.

114. Rumbold A, Duley L, Crowther CA, et al. Antioxidants for preventing pre-eclampsia. Cochrane Database Syst Rev. 2008;(1):CD004227.

115. Xu H, Perez-Cuevas R, Xiong X, et al. An international trial of antioxidants in the prevention of preeclampsia (INTAPP). Am J Obstet Gynecol. 2010;202(3):239. e1-239.e10.

116. Roberts JM, Myatt L, Spong CY, et al. Vitamins C and E to prevent complications of pregnancy-associated hypertension. N Engl J Med. 2010;362(14):1282-91.

117. Poston L, Briley AL, Seed PT, et al. Vitamin C and vitamin E in pregnant women at risk for pre-eclampsia (VIP trial): randomised placebo-controlled trial. Lancet. 2006;367(9517):1145-54.

118. Mistry HD, Broughton Pipkin F, Redman CW, et al. Selenium in reproductive health. Am J Obstet Gynecol. 2012;206(1):21-30.

119. Mistry HD, Williams PJ. The importance of antioxidant micronutrients in pregnancy. Oxid Med Cell Longev. 2011;2011:841749.

120. Oster O, Prellwitz W. Selenium and cardiovascular disease. Biol Trace Elem Res. 1990;24(2):91-103.

121. Rayman MP, Abou-Shakra FR, Ward NI, et al. Comparison of selenium levels in pre-eclamptic and normal pregnancies. Biol Trace Elem Res. 1996;55(1-2):9-20.

122. Hayman R, Brockelsby J, Kenny L, et al. Preeclampsia: the endothelium, circulating factor(s) and vascular endothelial growth factor. J Soc Gynecol Investig. 1999;6(1):3-10.

123. Roberts JM. Endothelial dysfunction in preeclampsia. Semin Reprod Endocrinol. 1998;16(1):5-15.

124. Roberts JM, Taylor RN, Goldfien A. Clinical and biochemical evidence of endothelial cell dysfunction in the pregnancy syndrome preeclampsia. Am J Hypertens. 1991;4(8):700-8.

125. Roberts JM, Hubel CA. Is oxidative stress the link in the two-stage model of pre-eclampsia? Lancet. 1999;354(9181):788-9.

126. Chappell S, Morgan L. Searching for genetic clues to the causes of pre-eclampsia. Clin Sci (Lond). 2006;110(4):443-58.

127. Ylikorkala O, Pekonen F, Viinikka L. Renal prostacyclin and thromboxane in normotensive and preeclamptic pregnant women and their infants. J Clin Endocrinol Metab. 1986;63(6):1307-12.

128. Mills JL, DerSimonian R, Raymond E, et al. Prostacyclin and thromboxane changes predating clinical onset of preeclampsia: a multicenter prospective study. JAMA. 1999;282(4):356-62.

129. Fitzgerald DJ, Entman SS, Mulloy K, et al. Decreased prostacyclin biosynthesis preceding the clinical manifestation of pregnancy-induced hypertension. Circulation. 1987;75(5):956-63.

130. Wang Y, Walsh SW, Kay HH. Placental lipid peroxides and thromboxane are increased and prostacyclin is decreased in women with preeclampsia. Am J Obstet Gynecol. 1992;167(4 Pt 1):946-9.

131. Klockenbusch W, Goecke TW, Krüssel JS, et al. Prostacyclin deficiency and reduced fetoplacental blood flow in pregnancy-induced hypertension and preeclampsia. Gynecol Obstet Invest. 2000;50:103-7.

132. Walsh SW. Preeclampsia: an imbalance in placental prostacyclin and thromboxane production. Am J Obstet Gynecol. 1985;152(3):335-40.

133. Wallenburg HC, Rotmans N. Enhanced reactivity of the platelet thromboxane pathway in normotensive and hypertensive pregnancies with insufficient fetal growth. Am J Obstet Gynecol. 1982;144(5):523-8.

134. Furchgott RF, Zawadzki JV. The obligatory role of endothelial cells in the relaxation of arterial smooth muscle by acetylcholine. Nature. 1980; 288(5789):373-6.

135. Palmer RM, Ashton DS, Moncada S. Vascular endo-thelial cells synthesize nitric oxide from L-arginine. Nature. 1988;333(6174):664-6.

136. Noori M, Savvidou M, Williams DJ. In: Lyall F, Belfort M (Eds). Pre-eclampsia: Etiology and Clinical Practice. New York: Cambridge University Press; 2007.

137. Broughton Pipkin F. In: Lyall F, Belfort M (Eds). Pre-eclampsia: Etiology and Clinical Practice, Cambridge: Cambridge University Press; 2007.

138. Broughton Pipkin F, Morrison R, O'Brien PM. Prostacyclin attenuates both the pressor and adrenocortical response to angiotensin II in human pregnancy. Clin Sci (Lond). 1989;76(5):529-34.

139. Clark BA, Halvorson L, Sachs B, et al. Plasma endothelin levels in preeclampsia: elevation and correlation with uric acid levels and renal impairment. Am J Obstet Gynecol. 1992;166(3): 962-8.

140. Dekker GA, Kraayenbrink AA, Zeeman GG, et al. Increased plasma levels of the novel vasoconstrictor peptide endothelin in severe pre-eclampsia. Eur J Obstet Gynecol Reprod Biol. 1991;40(3):215-20.

141. Taylor RN, Varma M, Teng NN, et al. Women with preeclampsia have higher plasma endothelin levels than women with normal pregnancies. J Clin Endocrinol Metab. 1990;71(6):1675-7.

142. McCarthy AL, Woolfson RG, Raju SK, et al. Abnormal endothelial cell function of resistance arteries from women with preeclampsia. Am J Obstet Gynecol. 1993;168(4):1323-30.

143. Cockell AP, Poston L. Flow-mediated vasodilatation is enhanced in normal pregnancy but reduced in preeclampsia. Hypertension. 1997;30(2 Pt 1):247-51.

144. Chambers JC, Fusi L, Malik IS, et al. Association of maternal endothelial dysfunction with preeclampsia. JAMA. 2001;285(12):1607-12.

145. Torry DS, Hinrichs M, Torry RJ. Determinants of placental vascularity. Am J Reprod Immunol. 2004;51(4):257-68.

146. Torry DS, Mukherjea D, Arroyo J, et al. Expression and function of placenta growth factor: implications for abnormal placentation. J Soc Gynecol Investig. 2003;10(4):178-88.

147. Levine RJ, Maynard SE, Qian C, et al. Circulating angiogenic factors and the risk of preeclampsia. N Engl J Med. 2004;350(7):672-83.

148. Maynard SE, Min JY, Merchan J, et al. Excess placental soluble fms-like tyrosine kinase 1 (sFlt1) may contribute to endothelial dysfunction, hypertension, and proteinuria in preeclampsia. J Clin Invest. 2003;111(5):649-58.

149. Higgins JR, Papayianni A, Brady HR, et al. Circulating vascular cell adhesion molecule-1 in pre-eclampsia, gestational hypertension, and normal pregnancy: evidence of selective dysregulation of vascular cell adhesion molecule-1 homeostasis in pre-eclampsia. Am J Obstet Gynecol. 1998;179(2):464-9.

150. Musci TJ, Roberts JM, Rodgers GM, et al. Mitogenic activity is increased in the sera of preeclamptic women before delivery. Am J Obstet Gynecol. 1988;159(6):1446-51.

151. Schlembach D, Wallner W, Sengenberger R, et al. Angiogenic growth factor levels in maternal and fetal blood: correlation with Doppler ultrasound parameters in pregnancies complicated by pre-eclampsia and intrauterine growth restriction. Ultrasound Obstet Gynecol. 2007;29(4):407-13.

152. Tjoa ML, Levine RJ, Karumanchi SA. Angiogenic factors and preeclampsia. Front Biosci. 2007;12:2395-402.

153. Lee ES, Oh MJ, Jung JW, et al. The levels of circulating vascular endothelial growth factor and soluble Flt-1 in pregnancies complicated by preeclampsia. J Korean Med Sci. 2007;22(1):94-8.

154. Sane DC, Anton L, Brosnihan KB. Angiogenic growth factors and hypertension. Angiogenesis. 2004;7(3):193-201.

155. Khaliq A, Dunk C, Jiang J, et al. Hypoxia down-regulates placenta growth factor, whereas fetal growth restriction up-regulates placenta growth factor expression: molecular evidence for "placental hyperoxia" in intrauterine growth restriction. Lab Invest. 1999;79(2):151-70.

156. Caniggia I, Winter JL. Adriana and Luisa Castellucci Award lecture 2001. Hypoxia inducible factor-1: oxygen regulation of trophoblast differentiation in normal and pre-eclamptic pregnancies—a review. Placenta. 2002;23 Suppl A:S47-57.

157. Kingdom J, Huppertz B, Seaward G, et al. Development of the placental villous tree and its consequences for fetal growth. Eur J Obstet Gynecol Reprod Biol. 2000;92(1):35-43.

158. Borzychowski AM, Croy BA, Chan WL, et al. Changes in systemic type 1 and type 2 immunity in normal pregnancy and pre-eclampsia may be mediated by natural killer cells. Eur J Immunol. 2005;35(10):3054-63.

159. Dekker GA, Sibai BM. Etiology and pathogenesis of preeclampsia: current concepts. Am J Obstet Gynecol. 1998;179(5):1359-75.

160. Faas MM, Schuiling GA. Pre-eclampsia and the inflammatory response. Eur J Obstet Gynecol Reprod Biol. 2001;95(2):213-7.

161. Le Bouteiller P, Pizzato N, Barakonyi A, et al. HLA-G, pre-eclampsia, immunity and vascular events. J Reprod Immunol. 2003;59(2):219-34.

162. Moffett A, Loke YW. The immunological paradox of pregnancy: a reappraisal. Placenta. 2004;25(1):1-8.

163. Yie SM, Li LH, Li YM, et al. HLA-G protein concentrations in maternal serum and placental tissue are decreased in preeclampsia. Am J Obstet Gynecol. 2004;191(2):525-9.

164. Goldman-Wohl DS, Ariel I, Greenfield C, et al. Lack of human leukocyte antigen-G expression in extravillous trophoblasts is associated with pre-eclampsia. Mol Hum Reprod. 2000;6(1):88-95.

165. Wallukat G, Homuth V, Fischer T, et al. Patients with preeclampsia develop agonistic autoantibodies against the angiotensin AT1 receptor. J Clin Invest. 1999;103(7):945-52.

166. Xia Y, Wen H, Bobst S, et al. Maternal autoantibodies from preeclamptic patients activate angiotensin receptors on human trophoblast cells. J Soc Gynecol Investig. 2003;10(2):82-93.

167. Xia Y, Zhou CC, Ramin SM, et al. Angiotensin receptors, autoimmunity, and preeclampsia. J Immunol. 2007;179(6):3391-5.

168. Sacks GP, Studena K, Sargent K, et al. Normal pregnancy and preeclampsia both produce inflammatory changes in peripheral blood leukocytes akin to those of sepsis. Am J Obstet Gynecol. 1998;179(1):80-6.

169. Esteve JM, Mompo J, Garcia de la Asuncion J, et al. Oxidative damage to mitochondrial DNA and glutathione oxidation in apoptosis: studies in vivo and in vitro. Faseb J. 1999;13(9):1055-64.

170. Hampton MB, Fadeel B, Orrenius S. Redox regulation of the caspases during apoptosis. Ann N Y Acad Sci. 1998;854:328-35.

171. Goswami D, Tannetta DS, Magee LA, et al. Excess syncytiotrophoblast microparticle shedding is a feature of early-onset pre-eclampsia, but not normotensive intrauterine growth restriction. Placenta. 2006;27(1):56-61.

172. Knight M, Redman CW, Linton EA, et al. Shedding of syncytiotrophoblast microvilli into the maternal circulation in pre-eclamptic pregnancies. Br J Obstet Gynaecol. 1998;105(6):632-40.

173. Eskenazi B, Harley K. Commentary: Revisiting the primipaternity theory of pre-eclampsia. Int J Epidemiol. 2001;30(6):1323-24.

174. Need JA. Pre-eclampsia in pregnancies by different fathers: immunological studies. Br Med J. 1975;1(5957):548-9.

175. Feeney JG, Scott JS. Pre-eclampsia and changed paternity. Eur J Obstet Gynecol Reprod Biol. 1980;11(1):35-8.

176. Li DK, Wi S. Changing paternity and the risk of preeclampsia/eclampsia in the subsequent pregnancy. Am J Epidemiol. 2000;151(1):57-62.

177. Williams PJ, Broughton Pipkin F. The genetics of pre-eclampsia and other hypertensive disorders of pregnancy. Best Pract Res Clin Obstet Gynaecol. 2011;25(4):405-17.

178. Chesley LC, Annitto JE, Cosgrove RA. The familial factor in toxemia of pregnancy. Obstet Gynecol. 1968;32(3):303-11.

179. Arngrimsson R, Björnsson S, Geirsson RT, et al. Genetic and familial predisposition to eclampsia and pre-eclampsia in a defined population. Br J Obstet Gynaecol. 1990:97(9);762-9.

180. Cincotta RB, Brennecke SP. Family history of pre-eclampsia as a predictor for pre-eclampsia in primigravidas. Int J Gynaecol Obstet. 1998;60(1):23-7.

181. Sutherland A, Cooper DW, Howie PW, et al. The incidence of severe pre-eclampsia amongst mothers and mothers-in-law of pre-eclamptics and controls. Br J Obstet Gynaecol. 1981;88:785-91.

182. Graves JA. Genomic imprinting, development and disease--is pre-eclampsia caused by a maternally imprinted gene? Reprod Fertil Dev. 1998;10(1):23-9.

183. Lander ES, Schork NJ. Genetic dissection of complex traits. Science. 1994;265(5181):2037-48.

184. Harrison GA, Humphrey KE, Jones N, et al. A genomewide linkage study of preeclampsia/eclampsia reveals evidence for a candidate region on 4q. Am J Hum Genet. 1997;60(5):1158-67.

185. Rubin PC. Hypertension in pregnancy. In: Rubin PC (Ed). Handbook of Hypertension. Amsterdam: Elsevier Science; 1988.

186. Lindheimer MD, Roberts JM, Cunningham FG, et al. In: Lindheimer MD, Roberts JM, Cunningham FG (Eds). Chesley's Hypertensive Disorders in Pregnancy. New York: Elsevier Academic Press; 2009.

3 Prediction of Preeclampsia: Biochemical and Biophysical Parameters

Vikram Sinai Talaulikar, Sabaratnam Arulkumaran

■ INTRODUCTION

Despite extensive scientific research for several decades, the etiology of preeclampsia still remains poorly understood. This serious vascular complication of pregnancy occurs in 2–8% of pregnancies, and is one of the leading causes of maternal and perinatal morbidity and mortality throughout the world. Preeclampsia is also associated with long-term consequences such as a high risk of cardiovascular diseases later in life.[1]

Availability of accurate predictive tests for preeclampsia can potentially have a great impact on maternal health. Several biophysical and biochemical markers have been suggested. These include angiogenic/antiangiogenic factors, placental proteins, free fetal nucleic acids, renal markers, Doppler ultrasound of uterine artery flow and maternal risk factors. The most promising tests combine biochemical and biophysical parameters for assessment of both placentation and maternal disease susceptibility. Screening pregnant women with accurate predictive tests for preeclampsia in early pregnancy could reduce unnecessary suffering and health care costs by early stratification of mothers based on their risk of developing the disease. This could lead to timely institution of preventive strategies and increased vigilance in those at high risk as well as avoid unnecessary intervention in low-risk women.

■ PREECLAMPSIA AS A SPECTRUM OF DISEASE AND "EARLY" VERSUS "LATE" ONSET PREECLAMPSIA

It has been evident over the past few decades that preeclampsia may not be a single disease entity but a spectrum of disorders with varying severity and time of onset. Preeclampsia may have an early onset (before 34 weeks gestation) or late onset (after 34 weeks). There are important differences in the pathophysiology of early versus late onset preeclampsia.[2] Early onset disease is typically characterized by impaired placentation and fetal growth restriction while late onset preeclampsia appears to be related to maternal factors, associated with adequate fetal growth and is thought to occur when hemodynamic and metabolic changes overwhelm the maternal response to maintain homeostasis. Most predictive tests for preeclampsia are accordingly based on the two major underlying processes involved in the pathogenesis: (1) inadequate invasion of the maternal spiral uterine arteries by placental extravillous trophoblast cells in the first trimester and (2) widespread endothelial cell dysfunction and/or vascular vasoconstriction.

■ PREDICTIVE TESTS FOR PREECLAMPSIA

The World Health Organization (WHO) has set standards for selecting biomarkers to diagnose/predict a disease.[3,4] The criteria includes: (1) well defined disorder; (2) known prevalence; (3) medically important disorder for which there is an effective and socially accepted remedy; (4) screening should be cost effective; (5) test should use available infrastructure and be easily introduced; (6) after identifying the high-risk group, follow-up methods should be acceptable to healthcare professionals, patients and society; (7) tests should be simple and safe; (8) distribution of test values in affected and unaffected populations is known, extent of overlap is small, a suitable cut-off point is definable; (9) all people who may benefit should have access. Preeclampsia, as a disorder, meets the majority of these criteria; however, the accuracy, desired detection rates and cost effectiveness of the biomarkers is not yet established for preeclampsia.[4]

In 2004, a large systematic review of predictive tests for preeclampsia identified over 50 proposed screening tests but many of these, including commonly used serum uric acid or roll over test, had low predictive values and were not clinically useful.[5,6] Only uterine artery Doppler, antiphospholipid antibodies and urinary kallikrein were of moderate predictive value in low-risk women. The authors concluded that, as of 2004, there was no clinically useful screening test for prediction of preeclampsia.[5]

Predictive tests for preeclampsia can be classified into:
- Biophysical parameters
  - Clinical factors (history and examination)
  - Doppler ultrasound of uteroplacental circulation
  - Microcirculation (capillary) changes in preeclampsia
- Biochemical parameters
  - Free fetal nucleic acids
  - Pregnancy associated protein A (PAPP-A)
  - Placental protein 13 (PP13)
  - Cystatin C
  - Fetal hemoglobin (HbF) and alpha-1-microglobulin (A1M)
  - Pentraxin 3 (PTX3)
  - Markers related to angiogenesis
  - Other markers

A summary of common biophysical and biochemical markers is presented in Table 3.1.

■ BIOPHYSICAL PARAMETERS

Clinical Factors (Maternal History and Examination)

Clinical History

Several maternal clinical characteristics have been identified as risk factors for developing preeclampsia. The most important of these are

Table 3.1: Common biophysical and biochemical markers used in various tests for prediction of preeclampsia

Markers	Predictive Value
Clinical factors (history and examination)	• Ethnicity, age (risk doubles above 40), parity (three times risk in nulliparas), multiple pregnancy (three times increased risk), history of preeclampsia in earlier pregnancies (seven times increased risk), family history of preeclampsia (three times increased risk) and associated medical conditions are risk factors • Have a combined prediction rate of only about 30% • In the first or second trimester of pregnancy, the mean arterial pressure (MAP) is a better predictor than systolic blood pressure, diastolic blood pressure or an increase of blood pressure. • MAP in combination with maternal variables has a better predictive accuracy, detection rate of 62.5% for preeclampsia and 40% for gestational hypertension at a 10% false-positive rate
Serum uric acid, microalbuminuria, roll-over test, midtrimester diastolic blood pressure and urinary calcium excretion	• Low predictive value thus not clinically useful
Doppler ultrasound of uteroplacental circulation	• Abnormal waveforms in the uterine artery such as increased pulsatility index with notching have been reported to be a good predictor in high-risk women • In the prediction of preeclampsia requiring delivery before 34 weeks, second trimester Doppler performs well, with detection rates of about 80% • For term disease in unselected populations, use remains controversial
Free fetal nucleic acids	• Significantly increased in preeclampsia beginning in early pregnancy • Their role merits further evaluation and validation by larger studies

Contd...

Contd...

Markers	Predictive Value
Pregnancy associated protein A (PAPP-A)	• When used as a single biochemical marker, prediction rates of only 10–20%. But when combined with Doppler ultrasound, prediction rates of 70% at false-positive rates of 5%
Placental protein 13 (PP13)	• At false-positive rates of 5–10%, detection rates of 37.5–69% as a single biochemical marker • When combined with Doppler ultrasound, the prediction rate increases to 71% at a false-positive rate of 10%
Fetal hemoglobin (HbF) and alpha-1-microglobulin (A1M)	• Significantly increased at 10–16 weeks gestation in women who subsequently developed the disease • At a false-positive rate of 5%, the prediction rate was 69%
Pentraxin 3	• Significantly higher in women with established preeclampsia in the third trimester and promising even as a single marker • Combination with history, midarterial pressure, Doppler or placental growth factor levels leads to better performance at 11–13 weeks
Markers related to angiogenesis	• Proangiogenic markers decrease and antiangiogenic markers increase in preeclampsia • Serum levels of placental growth factor (PIGF) and vascular endothelial growth factor are lower while soluble fms-like tyrosine kinase 1 (sFlt-1) and soluble endoglin levels are raised • Ratio of PIGF/sFlt-1 appears to be a promising marker. Several studies have shown the predictive power of PIGF/sFlt-1 ratio from the second trimester. The prediction rate is about 89%
Combined models of testing with biophysical and biochemical markers	• Combined screening appears to give better predictive accuracy with the sensitivity and specificity for early preeclampsia reaching 94.1% and 94.3% respectively

ethnicity, age, parity, multiple pregnancy and a history of preeclampsia in earlier pregnancies. Associated medical conditions, such as obesity, diabetes mellitus, chronic hypertension, renal disease, antiphospholipid syndrome and certain autoimmune diseases, also increase the risk of preeclampsia.[7] But, none of these alone or in combination predict preeclampsia sufficiently, as they are reported to have a combined prediction rate of about 30%.[8]

A systematic review of studies (2005) by Duckitt and Harrington[7] showed that the risk of preeclampsia almost doubled in women over 40 years of age [relative risk (RR), 1.7; 95% confidence interval (CI), 1.2–2.3 in primiparous women and RR, 2; 95% CI, 1.3–2.9 in multiparous women]. The risk of preeclampsia tripled in nulliparous women (RR, 2.9; 95% CI, 1.3–6.6), women with a family history of preeclampsia (RR, 2.9; 95% CI, 1.7–4.9) and in women with multiple pregnancies (RR, 2.9; 95% CI, 2.0–4.2 in twins and RR, 2.8; 95% CI, 1.3–6.4 in triplet pregnancy). In women with insulin-dependent diabetes, the risk of developing preeclampsia was quadrupled (RR, 3.6; 95% CI, 2.5–5).[7] However, body mass index (BMI) (at any cut-off), prepregnancy or at booking, was a fairly weak predictor for preeclampsia.[9]

Clinical Examination

Risk of preeclampsia is increased with elevated first trimester mean arterial blood pressure.[7,10] Since different hospital guidelines or protocols vary in their methodology of blood pressure measurements, a standardized approach is recommended. Blood pressure should be measured with the patient in a sitting position with an appropriately sized blood pressure cuff and with the hands level with the heart to provide accurate and reliable values. In the United Kingdom (UK), the National Institute for Health and Clinical Excellence (NICE) recommends a single reading, using the correct cuff size at heart level and Korotkoff phase V sounds.[11]

In their systematic review and meta-analysis, Cnossen et al.[10] found that when blood pressure is measured in the first or second trimester of pregnancy, the mean arterial pressure (MAP) is a better predictor for preeclampsia than systolic blood pressure, diastolic blood pressure or an increase of blood pressure. MAP is simple, cheap and noninvasive measurement that can be easily performed in all women at their first routine antenatal visit. A mean arterial pressure of 90 mm Hg or more showed a pooled sensitivity of 62% (95% CI, 35–89%) and a pooled specificity of 82% (95% CI, 72–92%), which corresponds with derived likelihood ratio of a positive test 3.5 (95% CI, 2–5) and likelihood ratio of a negative test of 0.46 (95% CI, 0.16–0.75). For a specificity of 90%, the sensitivities of diastolic blood pressure and systolic blood pressure were 35% and 24% respectively. In high-risk populations, a diastolic blood pressure of 75 mm Hg or more at 13–20 weeks gestation best predicted preeclampsia, although the accuracy of prediction was modest (likelihood ratio of positive and negative test of 2.8 and 0.39 respectively).[9,10] Poon et al.[12] evaluated the performance of MAP at 11–13+6 weeks gestation in combination with maternal variables in the prediction of preeclampsia in a prospective study of 5,193 women with singleton pregnancies. They found that MAP in combination with maternal variables (ethnic origin, BMI, history of preeclampsia) had a better predictive accuracy than MAP alone. Combination testing could identify 62.5% of those women who would develop preeclampsia and 40% of those who would develop gestational hypertension, at a 10% false-positive rate.[12] Women with higher blood pressures in early pregnancy also appear to have a heightened sensitivity to the circulating antiangiogenic factors and as a consequence develop preeclampsia at lower concentrations of these factors.[13]

Doppler Ultrasound of Uteroplacental Circulation

In normal pregnancies, Doppler measurements show decreased impedance to blood flow in the uterine arteries. This ensures adequate transfer of oxygen and nutrients to the fetoplacental unit. In early preeclampsia and fetal growth restriction, Doppler findings reveal increased impedance to the blood flow, which often predate the onset of the clinical disease by several weeks. These findings reflect the inadequate transformation of

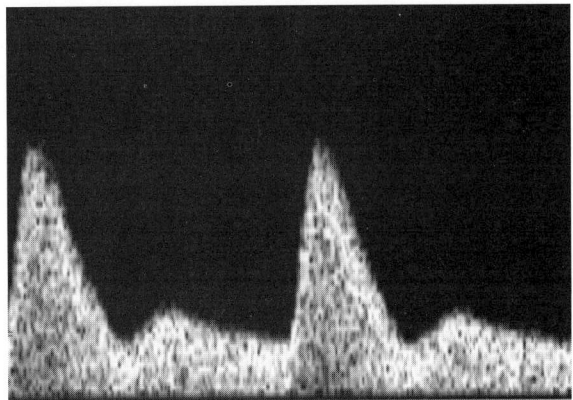

Fig. 3.1: Abnormal waveforms in the uterine artery, such as increased pulsatility index with persistent notching on Doppler ultrasound suggesting increased resistance to the uteroplacental blood flow

uterine spiral arteries by the invading extravillous trophoblast during early pregnancy. However, in the late onset form of preeclampsia such changes in uterine circulation are absent or mild. Most obstetric units now perform second trimester Doppler assessment of uterine circulation for prediction of preeclampsia.

Abnormal waveforms in the uterine artery (Fig. 3.1), such as increased pulsatility index (PI) with notching on Doppler ultrasound have been reported to be a good predictor of preeclampsia in high-risk women (positive likelihood ratio, 21).[14,15] Bilateral uterine artery notching or a mean PI above the 95th centile of the normal range indicates increased impedance of blood flow. It is known that the presence of either of these two factors at 23–24 weeks gestation in a routine antenatal population identifies 40% of women who later develop preeclampsia.[16] Evidence is also emerging on the possibility of use of Doppler for prediction of preeclampsia as early as 11 weeks gestation.[17] A large study of uterine artery Dopplers in 6,015 women at 11–13+6 weeks revealed a sensitivity of 82% for prediction of preeclampsia requiring delivery before 34 weeks at a 10% false-positive rate.[18] Yet another prospective study of 3,058 singleton pregnancies found that abnormal uterine artery Doppler at 11–14 weeks was significantly associated with preterm preeclampsia.[19]

In low-risk women and for term preeclampsia, however, the evidence supporting use of routine uterine artery Doppler screening is not strong and its use in the low-risk population remains controversial. A Cochrane review assessed the effects on pregnancy outcome, and obstetric practice, of routine uteroplacental Doppler ultrasound in first and second trimester of pregnancy in women at high and low risk of hypertensive complications. Two studies involving 4,993 participants were included. Both studies included women at low risk for hypertensive disorders, with Doppler ultrasound of the uterine arteries performed in the second trimester of pregnancy. In both studies, pathological finding of uterine arteries was followed by low dose aspirin administration. There was no difference in short-term maternal and fetal clinical outcomes. There was no benefit to either the baby or the mother when uteroplacental Doppler ultrasound was used in the second trimester of pregnancy in women at low risk for hypertensive disorders.[20] Another Cochrane review was conducted to assess the effects on obstetric practice and pregnancy outcome of routine fetal and umbilical Doppler ultrasound in unselected and low-risk pregnancies. Five controlled trials of Doppler ultrasound for the investigation of umbilical and fetal vessels waveforms in unselected pregnancies compared to no Doppler were included (n = 14,185 women). Routine fetal and umbilical Doppler ultrasound examination in low-risk or unselected populations did not result in increased antenatal, obstetric and neonatal interventions, and no overall differences were detected for substantive short-term clinical outcomes such as perinatal mortality.[21]

The detection rates of preeclampsia with uterine artery Doppler are better for the preterm and/or early onset disease than for the term severe or mild disease. The second trimester uterine artery Doppler studies show detection rates of 70–80% for preterm preeclampsia, while the detection rates are 30–40% for preeclampsia at any gestational age, with false-positive rates between 5% and 7%.[22]

A new approach that is being considered is 3D power Doppler of the uteroplacental circulation. In a recent prospective nonintervention study of 277 women at 10–13 weeks, the women (n = 24) who later presented with preeclampsia had significantly reduced indices of uteroplacental vascularization and blood flow.[23]

Structural Capillary Rarefaction and the Onset of Preeclampsia

Based on the findings in hypertensive nonpregnant patients, a recent study assessed, whether reduced capillary density (capillary rarefaction) preceded the onset of preeclampsia and could play a role in its pathogenesis. In this longitudinal cohort study including 305 women, intravital video microscopy was used to measure basal and maximal skin capillary densities, and levels of plasma angiogenic and antiangiogenic factors were measured. Women were studied at five consecutive predetermined visits. Preeclampsia occurred in 16 women (mean onset at 35.6 ± 4.8 weeks gestation), 272 women had normal pregnancies, eight had hypertension and nine pregnancies were complicated by fetal growth restriction. In women with a normal pregnancy, significant reduction in maximal capillary density occurred at 27–32 weeks but had resolved by the puerperium. In contrast, in women who later developed preeclampsia, structural rarefaction was greater and occurred earlier at 20–24 weeks of gestation and persisted into the puerperium. The change in soluble endoglin (antiangiogenic) from 11 weeks to 16 weeks gestation to 27–32 weeks gestation correlated significantly with the change in structural capillary density. The authors concluded that significant structural capillary rarefaction precedes the onset of preeclampsia and could play a role in its pathogenesis. These findings appear interesting and could hold a promise for development of novel predictive tests for preeclampsia in the future.[24]

■ BIOCHEMICAL PARAMETERS

Using new research technologies such as genomics and proteomics, several new pathways and bioactive factors have been described in the pathogenesis of preeclampsia.[25] Some of these markers are products of the trophoblast or adjacent decidua and reflect the placental dysfunction, while others represent the maternal systemic inflammatory response and widespread endothelial dysfunction.

The chemical structure and tissue origin of a marker influences its appearance in maternal blood. The time window in which the difference between the blood levels in women who will develop preeclampsia and those who will not, can also vary between markers. It is important to note that many of the markers show significant variation during normal pregnancy and may not always be discriminative enough to be clinically useful.[26]

Free Fetal Nucleic Acids

Fetal nucleic acids (fetal DNA and mRNA) are mainly of placental origin and they can now be readily detected and quantified in the maternal plasma using techniques such as real-time polymerase chain reaction and fluorescence in situ hybridization. Unlike free fetal DNA (ffDNA) [the amount of which is routinely determined by quantifying Y chromosome specific sequences, e.g. sex determining region Y (SRY)], the mRNA has the advantage of being a fetal marker that could be used in pregnancies with both male and female fetuses. Free fetal DNA is detected in maternal plasma as early as the 4th week of gestation and its concentration increases with gestational age. It is rapidly cleared from maternal plasma following delivery of the placenta. Trophoblastic apoptosis from placenta appears to be the main source of ffDNA in the maternal circulation.[27] A number of studies have demonstrated elevated levels of fetal nucleic acids (ffDNA and mRNA) in preeclampsia. Lo et al. showed a five-fold increase in the median concentration of circulating fetal DNA in women with preeclampsia compared with normal pregnancies matched for gestational age.[28] Alberry et al.[29] found that in pregnancies with either preeclampsia or fetal growth restriction, there were higher levels of ffDNA than in normal pregnancy. Shimada et al.[30] found an increased ffDNA concentration in placental complications such as preeclampsia, placenta previa and premature placental separation.

In a large study performed on 2,156 pregnancies with male fetuses, Levine et al.[31] demonstrated an elevation of ffDNA in maternal plasma at two time points in pregnancy - between 17 weeks and 28 weeks of gestation followed by a second elevation 3 weeks before the onset of symptoms and recent studies suggest that levels are high as early as the first trimester of pregnancy in women who develop early and severe preeclampsia.[32,33] Free fetal DNA levels have also been correlated with the severity of the disease.[34]

Maternal plasma mRNA for plasminogen activator inhibitor-1 and tissue-type plasminogen activator was found to be significantly increased in women with preeclampsia and positively correlated with the severity.[35] Farina et al.[36] compared the concentration of seven mRNA markers [inhibin A, plasminogen activator inhibitor-1, selectin-P, KISS1, human placental lactogen, pregnancy-associated plasma protein-A and vascular endothelial growth factor receptor (VEGF)] between normal pregnancy and preeclampsia, and demonstrated a significant increase in fetal DNA and mRNA in the preeclampsia group. The role of fetal nucleic acids as potential markers for preeclampsia prediction looks promising and merits further evaluation and validation by larger studies.

Pregnancy Associated Protein A

Pregnancy associated protein A is a glycoprotein synthesized in the placenta and its maternal plasma concentration increases throughout the pregnancy. It is a protease for the insulin-like growth factor binding protein-4 (IGFBP-4). PAPP-A has been used in combination with beta human chorionic gonadotropin (β hCG) and nuchal translucency thickness for trisomy 21 screening towards the end of first trimester. Decreased levels of PAPP-A in the first trimester have been associated with increased risk for preeclampsia, fetal growth restriction and preterm delivery.[37-40]

When PAPP-A is used as a single biochemical marker for preeclampsia screening, it fares poorly, with prediction rates of only 10–20%.[41-43] But when combined with Doppler ultrasound, PAPP-A has prediction rates of 70% at false-positive rates of 5%.[25]

Placental Protein 13

Placental protein 13 is a member of the galectin family and is produced by the placental trophoblast cells.

In normal pregnancies, serum levels of PP13 slowly rise with advancing gestation. Several studies have shown lower serum levels of PP13 in the first trimester in pregnancies that subsequently developed preeclampsia.[44,45] At false-positive rates of 5–10% they found detection rates of 37.5–69%, using PP13 as a single biochemical marker. When serum screening was combined with the Doppler ultrasound, the prediction rate increased to 71% at a false-positive rate of 10%.[45]

Romero et al.[46] in their study of 300 patients, 50 of whom developed preeclampsia, showed a detection rate of 36% for all types of preeclampsia at false-positive rate of 20% using PP13 screening. While the prediction rate for early onset pre-eclampsia (< 34 weeks) was 100% and preterm preeclampsia (< 37 weeks) 85%, the prediction rate for severe preeclampsia at term was 24%. PP13 therefore appears to be a reasonable biochemical marker for early onset and preterm disease but a weak marker for term preeclampsia. Nicolaides et al.[47] also studied PP13 as a biochemical marker for early onset preeclampsia at 11–13+6 weeks gestation. At a false-positive rate of 10%, PP13 showed a prediction rate of 80% as a single marker and in combination with Doppler ultrasound, the prediction rate increased to 90%.

Cystatin C

Cystatin C is a protease inhibitor and marker for renal function. The maternal plasma level of cystatin C is increased in women with preeclampsia and level of cystatin C is a reliable diagnostic marker for preeclampsia.[48,49] Cystatin C may prove useful in combination with other biomarkers in prediction of preeclampsia.

Fetal Hemoglobin and Alpha1-Microglobulin

Increased mRNA levels of HbF in the placental tissue and free HbF protein in the placental vascular lumen have been described in women with preeclampsia.[25,50] Hemoglobin and its metabolites are highly reactive and could result in cell membrane and DNA damage and inactivation of nitric oxide (NO) by generation of reactive oxygen species.[51,52] The plasma and tissue protein A1M has been shown to bind and degrade heme, have radical-scavenger properties and protect cells.[25,53,54]

In a study of 96 patients (60 of whom developed preeclampsia) the serum concentrations of HbF and A1M were significantly increased at 10–16 weeks gestation in women who subsequently developed the disease. At a false-positive rate of 5%, the prediction rate was 69%. Optimal prediction rate was 90% for a false-positive rate of 23%.[55]

Pentraxin 3

Pentraxin 3 (PTX3) is an inflammatory molecule belonging to the pentraxin family and is expressed in response to inflammatory stimuli by a variety of cells, including endothelial cells, monocytes, macrophages and fibroblasts.[56] Studies have shown that maternal PTX3 levels are significantly higher in women with established preeclampsia in the third trimester when compared to those with normal pregnancies.[57,58] Abnormally high maternal serum PTX3 levels in early pregnancy appear to be associated with subsequent development of preterm preeclampsia.[59,60] Poon et al. have shown that combination of PTX3 with other information, such as history, mean arterial pressure, Doppler or placental growth factor levels, leads to better performance in patients at 11–13 weeks gestation than as a single marker.[61]

Markers Related to Angiogenesis

Preeclampsia is characterized by an antiangiogenic state and angiogenic markers can be utilized to predict preeclampsia a few weeks before the onset of clinical symptoms. The difficulties associated with the use of these markers, is their variability and that they are not specific for preeclampsia but show similar changes in intrauterine growth restriction not associated with preeclampsia.[62]

In normal pregnancy, a proangiogenic state exists, with low levels of antiangiogenic factors until the end of the second trimester and high levels of angiogenic factors. But toward the end of pregnancy these ratios gradually begin to reverse. Women with preeclampsia show alterations in these angiogenic profiles, with an earlier shift to an antiangiogenic state with endothelial dysfunction. In preeclampsia, serum levels of placental growth factor (PlGF) and VEGF are lower while soluble fms-like tyrosine kinase 1 (sFlt-1) and soluble endoglin (sEng) levels are raised.[63,64]

Vascular Endothelial Growth Factor

Vascular endothelial growth factor is the principal promoter of angiogenesis. It stimulates endothelial cell migration and sprouting of new blood vessels. First trimester $VEGF_{165}b$ concentrations are significantly reduced in the plasma of women who later develop preeclampsia.[15]

Soluble fms-like Tyrosine Kinase 1

Soluble fms-like tyrosine kinase 1 is a splice variant of the VEGF receptor which is inhibitory to VEGF. This antiangiogenic molecule is produced by the placenta and binds to VEGF, preventing it from exerting its physiological effects. Increased levels of sFlt-1 have been described in early onset preeclampsia.[63,65-67] Administration of sFlt-1 to pregnant rats resulted in hypertension and proteinuria.[68] High concentrations have been detected in the maternal circulation 5 weeks before the onset of clinical disease.[65] Other authors have also reported that high sFlt-1 levels early in pregnancy may be predictive of subsequent preeclampsia.[69,70]

Placental Growth Factor

Placental growth factor is a proangiogenic molecule from the VEGF family. It is expressed in large amounts by the syncytiotrophoblast. Serum levels of PlGF are lower in preeclampsia and the ratio of PlGF/sFlt-1 appears to be a promising marker for prediction of preeclampsia. Several studies have shown the predictive power of PlGF/sFlt-1 ratio from the second trimester.[71-73] The prediction rate is about 89%.[25,73] For a diagnostic cut-off of 38.46 for sFlt-1/PlGF ratio, the positive and negative predictive values were 88.5%, positive likelihood ratio was 7.7 and negative likelihood ratio was 0.13.[73] For a cut-off value of 85 for sFlt-1/PlGF ratio, the highest sensitivity was 82% and specificity was 95%.[72]

Soluble Endoglin

Endoglin is a coreceptor for transforming growth factor beta 1 and beta 3 and is expressed by placental trophoblasts. A soluble form of this molecule is elevated in the serum from 17 weeks of gestation in women who develop preeclampsia[63] and contributes to the endothelial dysfunction. Its concentration is correlated with disease severity and along with sFlt-1, it has been shown to increase microvascular permeability.[74] When sEng is used in the first trimester in combination with Doppler ultrasound and PlGF, the prediction rate for early onset preeclampsia is 77.8% at a false-positive rate of 5%.[75]

Other Markers

A number of other biomarkers including maternal serum alpha-fetoprotein, HCG, serum ischemia modified albumen, serum neutrophil gelatinase-associated lipocalin, serum P selectin and plasma fibronectin have been evaluated in single or combined screening models and some appear to hold promise for development of screening strategies in the future. Urinary kallikrein excretion is another example of a test that seems to offer the promise of both high sensitivity (greater than 80%) and specificity (greater than 90%), and requires further investigation.[9] The excretion of urinary kallikrein is lower in preeclampsia than in the normotensive pregnancy.

■ COMBINING BIOPHYSICAL AND BIOCHEMICAL MARKERS FOR PREECLAMPSIA PREDICTION

Given the variation in onset and severity of preeclampsia in different women, and the wide range of markers available, it appears that combination testing rather than single marker approach may be more accurate and reliable for prediction of preeclampsia.

The combination of maternal history and uterine artery Doppler assessment at 23 weeks resulted in the prediction of 67.5% of women who subsequently developed preeclampsia.[76] However, the false-positive rate for this method was 25%. Crispi et al.[77] found that at 24 weeks of gestation, combined uterine artery PI and maternal PlGF accurately predicted 89.5% of early onset preeclampsia with a specificity of 95%. Diab et al.[78] quantified sFlt-1 and PIGF concentrations in 108 pregnant women with abnormal uterine artery waveforms at 23 weeks: sFlt-1 concentration was significantly higher and PIGF lower in the serum of women developing preeclampsia later in the pregnancy. The addition of the sFlt-1/PIGF ratio to Doppler ultrasound analysis further improved the power to predict preeclampsia in the second trimester, with a sensitivity and specificity of 98% and 95% respectively.

In another study of 63 pregnancies with abnormal uterine perfusion at 21 weeks of gestation, sFlt-1 and uterine artery PI combination had a sensitivity of 83% and a specificity of 95% in preeclampsia prediction.[79]

Nicolaides et al.[47] have shown that low PP13 and elevated median uterine artery PI at 11+0–13+6 weeks of gestation can identify 90% of cases of future preeclampsia (with a 10% false-positive rate). Akolekar et al.[8] combined maternal characteristics, PI and MAP with serum levels of PAPP-A, PlGF, PP13, inhibin-A, activin-A, sEng, pentraxin 3 and P-selectin in a large study at 11–13+6 weeks gestation. The prediction rates, at a false-positive rate of 5%, were 91% for early onset, 79.4% for intermediate onset and 60.9% for late onset preeclampsia. Wortelboer et al.[80] also developed a model based on the first trimester biochemical markers, PAPP-A, β hCG, PlGF, disintegrin and ADAM metallopeptidase domain 12 (ADAM12). Their prediction of all preeclampsia was 44% at a 5% false-positive rate.

A first trimester model based on maternal characteristics, PI and the biochemical markers PAPP-A, inhibin-A, PP13, ADAM12, free β hCG and PlGF has been developed by Audibert et al. who showed a 100% prediction rate for early onset preeclampsia at a false-positive rate of 10%.[81] Poon et al.[82] evaluated 7,797 women with singleton, first trimester pregnancies with a predictive model incorporating maternal variables, uterine artery Doppler, maternal MAP, PAPP-A and PlGF. At a 5% false-positive rate, the sensitivity and specificity for early preeclampsia were 94.1% and 94.3% respectively. The likelihood ratio for a positive test was 16.5 and the negative likelihood ratio was 0.06.

SCREENING—NEED FOR SIMPLICITY AS WELL AS ACCURACY

Preeclampsia is still responsible for a large number of maternal deaths in the less resourced countries of the world, where it is often first diagnosed when the woman presents with complications such as eclampsia or placental abruption. Some of these women do not even have an access to the most basic antenatal services such as regular blood pressure monitoring, ultrasound examinations or care by doctors. These factors are important to be considered if a useful biomarker is to be developed for use in such settings for preeclampsia prediction. Simplicity and accuracy of prediction are both equally desired aspects of predictive tests for preeclampsia, which could prove life saving for mothers in under resourced settings.

CONCLUSION

Early prediction of development of preeclampsia is important as it could lead to appropriate allocation of health care resources with increased surveillance in women at high risk while avoiding unnecessary intervention in those at low risk. The UK, NICE guidelines require that at the first clinical visit of a pregnant woman, a risk assessment for preeclampsia be performed and plan made regarding further antenatal care on its basis. Most obstetric units presently rely on clinical history, blood pressure examination and urinary protein testing for prediction of preeclampsia. However, a large number of potential biophysical and biochemical markers have been identified in the recent times for accurate prediction of the risk of developing preeclampsia. Fetal nucleic acids, angiogenic vascular markers and placental proteins hold promise for future, either alone or in combination with uterine artery Doppler. Presently, the results seem more accurate for prediction of early onset preeclampsia which accounts for a small number of cases but is responsible for majority of fetal and maternal morbidity and mortality. However, research also needs to continue into developing preventive strategies and its benefit needs to be demonstrated, before screening can be universally recommended.

REFERENCES

1. McDonald SD, Malinowski A, Zhou Q, et al. Cardiovascular sequelae of preeclampsia/eclampsia: a systematic review and meta-analyses. Am Heart J. 2008;156(5):918-30.

2. Raymond D, Peterson E. A critical review of early-onset and late-onset preeclampsia. Obstet Gynecol Surv. 2011;66(8):497-506.

3. Wilson JM, Jungner YG. Principles and practice of screening for disease. Public health Papers no. 34, vol. 22. Geneva: World Health Organization; 1968. pp. 1-163.

4. Cetin I, Huppertz B, Burton G, et al. Pregenesys pre-eclampsia markers consensus meeting: What do we require from markers, risk assessment and model systems to tailor preventive strategies? Placenta. 2011;32 Suppl:S4-16.

5. Conde-Agudelo A, Villar J, Lindheimer M. World Health Organization systematic review of screening tests for preeclampsia. Obstet Gynecol. 2004;104(6):1367-91.

6. Leslie K, Thilaganathan B, Papageorghiou A. Early prediction and prevention of pre-eclampsia. Best Pract Res Clin Obstet Gynaecol. 2011;25(3):343-54.

7. Duckitt K, Harrington D. Risk factors for pre-eclampsia at antenatal booking: systematic review of controlled studies. BMJ. 2005;330(7491):565.

8. Akolekar R, Syngelaki A, Sarquis R, et al. Prediction of early, intermediate and late pre-eclampsia from maternal factors, biophysical and biochemical markers at 11-13 weeks. Prenat Diagn. 2011;31(1): 66-74.

9. Thangaratinam S, Langenveld J, Mol BW, et al. Prediction and primary prevention of preeclampsia. Best Pract Res Clin Obstet Gynaecol. 2011;25(4): 419-33.

10. Cnossen JS, Vollebregt KC, de Vrieze N, et al. Accuracy of mean arterial pressure and blood pressure measurements in predicting pre-eclampsia: systematic review and meta-analysis. BMJ. 2008;336(7653):1117-20.

11. National Collaborating Centre for Women's and Children's Health (2008). NICE Guideline. Antenatal care: routine care for the healthy pregnant woman CG62 [online] Available from www.nice.org.uk [Accessed April 2013]

12. Poon LC, Kametas NA, Pandeva I, et al. Mean arterial pressure at 11(+0) to 13(+6) weeks in the prediction of preeclampsia. Hypertension. 2008;51(4):1027-33.

13. Noori M, Donald AE, Angelakopoulou A, et al. Prospective study of placental angiogenic factors and maternal vascular function before and after preeclampsia and gestational hypertension. Circulation. 2010;122(5):478-87.

14. Cnossen JS, Morris RK, ter Riet G, et al. Use of uterine artery Doppler ultrasonography to predict pre-eclampsia and intrauterine growth restriction: a systematic review and bivariable meta-analysis. CMAJ. 2008;178(6):701-11.

15. Alberry M, Bills V, Soothill P. An update on pre-eclampsia prediction research. The Obstetrician & Gynaecologist. 2011;13:79-85.

16. Papageorghiou AT, Yu CK, Cicero S, et al. Second trimester uterine artery Doppler screening in unselected populations: a review. J Matern Fetal Neonatal Med. 2002;12(2):78-88.

17. Plasencia W, Maiz N, Poon L, et al. Uterine artery Doppler at 11 + 0 to 13 + 6 weeks and 21 + 0 to 24 + 6 weeks in the prediction of pre-eclampsia. Ultrasound Obstet Gynecol. 2008;32(2):138-46.

18. Plasencia W, Maiz N, Bonino S, et al. Uterine artery Doppler at 11 to 13+6 weeks in the prediction of pre-eclampsia. Ultrasound Obstet Gynecol. 2007; 30:742-9.

19. Melchiorre K, Wormald B, Leslie K, et al. First-trimester uterine artery Doppler indices in term and preterm pre-eclampsia. Ultrasound Obstet Gynecol. 2008;32(2):133-7.

20. Stampalija T, Gyte GM, Alfirevic Z. Utero-placental Doppler ultrasound for improving pregnancy outcome. Cochrane Database Syst Rev. 2010;(9):CD008363.

21. Alfirevic Z, Stampalija T, Gyte GM. Fetal and umbilical Doppler ultrasound in normal pregnancy. Cochrane Database Syst Rev. 2010;(8):CD001450.

22. Spencer K, Cowans NJ, Chefetz I, et al. First-trimester maternal serum PP-13, PAPP-A and second-trimester uterine artery Doppler pulsatility index as markers of pre-eclampsia. Ultrasound Obstet Gynecol. 2007;29(2):128-34.

23. Dar P, Gebb J, Reimers L, et al. First-trimester 3-dimensional power Doppler of the uteroplacental circulation space: a potential screening method for preeclampsia. Am J Obstet Gynecol. 2010;203(3): 238.e1-7.

24. Nama V, Manyonda IT, Onwude J, et al. Structural capillary rarefaction and the onset of preeclampsia. Obstet Gynecol. 2012;119(5):967-74.

25. Anderson UD, Olsson MG, Kristensen KH, et al. Review: Biochemical markers to predict pre-eclampsia. Placenta. 2012;33 Suppl:S42-7.

26. Baumann MU, Bersinger NA, Surbek DV. Serum markers for predicting pre-eclampsia. Mol Aspects Med. 2007;28(2):227-44.

27. Ishihara N, Matsuo H, Murakoshi H, et al. Increased apoptosis in the syncytiotrophoblast in human term placentas complicated by either preeclampsia or intrauterine growth retardation. Am J Obstet Gynecol. 2002;186(1):158-66.

28. Lo YM, Leung TN, Tein MS, et al. Quantitative abnormalities of fetal DNA in maternal serum in PET. Clin Chem. 1999;45(2):184-8.

29. Alberry MS, Maddocks DG, Hadi MA, et al. Quantification of cell free fetal DNA in maternal plasma in normal pregnancies and in pregnancies with placental dysfunction. Am J Obstet Gynecol. 2009;200(1):98.e1-6.

30. Shimada K, Murakami K, Shozu M, et al. Sex-determining region Y levels in maternal plasma: evaluation in abnormal pregnancy. J Obstet Gynaecol Res. 2004;30(2):148-54.

31. Levine RJ, Qian C, Leshane ES. Two-stage elevation of cell-free fetal DNA in maternal sera before onset of preeclampsia. Am J Obstet Gynecol. 2004;190(3):707-13.

32. Illanes S, Parra M, Trebilcock J, et al. Increased free fetal DNA (ffDNA) levels in the plasma of pregnant women in early pregnancy are observed in patients who subsequently develop severe placental disease. Ultrasound Obstet Gynecol. 2007;30:431.

33. Illanes S, Parra M, Serra R, et al. Increased free fetal DNA levels in early pregnancy plasma of

women who subsequently develop preeclampsia and intrauterine growth restriction. Prenat Diagn. 2009;29(12):1118-22.

34. Swinkels DW, de Kok JB, Hendriks JC, et al. Hemolysis, elevated liver enzymes and low platelet count (HELLP) syndrome as a complication of preeclampsia in pregnant women increases the amount of cell-free fetal and maternal DNA in maternal plasma and serum. Clin Chem. 2002;48(4):650-3.

35. Purwosunu Y, Sekizawa A, Koide K, et al. Cell-free mRNA concentrations of plasminogen activator inhibitor-1 and tissue-type plasminogen activator are increased in the plasma of pregnant women with preeclampsia. Clin Chem. 2007;53(3):399-404.

36. Farina A, Sekizawa A, Purwosunu Y, et al. Quantitative distribution of a panel of circulating mRNA in preeclampsia versus controls. Prenat Diagn. 2006;26(12):1115-20.

37. Ranta JK, Raatikainen K, Romppanen J, et al. Decreased PAPP-A is associated with preeclampsia, premature delivery and small for gestational age infants but not with placental abruption. Eur J Obstet Gynecol Reprod Biol. 2011;157(1):48-52.

38. Odibo AO, Zhong Y, Longtine M, et al. First-trimester serum analytes, biophysical tests and the association with pathological morphometry in the placenta of pregnancies with preeclampsia and fetal growth restriction. Placenta. 2011;32(4):333-8.

39. Spencer K, Yu CK, Cowans NJ, et al. Prediction of pregnancy complications by first-trimester maternal serum PAPP-A and free beta-hCG and with second-trimester uterine artery Doppler. Prenat Diagn. 2005;25(10):949-53.

40. Smith GC, Stenhouse EJ, Crossley JA, et al. Early pregnancy levels of pregnancy-associated plasma protein a and the risk of intrauterine growth restriction, premature birth, preeclampsia, and stillbirth. J Clin Endocrinol Metab. 2002;87(4):1762-7.

41. Goetzinger KR, Singla A, Gerkowicz S, et al. Predicting the risk of pre-eclampsia between 11 and 13 weeks' gestation by combining maternal characteristics and serum analytes, PAPP-A and free β-hCG. Prenat Diagn. 2010;30(12-13):1138-42.

42. Poon LC, Maiz N, Valencia C, et al. First-trimester maternal serum pregnancy-associated plasma protein-A and pre-eclampsia. Ultrasound Obstet Gynecol. 2009;33(1):23-33.

43. Spencer K, Cowans NJ, Nicolaides KH. Low levels of maternal serum PAPP-A in the first trimester and the risk of pre-eclampsia. Prenat Diagn. 2008;28(1):7-10.

44. Akolekar R, Syngelaki A, Beta J, et al. Maternal serum placental protein 13 at 11-13 weeks of gestation in preeclampsia. Prenat Diagn. 2009;29(12):1103-8.

45. Khalil A, Cowans NJ, Spencer K, et al. First trimester markers for the prediction of pre-eclampsia in women with a-priori high risk. Ultrasound Obstet Gynecol. 2010;35(6):671-9.

46. Romero R, Kusanovic JP, Than NG, et al. First trimester maternal serum PP13 in the risk assessment for preeclampsia. Am J Obstet Gynecol. 2008;199(2):122.e1-122.e11.

47. Nicolaides KH, Bindra R, Turan OM, et al. A novel approach to first-trimester screening for early pre-eclampsia combining serum PP-13 and Doppler ultrasound. Ultrasound Obstet Gynecol. 2006;27(1):13-7.

48. Kristensen K, Wide-Swensson D, Schmidt C, et al. Cystatin C, beta-2-microglobulin and beta-trace protein in pre-eclampsia. Acta Obstet Gynecol Scand. 2007;86(8):921-6.

49. Strevens H, Wide-Swensson D, Grubb A. Serum cystatin C is a better marker for preeclampsia than serum creatinine or serum urate. Scand J Clin Lab Invest. 2001;61(7):575-80.

50. Centlow M, Carninci P, Nemeth K, et al. Placental expression profiling in preeclampsia: local overproduction of hemoglobin may drive pathological changes. Fertil Steril. 2008;90(5):1834-43.

51. Tsemakhovich VA, Bamm VV, Shaklai M, et al. Vascular damage by unstable hemoglobins: the role of heme-depleted globin. Arch Biochem Biophys. 2005;436(2):307-15.

52. Kim-Shapiro DB, Schechter AN, Gladwin MT. Unraveling the reactions of nitric oxide, nitrite, and hemoglobin in physiology and therapeutics. Arterioscler Thromb Vasc Biol. 2006;26(4):697-705.

53. Allhorn M, Berggård T, Nordberg J, et al. Processing of the lipocalin alpha(1)-microglobulin by hemoglobin induces heme-binding and heme-degradation properties. Blood. 2002;99(6):1894-901.

54. Akerström B, Maghzal GJ, Winterbourn CC. The lipocalin alpha1- microglobulin has radical scavenging activity. J Biol Chem. 2007;282(43):31493-503.

55. Anderson UD, Olsson MG, Rutardóttir S, et al. Fetal hemoglobin and α(1)-microglobulin as first- and early second trimester predictive biomarkers for preeclampsia. Am J Obstet Gynecol. 2011;204(6):520.e1-5.

56. Garlanda C, Bottazzi B, Bastone A, et al. Pentraxins at the crossroads between innate immunity, inflammation, matrix deposition, and female fertility. Annu Rev Immunol. 2005;23:337-66.

57. Cetin I, Cozzi V, Pasqualini F, et al. Elevated maternal levels of the long pentraxin 3 (PTX3) in preeclampsia and intrauterine growth restriction. Am J Obstet Gynecol. 2006;194(5):1347-53.

58. Rovere-Querini P, Antonacci S, Dell'Antonio G, et al. Plasma and tissue expression of the long pentraxin 3 during normal pregnancy and preeclampsia. Obstet Gynecol. 2006;108(1):148-55.

59. Cetin I, Cozzi V, Papageorghiou AT, et al. First trimester PTX3 levels in women who subsequently develop preeclampsia and fetal growth restriction. Acta Obstet Gynecol Scand. 2009;88(7):846-9.

60. Akolekar R, Casagrandi D, Livanos P, et al. Maternal plasma pentraxin 3 at 11 to 13 weeks of gestation in hypertensive disorders of pregnancy. Prenat Diagn. 2009;29(10):934-8.

61. Poon LC, Akolekar R, Lachmann R, et al. Hypertensive disorders in pregnancy: screening by biophysical and biochemical markers at 11-13 weeks. Ultrasound Obstet Gynecol. 2010;35(6):662-70.

62. Stepan H, Krämer T, Faber R. Maternal plasma concentrations of soluble endoglin in pregnancies with intrauterine growth restriction. J Clin Endocrinol Metab. 2007;92(7):2831-4.

63. Levine RJ, Lam C, Qian C, et al. Soluble endoglin and other circulating antiangiogenic factors in preeclampsia. N Engl J Med. 2006;355(10):992-1005.

64. Rana S, Karumanchi SA, Levine RJ, et al. Sequential changes in antiangiogenic factors in early pregnancy and risk of developing preeclampsia. Hypertension. 2007;50(1):137-42.

65. Levine RJ, Maynard SE, Qian C, et al. Circulating angiogenic factors and the risk of preeclampsia. N Engl J Med. 2004;350(7):672-83.

66. Maynard SE, Min JY, Merchan J, et al. Excess placental soluble fms-like tyrosine kinase 1 (sFlt1) may contribute to endothelial dysfunction, hypertension, and proteinuria in preeclampsia. J Clin Invest. 2003;111(5):649-58.

67. Wikstrom AK, Larsson A, Eriksson UJ, et al. Placental growth factor and soluble FMS-like tyrosine kinase-1 in early-onset and late-onset preeclampsia. Obstet Gynecol. 2007;109(6):1368-74.

68. Ferrara N. Vascular endothelial growth factor: basic science and clinical progress. Endocr Rev. 2004;25(4):581-611.

69. Wathén KA, Tuutti E, Stenman UH, et al. Maternal serum-soluble vascular endothelial growth factor receptor-1 in early pregnancy ending in preeclampsia or intrauterine growth retardation. J Clin Endocrinol Metab. 2006;91(1):180-4.

70. Thadhani R, Mutter WP, Wolf M, et al. First trimester placental growth factor and soluble fms-like tyrosine kinase 1 and risk for preeclampsia. J Clin Endocrinol Metab. 2004;89(2):770-5.

71. Akolekar R, de Cruz J, Foidart JM, et al. Maternal plasma soluble fms-like tyrosine kinase-1 and free vascular endothelial growth factor at 11 to 13 weeks of gestation in preeclampsia. Prenat Diagn. 2010;30(3):191-7.

72. Verlohren S, Galindo A, Schlembach D, et al. An automated method for the determination of the sFlt-1/PlGF ratio in the assessment of preeclampsia. Am J Obstet Gynecol. 2010;202(2):161.e1-161.e11.

73. De Vivo A, Baviera G, Giordano D, et al. Endoglin, PlGF and sFlt-1 as markers for predicting preeclampsia. Acta Obstet Gynecol Scand. 2008; 87(8):837-42.

74. Venkatesha S, Toporsian M, Lam C, et al. Soluble endoglin contributes to the pathogenesis of preeclampsia. Nat Med. 2006;12(6):642-9.

75. Foidart JM, Munaut C, Chantraine F, et al. Maternal plasma soluble endoglin at 11-13 weeks' gestation in pre-eclampsia. Ultrasound Obstet Gynecol. 2010;35(6):680-7.

76. Papageorghiou AT, Yu CK, Erasmus IE, et al. Assessment of risk for the development of pre-eclampsia by maternal characteristics and uterine artery Doppler. BJOG. 2005;112(6):703-9.

77. Crispi F, Llurba E, Domínguez C, et al. Predictive value of angiogenic factors and uterine artery Doppler for early- versus late-onset pre-eclampsia and intrauterine growth restriction. Ultrasound Obstet Gynecol. 2008:31(3):303-9.

78. Diab AE, El-Behery MM, Ebrahiem MA, et al. Angiogenic factors for the prediction of pre-eclampsia in women with abnormal midtrimester uterine artery Doppler velocimetry. Int J Gynaecol Obstet. 2008:102(2);146-51.

79. Stepan H, Unversucht A, Wessel N, et al. Predictive value of maternal angiogenic factors in second trimester pregnancies with abnormal uterine perfusion. Hypertension. 2007;49(4):818-24.

80. Wortelboer EJ, Koster MP, Cuckle HS, et al. First-trimester placental protein 13 and placental growth factor: markers for identification of women destined to develop early-onset pre-eclampsia. BJOG. 2010; 117(11):1384-9.

81. Audibert F, Boucoiran I, An N, et al. Screening for preeclampsia using first-trimester serum markers and uterine artery Doppler in nulliparous women. Am J Obstet Gynecol. 2010;203(4):383.e1-8.

82. Poon LC, Kametas NA, Maiz N, et al. First trimester prediction of hypertensive disorders in pregnancy. Hypertension. 2009;53(5):812-8.

4 Prevention Strategies in Preeclampsia

Gita Arjun

INTRODUCTION

Preeclampsia, as a complication of pregnancy, has been known for the past 2,000 years. In spite of strides in medical care, it continues to be a major cause of maternal and perinatal mortality, especially in developing countries. According to the World Health Organization (WHO), worldwide, over 100,000 women die from preeclampsia each year, and the condition continues to be responsible for maternal deaths even in developed countries.[1] The prevalence of the condition varies between 5% and 10%, but could be as high as 18% in developing countries.[2] An estimated 10–15% of the maternal deaths in developing countries are associated with hypertensive disorders of pregnancy. Perinatal mortality has also been reported as being increased in infants of these women.

Preeclampsia refers to a syndrome of new onset of *hypertension and proteinuria* after 20 weeks of gestation in a previously normotensive woman. The syndrome is called superimposed preeclampsia when accelerating hypertension and proteinuria develop after 20 weeks in a woman with pre-existing hypertension.

IDENTIFYING RISK FACTORS FOR DEVELOPING PREECLAMPSIA

The search has been on for a therapeutic intervention that could prevent preeclampsia from developing. In order to initiate therapy, the women who are at risk for developing preeclampsia have to be identified.

In a systematic review of controlled studies, Duckitt and Harrington[3] listed the following as risk factors for developing preeclampsia:
- Presence of antiphospholipid antibodies
- History of preeclampsia
- Pre-existing diabetes
- Multiple pregnancy
- Family history
- Nulliparity
- Raised BMI before pregnancy or at booking
- Maternal age more than 40
- Renal disease
- Hypertension
- Greater than or equal to 10 years since the last pregnancy
- Raised blood pressure at booking

SCREENING TESTS FOR PREECLAMPSIA

The American College of Obstetricians and Gynecologists (ACOG) does not consider any single screening test for preeclampsia to be reliable and cost effective.[4]

Studies have shown that Doppler evaluation of the uterine arteries may be used as a predictor of preeclampsia. The presence of bilateral uterine artery notching between 23 weeks and 25 weeks of gestation is an independent risk factor for the development or preeclampsia and the delivery of a small for gestational age (SGA) neonate in the absence of preeclampsia.[5-8]

However, a systematic review of the Cochrane Database failed to show any benefit to either the baby or the mother when uteroplacental Doppler ultrasound was used in the second trimester of pregnancy in women at low risk for hypertensive disorders.[9]

Studies have shown that in the first trimester, a combined screening with uterine artery Doppler and biochemical markers is predictive of preeclampsia, especially early onset preeclampsia.[10,11] However, there are no clear guidelines advising routine screening with first trimester Doppler for nulliparas. Routine screening with this modality would increase cost of antenatal care, will require technical skills not universally available and may not be feasible in many parts of the developing world.

INTERVENTIONS FOR THE PREVENTION OF PREECLAMPSIA

Detailed history taking and meticulous antepartum care is a key in the early detection of developing preeclampsia. Close follow-up of high-risk women, particularly starting from the 20th week, will decrease the chances of missing early symptoms. Currently, medical interventions are not available that would prevent preeclampsia. However, early diagnosis followed by appropriate management may prevent the dangerous cascade of complications like eclampsia and multiorgan failure.

This chapter will review several interventions that have been evaluated for prevention of preeclampsia. There is no effective intervention for the low-risk gravida. *Low-dose aspirin is currently the only medical intervention that has been demonstrated to have some effect in women at high risk for developing preeclampsia.*

Antiplatelet Agents

The current understanding of the pathophysiology of preeclampsia includes two mechanisms:
1. Faulty implantation of the placenta early in pregnancy is considered to be the single most important precipitating factor for preeclampsia. In a normal pregnancy, there is trophoblastic invasion of the spiral arteries in the uterus during the second trimester. Failure of the trophoblast invasion leads to underperfusion of the circulation between uterus and placenta. This reduction in blood flow through the placenta leads to placental ischemia. The resulting placental damage is thought to lead to release of factors into the maternal circulation, which is responsible for the maternal syndrome.
2. Activation of platelets and the clotting system may occur early in the course of the disease. A number of prostanoids are considered to be essential in the pathopysiology of preeclampsia. Deficient intravascular production of *prostacyclin* (with vasodilator properties) and excessive production of *thromboxane* (a stimulant of platelet aggregation, along with vasoconstrictor properties) occur in preeclampsia.

The unraveling of the pathophysiology of preeclampsia led to the hypothesis that antiplatelet agents, and low-dose aspirin in particular, might prevent or delay the development of preeclampsia. Earlier, it was also hypothesized that in women who already have the disorder, the risk of adverse events might be reduced. This however has not proved to be true.

Acetylsalicylic acid (aspirin) in low doses (60–150 mg per day) is known to inhibit thromboxane-mediated vasoconstriction more than prostacyclin-mediated vasodilatation.[12,13] It was therefore postulated that it might offer protection against vasoconstriction and pathological blood coagulation in the placenta.

Studies of Aspirin Therapy in Prevention of Preeclampsia

The earliest studies done for this indication included small numbers of women and were done in highly selected at-risk women. Women who had developed severe early onset preeclampsia with fetal growth restriction or death,[14,15] women who had tested positive with an angiotensin II infusion test early in the third trimester and women with a positive "roll over" test were some of the subjects for these studies.

The Collaborative Low-dose Aspirin Study in Pregnancy (CLASP) trial was one of the early large trials. It included 9,364 women at 12–32 weeks of gestation at increased risk of developing preeclampsia or fetal growth restriction.[16]

The CLASP study included women with a previous history of preeclampsia or growth restriction, hypertension, renal disease, or other factors. The study did not show a significant benefit of low-dose aspirin (60 mg) therapy. The incidence of proteinuric preeclampsia was 6.7% in the treated group versus 7.6% in the placebo group. The incidence of preterm deliveries, however, was significantly lower in the treated group. This is due to the fact that aspirin seemed to cause a delay in the onset of preeclampsia to later gestational ages.[16]

A double-blind study[17] used low-dose aspirin versus placebo in high-risk women. The study showed no significant reduction of preeclampsia when aspirin was started between 13 weeks and 26 weeks of gestation in high-risk women.

Meta-analysis of Antiplatelet Therapy in Prevention of Preeclampsia

A systematic review of the Cochrane Database[18] showed an advantage to the administration of antiplatelet agents (aspirin and dipyridamole) in women at risk for developing preeclampsia. There is a 17% reduction in the risk for developing preeclampsia with these agents. In high-risk women, 19 women needed to be treated to prevent 1 case of preeclampsia. However, in women who are not at risk, 72 women need to be treated to prevent 1 case of preeclampsia.

Coomarasamy et al.[19] in a systematic review concluded that aspirin therapy benefits women who are historically at high risk for preeclampsia—women with previous severe or early onset pre-eclampsia, chronic hypertension, severe diabetes and moderate to severe renal disease. Since good history taking is all that is required in these women, these findings are particularly useful in developing countries where expensive diagnostic tests need not be done to identify women at risk.

Women Who Should Receive Aspirin

The ACOG practice bulletin does not recommend low-dose aspirin therapy for women at low risk for development of preeclampsia.[4]

The NICE guidelines[20] recommend administering aspirin in women with at least one of the following high risk factors:
- Hypertensive disease during a previous pregnancy
- Chronic kidney disease
- Autoimmune disease such as systemic lupus erythematosis or antiphospholipid syndrome

- Type 1 or type 2 diabetes
- Chronic hypertension

The NICE guidelines also recommend administering aspirin in women with at least *two* of the following moderate risk factors:
- Age greater than or equal to 40 years
- First pregnancy
- Multiple gestation
- More than 10 years between pregnancies
- Body mass index greater than or equal to 35 kg/m^2 at presentation
- Family history of preeclampsia

Low-dose aspirin appears to be of little or no benefit in women who already have developed pregnancy induced hypertension.[21] Aspirin, in the setting of pregnancy induced hypertension, does not prevent progression of the disease.

Dose of Aspirin

The optimum dose is unclear; studies have used 60–150 mg. Aspirin tablets of 75 mg and 81 mg strength are readily available in most countries and are therefore the easiest to prescribe.

Timing of Initiating Aspirin

If aspirin is used to prevent preeclampsia, treatment should be begun at 12–14 weeks of gestation.

The NICE guidelines[20] recommend that women at high risk of preeclampsia be administered 75 mg of aspirin daily from 12 weeks until the birth of the baby.

Bujold et al.,[22] in a systematic review and meta-analysis of the use of aspirin, also noted that the time of initiating aspirin had an impact on the occurrence of preeclampsia. In women with early abnormal uterine artery Doppler studies, they found a 52% reduction in the risk of preeclampsia compared with the control group, when aspirin therapy was started *before 16 weeks of gestation*. In a later meta-analysis,[23] they found that in women identified to be at risk for preeclampsia, the daily administration of low-dose aspirin, initiated before 16 weeks of gestation was associated with a significant decrease in the incidence of preeclampsia, severe preeclampsia, intrauterine growth restriction and preterm birth.

In a related paper, Lambers et al.,[24] found that the incidence of hypertensive complications was significantly lower in a group of women treated with low-dose aspirin throughout in vitro fertilization treatment and first trimester of pregnancy.

Discontinuing Aspirin

Aspirin is discontinued approximately 5–10 days before expected delivery to reduce the intrapartum risk of bleeding.[25]

Safety of Aspirin

The safety of aspirin in pregnancy is established. Several studies, (both observational studies and systematic reviews) have not shown any evidence of increase in placental abruption, fetal intraventricular hemorrhage, other neonatal bleeding, teratogenicity or long-term adverse effects of aspirin use in pregnancy.[18,19,26,27]

Low Molecular Weight Heparin

Anticoagulation is not recommended for reducing the risk of preeclampsia in either the general population or in those with preeclampsia in a previous pregnancy.[28]

There are no large randomized trials to evaluate the use of anticoagulation (unfractionated heparin, low molecular weight heparin) for prevention of preeclampsia in women with or without thrombophilias or in women with previous severe or preterm preeclampsia. In a small open-label trial, Mello and associates,[29] showed a clinically and statistically significant reduction in preeclampsia and its sequelae in a group of women with previous preeclampsia who have demonstrable thrombophilia and who had angiotensin-converting enzyme DD. Further research is required to find out if there is any place for anticoagulation outside of these very specific subgroups of women.

Calcium

There appears to be no benefit from calcium supplementation to prevent preeclampsia.[4]

Levine and associates,[30] in a double-blind study, gave either 2 g of calcium or placebo daily to 4,589 women from 13 weeks to 21 weeks of their pregnancy onward. They found no significant decreases in rates of hypertension or preeclampsia—even in women whose daily calcium consumption was comparable to the low consumption of women in developing countries.

In women whose calcium intake is known to be adequate, there is no statistically significant reduction in risk of developing preeclampsia with calcium supplementation.[31]

However, a systematic review of the Cochrane Database, Hofmeyr et al,[32] concluded that calcium supplementation appears to reduce the risk of preeclampsia approximately by half. It therefore also reduces the risk of preterm birth—the uncommon occurrence of the composite outcome "maternal death or serious morbidity". The benefits are greatest in women with deficient dietary calcium, which may be a problem in developing countries.

Villar and associates[33] conducted the largest trial of women with low baseline calcium intake. They did not demonstrate a substantial reduction in preeclampsia, but showed that it did reduce the severity of disease, maternal morbidity and neonatal mortality.

Antioxidant Therapy

One of the hypotheses for the development of preeclampsia is the presence of oxidative stress. Excessive amounts of chemicals called "free radicals" have been implicated in the pathophysiology of the disease. Antioxidants, such as vitamin C, vitamin E, selenium and lycopene, can neutralize free radicals.

Though many trials have been conducted to assess the effect of antioxidants in the prevention of preeclampsia, supplementation with vitamin C and/or E for prevention or treatment of pre-eclampsia is not recommended.

Spinnato and colleagues[34] conducted a randomized, placebo-controlled, double-blind clinical trial in four Brazilian sites. Women with chronic hypertension or a prior history of preeclampsia were randomly assigned to daily treatment with both vitamin C (1,000 mg) and vitamin E (400 IU) or placebo. The trial failed to demonstrate a benefit of antioxidant supplementation in reducing the rate of pre-eclampsia among this group of high-risk patients.

In a systematic review of the Cochrane Database,[35] there was no evidence to support the use of antioxidants to reduce the risk of preeclampsia. The review covered 10 trials, involving 6,533 women, and looked at several antioxidants. Overall the review found no reduction in preeclampsia, high blood pressure or preterm birth with the use of antioxidant supplements.

Nitric Oxide

Preeclampsia is associated with endothelial damage and nitric oxide mediates many functions of the endothelium, including vasodilatation and inhibition of platelet aggregation. Therefore, it has been hypothesized that nitric oxide donors (e.g. glyceryl trinitrate) and precursors (e.g. L-arginine) may prevent preeclampsia.

A systematic review of the Cochrane Database[36] concluded that there was "insufficient evidence to draw reliable conclusions about whether nitric oxide donors and precursors prevent preeclampsia or its complications".

The NICE guideline[31] recommends against using nitric oxide donors and precursors for the prevention of hypertensive disorders in pregnancy.

Other Measures

Rest, bed rest, restriction of salt intake, exercise, weight management and decrease in working hours have not been shown to have any effect on the development of preeclampsia.

CONCLUSION

Low-dose aspirin is currently the only medical intervention that has been demonstrated to have some effect in women at high risk for developing preeclampsia. The recommended dose is 75–81 mg and the medication should be started at 12 weeks to be effective. Only women at high risk will show any benefit. It is not recommended for the general obstetric population for this indication.

REFERENCES

1. WHO. Risking death to give life. Geneva: World Health Organization; 2005.
2. Geographic variation in the incidence of hypertension in pregnancy. World Health Organization International Collaborative Study of Hypertensive Disorders of Pregnancy. Am J Obstet Gynecol. 1988;158(1):80-3.
3. Duckitt K, Harrington D. Risk factors for preeclampsia at antenatal booking: systematic review of controlled studies. BMJ. 2005;330(7491):565.
4. ACOG Committee on Obstetric Practice. ACOG practice bulletin. Diagnosis and management of preeclampsia and eclampsia. Number 33, January 2002. American College of Obstetricians and Gynecologists. Int J Gynaecol Obstet. 2002;77(1): 67-75.
5. Harrington K, Cooper D, Lees C, et al. Doppler ultrasound of the uterine arteries: the importance of bilateral notching in the prediction of pre-eclampsia, placental abruption or delivery of a small-for-gestational-age baby. Ultrasound Obstet Gynecol. 1996;7(3):182-8.
6. Papageorghiou AT, Yu CK, Bindra R, et al. Multicenter screening for pre-eclampsia and fetal growth restriction by transvaginal uterine artery Doppler at 23 weeks of gestation. Ultrasound Obstet Gynecol. 2001;18(5):441-9.
7. Yu CK, Smith GC, Papageorghiou AT, et al. An integrated model for the prediction of preeclampsia using maternal factors and uterine artery Doppler velocimetry in unselected low-risk women. Am J Obstet Gynecol. 2005;193(2):429-36.
8. Espinoza J, Kusanovic JP, Bahado-Singh R, et al. Should bilateral uterine artery notching be used in the risk assessment for preeclampsia, small-for-gestational-age, and gestational hypertension? J Ultrasound Med. 2010;29(7):1103-15.
9. Stampalija T, Gyte GM, Alfirevic Z. Utero-placental Doppler ultrasound for improving pregnancy outcome. Cochrane Database Syst Rev. 2010;(9): CD008363.
10. Poon LC, Stratieva V, Piras S, et al. Hypertensive disorders in pregnancy: combined screening by uterine artery Doppler, blood pressure and serum PAPP-A at 11-13 weeks. Prenat Diagn. 2010; 30(3):216-23.
11. Audibert F, Boucoiran I, An N, et al. Screening for preeclampsia using first-trimester serum markers and uterine artery Doppler in nulliparous women. Am J Obstet Gynecol. 2010;203(4):383.e1-8.
12. Clarke RJ, Mayo G, Price P, et al. Suppression of thromboxane A2 but not of systemic prostacyclin by controlled-release aspirin. N Engl J Med. 1991; 325(16):1137-41.
13. Dekker GA, Sibai BM. Low-dose aspirin in the prevention of preeclampsia and fetal growth retardation: rationale, mechanisms, and clinical trials. Am J Obstet Gynecol. 1993;168(1 Pt 1):214-27.
14. Benigni A, Gregorini G, Frusca T, et al. Effect of low-dose aspirin on fetal and maternal generation of thromboxane by platelets in women at risk for pregnancy-induced hypertension. N Engl J Med. 1989;321(6):357-62.
15. Beaufils M, Uzan S, Donsimoni R, et al. Prevention of pre-eclampsia by early antiplatelet therapy. Lancet. 1985;1(8433):840-2.

16. CLASP: a randomised trial of low-dose aspirin for the prevention and treatment of pre-eclampsia among 9364 pregnant women. CLASP (Collaborative Low-dose Aspirin Study in Pregnancy) Collaborative Group. Lancet. 1994;343(8898):619-29.

17. Caritis S, Sibai B, Hauth J, et al. Low-dose aspirin to prevent preeclampsia in women at high risk. National Institute of Child Health and Human Development Network of Maternal-Fetal Medicine Units. N Engl J Med. 1998;338(11):701-5.

18. Duley L, Henderson-Smart DJ, Meher S, et al. Antiplatelet agents for preventing pre-eclampsia and its complications. Cochrane Database Syst Rev. 2007;(2):CD004659.

19. Coomarasamy A, Honest H, Papaioannou S, et al. Aspirin for prevention of preeclampsia in women with historical risk factors: a systematic review. Obstet Gynecol. 2003;101(6):1319-32.

20. Visintin C, Mugglestone MA, Almerie MQ, et al. Management of hypertensive disorders during pregnancy: summary of NICE guidance. BMJ. 2010;341:c2207.

21. Schiff E, Barkai G, Ben-Baruch G, et al. Low-dose aspirin does not influence the clinical course of women with mild pregnancy-induced hypertension. Obstet Gynecol. 1990;76(5 Pt 1):742-4.

22. Bujold E, Morency AM, Roberge S, et al. Acetylsalicylic acid for the prevention of preeclampsia and intra-uterine growth restriction in women with abnormal uterine artery Doppler: a systematic review and meta-analysis. J Obstet Gynaecol Can. 2009;31(9):818-26.

23. Bujold E, Roberge S, Lacasse Y, et al. Prevention of preeclampsia and intrauterine growth restriction with aspirin started in early pregnancy: a meta-analysis. Obstet Gynecol. 2010;116(2 Pt 1):402-14.

24. Lambers MJ, Groeneveld E, Hoozemans DA, et al. Lower incidence of hypertensive complications during pregnancy in patients treated with low-dose aspirin during in vitro fertilization and early pregnancy. Hum Reprod. 2009;24(10):2447-50.

25. Hirsh J, Guyatt G, Albers GW, et al. Executive summary: American College of Chest Physicians Evidence-Based Clinical Practice Guidelines (8th Edition). Chest. 2008;133(6 Suppl):71S-109S.

26. Slone D, Siskind V, Heinonen OP, et al. Aspirin and congenital malformations. Lancet. 1976; 1(7974):1373-5.

27. Klebanoff MA, Berendes HW. Aspirin exposure during the first 20 weeks of gestation and IQ at four years of age. Teratology. 1988;37(3):249-55.

28. August P. Prevention of preeclampsia. In: UpToDate, Lockwood, CJ (Ed). Waltham, MA: UpToDate; 2012.

29. Mello G, Parretti E, Fatini C, et al. Low-molecular-weight heparin lowers the recurrence rate of preeclampsia and restores the physiological vascular changes in angiotensin-converting enzyme DD women. Hypertension. 2005;45:(1)86-91.

30. Levine RJ, Hauth JC, Curet LB, et al. Trial of calcium to prevent preeclampsia. N Engl J Med. 1997;337(2):69-76.

31. NICE Clinical Guideline. Hypertension in pregnancy: the management of hypertensive disorders during pregnancy. London: National Institute for Health and Clinical Excellence; 2011.

32. Hofmeyr GJ, Lawrie TA, Atallah AN, et al. Calcium supplementation during pregnancy for preventing hypertensive disorders and related problems. Cochrane Database Syst Rev. 2010;(8):CD001059.

33. Villar J, Abdel-Aleem H, Merialdi M, et al. World Health Organization randomized trial of calcium supplementation among low calcium intake pregnant women. Am J Obstet Gynecol. 2006;194(3):639-49.

34. Spinnato JA, Freire S, Pinto E Silva JL, et al. Anti-oxidant therapy to prevent preeclampsia: a randomized controlled trial. Obstet Gynecol. 2007; 110(6):1311-8.

35. Rumbold A, Duley L, Crowther CA, et al. Antioxidants for preventing pre-eclampsia. Cochrane Database Syst Rev. 2008;(1):CD004227.

36. Meher S, Duley L. Nitric oxide for preventing pre-eclampsia and its complications. Cochrane Database Syst Rev. 2007;(2):CD006490.

5 Maternal Vascular Differences in Preeclampsia

Vikram Sinai Talaulikar, Isaac T Manyonda

INTRODUCTION

Preeclampsia (PE) is a multisystem disorder peculiar to human pregnancy that is characterized by widespread endothelial dysfunction and changes in the vascular system. It affects 4–5% of all pregnancies and remains a leading cause of maternal and perinatal morbidity and mortality. Despite decades of research, the pathophysiology of PE is not fully understood. It has become increasingly evident that, the disorder is not a single disease entity but rather represents a heterogenous spectrum of disease resulting from both placental and maternal factors. Two stages of vascular dysfunction appear to be involved. The first stage is characterized by inadequate trophoblast invasion of the uterine decidua leading to defective spiral artery remodeling in early pregnancy. Genetic and immunological factors as well as pre-existing vascular diseases appear to play an important role at this stage. The second stage is defined by widespread endothelial dysfunction with multiorgan involvement, and clinical signs and symptoms of the disease such as onset of hypertension.

EARLY VASCULAR CHANGES IN THE UTEROPLACENTAL CIRCULATION IN NORMAL PREGNANCY AND PREECLAMPSIA

Normal pregnancy is associated with significant hemodynamic changes and vasodilatation in the uterine and systemic circulation in order to meet the metabolic demands of the mother and developing fetus. The human placenta receives its blood supply from more than 100 uteroplacental arteries which have undergone the physiological remodeling of pregnancy due to invasion of the vessel wall by extravillous trophoblast (EVT) cells of the placenta.[1,2] The process of conversion of the spiral arteries of the nonpregnant uterus to the wide uteroplacental arteries is called the "physiological change" of pregnancy.[3] Cytotrophoblast cell columns originate from anchoring villi of the placenta and develop a shell, from which interstitial EVTs detach. These cells invade into the decidua and the superficial myometrium either through the decidua or via the distal ends of the spiral arteries (Figs 5.1A and B).[4] The interstitial trophoblasts will migrate in the direction of vessels and target

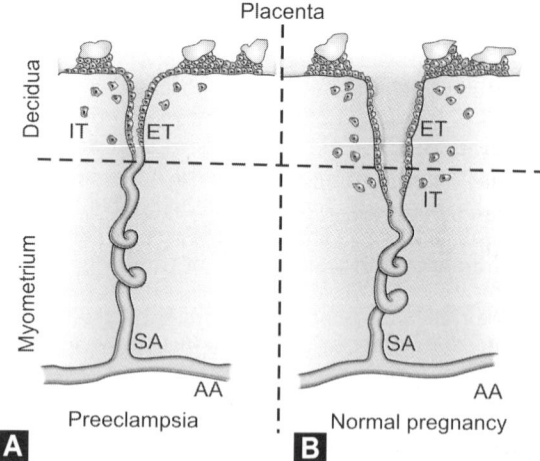

Figs 5.1A and B: Spiral artery (SA) remodeling in (A) preeclampsia compared to (B) normal pregnancy. Note the narrower lumen of the artery in preeclampsia. Also note the restricted invasion of the endovascular trophoblast (ET) and interstitial trophoblast (IT) only up to decidua in preeclamptic tissue as compared to superficial myometrium in normal pregnancy
(AA: Arcuate artery of uterus)

arteries rather than veins. The EVT cells invade the spiral vessels from their openings into the intervillous space right up to origin of these vessels in the inner one third of the myometrium in the first trimester of pregnancy progressively replacing endothelial cells, medial elastic tissue, smooth muscle and neural tissue. This process of remodeling transforms the arteries into wider, low resistance large capacitance vessels which are less responsive to vasoconstrictive agents, so that adequate blood supply is maintained to the fetoplacental unit.

Both pregnancy induced hormones and the EVTs account for vascular changes during decidual remodeling. The decidual vascular adaptation also continues from early to late first trimester and is represented by a decreasing vessel density and increasing luminal surface.[5] Such changes may occur due to vasodilatation or as an adaptive response to the increasing blood flow.[6,7] Maternal circulation to the placenta is extremely slow before the 8th week of pregnancy because of arterial plugs.[8] Circulation is gradually established over the next few weeks and by 12 weeks the blood flow to the intervillous space is complete. Various growth factors and cytokines, adhesion molecules, proteases, uterine natural killer (uNK) cells as well oxygen levels regulate the trophoblast invasion. The low oxygen environment protects the embryo from forceful maternal blood flow and oxygen overload.[9] Unplugging of the arteries from the periphery to the center generates a burst of oxidative stress. The increase in oxidative stress may serve an important physiological function in normal placental and decidual development by triggering differentiation pathways to regulate remodeling of villi, invasion of trophoblasts and production of angiogenic factors.[10]

However, in PE, the blood supply to the feto-placental unit is impaired due to defective spiral artery remodeling in early pregnancy. In most cases, the physiological vascular changes tend to be restricted to the decidual segments of the uteroplacental arteries leaving the myometrial segments unaltered in their musculoelastic architecture and thereby responsive to vasomotor influences.[2,11] Also, there may be a total absence of physiological changes in a proportion of spiral arteries decreasing the number of wide bore vessels available to maintain adequate blood supply to the fetus.[2]

Trophoblast invasion is regulated by a number of factors such as cytokines, growth factors, adhesion molecules, matrix metalloproteinases and oxygen tension.[12] Impaired endovascular trophoblast invasion may be a result of impaired decidualization, failure of trophoblasts to adopt a vascular phenotype, increased trophoblast apoptosis or abnormal maternal immune response (uNK cells and macrophages).[13-15] Hypoxia or hyperoxia can also alter trophoblast development. It has been suggested that premature loss of the arterial plugs that maintain low oxygen concentrations during early pregnancy could expose the trophoblast to hyperoxia resulting in defective trophoblast invasion.[16] Deplugging of the spiral arterioles starts in the center and spreads to the periphery. Insufficient lateral spread of the endovascular plugging could result in extensive chorionic regression, and a small placenta contributing to fetal growth restriction, PE or both.[17]

DOPPLER ASSESSMENT OF UTERINE VASCULATURE

Doppler assessment of impedance to uterine artery blood flow, serves as a proxy measure of the degree to which successful vascular remodeling has occurred in early pregnancy (Fig. 5.2). Histological examination of the placental tissue in pregnancies with high resistance uterine artery Doppler has shown deficient spiral artery remodeling as early as the first trimester.[18,19] Due to its low positive predictive values for term PE in unselected or low-risk pregnancies, the use of Doppler as a screening tool is still debated. However, in the prediction

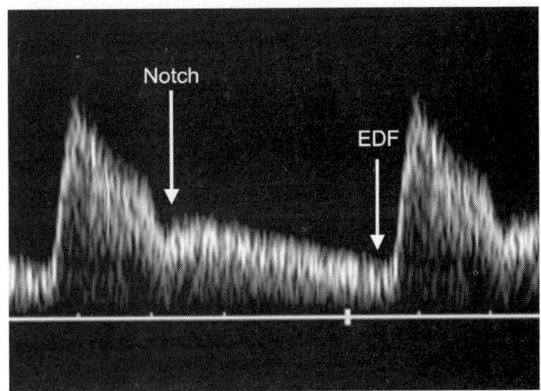

Fig. 5.2: Doppler findings of persistent diastolic notch and increased uterine artery resistance to blood flow beyond 22 weeks

of severe PE requiring delivery before 34 weeks, several large studies have reported a detection rate of about 80% with second trimester Doppler.[20,21]

■ MICROCIRCULATION IN NORMAL PREGNANCY AND PREECLAMPSIA

Microcirculation is the collective name given to the smallest components of the cardiovascular channels, arterioles, capillaries and venules. Anatomically, microcirculation is defined as all blood vessels with a diameter less than 150 microns.[22] A microcirculatory unit includes the feeding arterioles, its venular counterpart, and the branching between the two. Microcirculatory units control tissue perfusion, blood tissue exchange of nutrients and metabolic products and tissue blood volume. The arterioles contribute to the maintenance of systemic blood pressure by adjusting peripheral resistance through the intervention of neurologically mediated reflex stimuli. They also adjust the volume of blood flow into the tissue through local environmental factors and in response to circulating hormones. The capillaries are the major site for exchange of respiratory gases, fluids and metabolites between the circulating blood, and the surrounding tissues and tissue spaces. The network of capillaries, the capillary bed, varies greatly in its density, length, and three-dimensional architecture, depending on the organ and tissue. The endothelial cells are a major source for the formation of new channels by angiogenesis which involves activation and proliferation of endothelial cells, degradation of their basal membrane, migration though the surrounding extracellular matrix (ECM), attracting pericellular smooth muscle cells and maturation of vessels.[23,24] Deviations from a steady state in the growth and disappearance of microvessels can cause the microvascular density within a vascular bed to increase or decrease. The latter phenomenon is referred to as "rarefaction" of microvessels.

Changes in microcirculation have been reported in both essential hypertension as well as PE by various study groups. Patients with essential hypertension show reduced endothelial dependent microvascular dilator responses with acetylcholine.[25-27] In hypertension maximum vasodilatation is reduced resulting in a reduced vasodilator reserve and vasomotor responses are enhanced. This effect has been termed the vascular amplifier and is suggested as a mechanism by which the circulation can chronically maintain elevated resistance without excessive vasoconstriction.[28]

More consistent results of impaired endothelium dependent and endothelium independent vasodilatation have been found in women with history of PE by flow mediated dilatation studies. Flow mediated dilatation increased in pregnancy starting at around 10 weeks and continuing to 30 weeks and then decreasing gradually from 30 weeks until term.[29] The decrease may be due to the increasing diameter of the vessel or a decrease in reactive hyperemia. Venous occlusion plethysmography 100 showed endothelium dependent and independent vasodilatation was decreased in the preeclamptic group 4–5 years after delivery.[30,31]

There are numerous studies showing impaired capillary blood cell velocity, venoarterial reflex at the nutritive level of the venules and reduced resting blood flow in patients with PE or at an increased risk of developing PE.[32] These studies provide evidence that there is abnormality of the microcirculation in PE and this abnormality exists before the development of hypertension or proteinuria. The endothelial dysfunction in PE could therefore be either attributed to increased production of endothelium derived bioactive substances or increased sensitivity of the microcirculation. Underlying mechanisms could involve any of the following—mechanical changes in the arterial wall limiting the vasodilatory capacity, impaired bioavailability of nitric oxide (NO) or impaired cell signaling in the smooth muscle.

One of the most consistent finding at the level of the microcirculation in human essential hypertension is microvascular rarefaction. Microvascular rarefaction (arteriolar and capillary) not only alters systemic vascular resistance, but also alters blood flow distribution.[33,34] There are several hypotheses to account for the reduction in number of arterioles and capillaries in hypertensive subjects, including genetic programming, failure of angiogenesis during maturation, alterations in the renin-angiotensin system and long-term autoregulatory mechanisms.[35] The reduction in density not only results in increase in peripheral resistance but also plays an important role in determining the blood pressure. Reduction of microcirculatory units resulting from impaired angiogenesis is also implicated in the clinical syndrome of PE. Preliminary studies have shown a reduction in functional number of capillaries and also total or maximal number of capillaries.[36] Microvascular rarefaction may be either primary or secondary. Primary rarefaction is due to impaired angiogenesis during development or early intrauterine life while secondary rarefaction is due to functional shut-off or apoptosis of existing capillaries.

A study attempted to estimate whether capillary rarefaction preceded the onset of PE (N = 305) using video microscopy to measure basal and maximal skin capillary densities and plasma levels of angiogenic and antiangiogenic factors.[37] Preeclampsia occurred in 16 women (mean onset at 35.6 ± 4.8 weeks of gestation), 272 women had normal pregnancies, eight had hypertension and nine pregnancies were complicated by intrauterine growth restriction. In women with a normal pregnancy, significant reduction in maximal capillary density occurred at 27–32 weeks but had resolved by the puerperium. In contrast, in women who later developed PE, structural rarefaction was greater and occurred earlier at 20–24 weeks of gestation and persisted into the puerperium. It was also found that the change in soluble endoglin from 11–16 weeks of gestation to 27–32 weeks of gestation significantly correlated with the change in structural capillary density. Significant structural capillary rarefaction appeared to precede the onset of PE (Figs 5.3A and B).[37]

VASCULAR ENDOTHELIUM IN NORMAL PREGNANCY AND PREECLAMPSIA

The vascular endothelium performs an extensive range of homeostatic functions in the human body. It regulates the vascular tone, blood pressure, blood flow, coagulation, fibrinolysis, angiogenesis as well as inflammatory processes.[38] It releases a number of factors which function as relaxing, contracting, growth or regulatory molecules and an imbalance in these factors can contribute to the pathophysiology of PE (Box 5.1).

Endothelium derived vasoactive factors influence vascular tone through prostaglandins. These can be either vasoconstrictors, such as thromboxane and endothelins, or vasodilators such as prostacycline and nitric oxide (NO). In normal pregnancy, one of the earliest circulatory changes is the fall in peripheral vascular resistance. This is evident as early as 5 weeks and falls by about 40% in the first trimester. This fall in peripheral resistance is mainly brought about by vasoactive substances and changes in autonomic nervous system.[39] Animal studies have also suggested increased NO activity as a contributory factor.[40]

Endothelial dysfunction associated with PE is characterized by increased capillary permeability, platelet thrombosis and increased vascular tone. There is an abnormal sensitivity of blood vessels to vasopressors such as angiotensin, reversal of the physiologic vasodilatation and widespread activation of coagulation system. Elevated levels of fibronectin and factor VIII related antigen in early pregnancy suggest endothelial cell damage.[41]

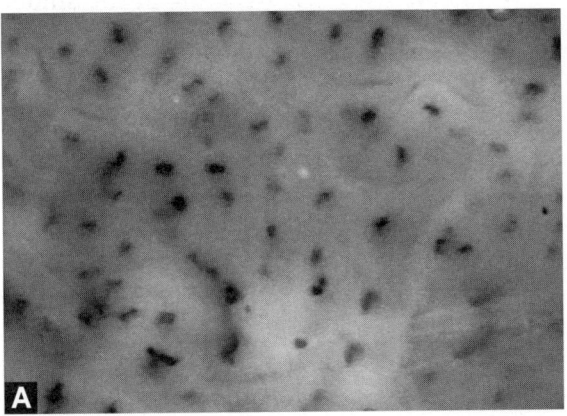 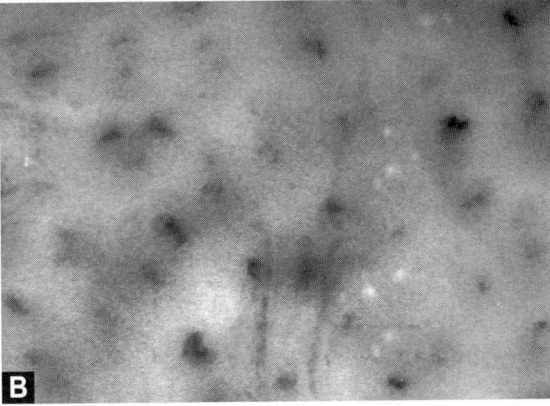

Figs 5.3A and B: Measurement of capillary rarefaction in (A) controls and (B) women who developed preeclampsia. Note the reduction in capillary density in preeclampsia

> **Box 5.1:** Major bioactive factors derived from the vascular endothelium
>
> - Vasoconstrictors
>   - Angiotensin II
>   - Urotensin II
>   - Endothelin 1
>   - Thromboxane A2
> - Vasodilators
>   - Nitric oxide
>   - Prostacycline (PGI$_2$)
>   - Hyperpolarizing factor
> - Acute phase reactants and mediators of inflammation
>   - Interleukin- 1
>   - Interleukin- 6
>   - Interleukin- 8
>   - Colony stimulating factor
>   - Chemotactic factor
> - Angiogenesis and fibrinolysis regulators
>   - Tissue plasminogen activator
>   - Plasminogen activator inhibitor
>   - Soluble fms-like tyrosine kinase-1
>   - Vascular endothelial growth factor

Glomerular endotheliosis and acute atherosis in uteroplacental arteries provide the morphological evidence of such endothelial damage.[39]

It is also thought that PE and its complications, such as HELLP syndrome (hemolysis, elevated liver enzymes and low platelets), may be associated with generalized endotheliosis and abnormal proliferation of endothelial cells.[42] The PE associated glomerular endotheliosis in the kidney could result in renal injury. In PE, the endothelial cells lining the glomerular capillaries are swollen and hypertrophied, leaving less space for erythrocytes, and glomerular endotheliosis could be manifested as a decrease in both glomerular filtration rate and renal plasma flow, resulting in increased blood urea nitrogen and creatinine levels similar to that of nonpreganant women.[42] The decrease in vascular endothelial growth factor (VEGF) levels is partly responsible for glomerular endotheliosis. Generalized endotheliosis could also affect the systemic blood vessels leading to increased vascular resistance and hypertension. More specifically, it could affect the blood vessels of the brain leading to seizures or the blood vessels of the liver leading to HELLP syndrome.[42]

The endothelium may be activated by pro-inflammatory cytokines such as tumor necrosis factor alpha (TNF α) and interleukin-1 (IL-1).[43] The placenta is an important source of cytokines and hypoxia has been reported to increase TNF α and IL-1 production by term villous cells in culture.[44] Faas et al.[45] using ultra low dose endotoxin infusion (induces strong TNF α production), observed a significant increase in blood pressure, urinary albumin excretion, platelet coagulopathy and glomerular fibrinogen deposits in pregnant rats.

Endothelial injury is also associated with increased secretion of the vasoconstrictor agents thromboxane A2 and endothelins.[46-48] In pregnant sheep, continuous exogenous endothelin 1 administration produces cardiovascular and hemodynamic changes that strongly resemble those found in preeclamptic women.[48,49]

Role of Nitric Oxide, Prostacyclins and Other Molecules

Preeclampsia is associated with decreased vasodilator mediators such as nitric oxide, prostacyclins and increased vasoconstrictor mediators such as endothelin, angiotensin II and thromboxane A2.[42] Studies have also reported enhanced mechanisms of vascular smooth muscle contraction including intracellular free Ca^{2+} concentration and calcium sensitization pathways such as protein kinase C, Rho-kinase and mitogen-activated protein kinase.[42] Although reduced prostacyclin production leading to imbalance in the thromboxane/prostacyclin ratio has been shown in PE, the role of this disorder in the initiating events leading to PE remains imprecise. A study measured urinary excretion of thromboxane B2 metabolites as markers of thromboxane A2 synthesis in eight patients with moderate to severe pregnancy induced hypertension and in six normotensive pregnant women at term.[50] Excretion of thromboxane B2 metabolites was significantly higher in the patients with pregnancy induced hypertension than in the normotensive pregnant group. Thromboxane metabolite excretion correlated with mean arterial blood pressure, plasma lactate dehydrogenase and platelet count which are indices of the severity of pregnancy induced hypertension. Excretion of both metabolites fell rapidly postpartum in parallel with resolution of clinical signs.[50] Another study[51] examined 6-keto-prostaglandin F(1)(alpha) and thromboxane B2 plasma levels throughout normotensive and preeclamptic pregnancies. Blood samples were collected from 30 healthy, nonpregnant women and at 4 weeks interval from a cohort of nulliparous women who were recruited before 16 weeks of gestation. Preeclampsia developed in 26 patients; 52 normotensive control subjects were matched from the same cohort. The 6-keto-prostaglandin F(1)(alpha) and thromboxane B2 were assayed by radioimmunoassay. Trends were compared between pregnancy groups and with the nonpregnant women. The 6-keto-prostaglandin F(1)(alpha)/thromboxane B2 ratio decreased throughout pregnancy in women with PE; there were no significant changes in normotensive women. The study found higher thromboxane B2 levels within the group with PE during the first gestational trimester. During the third trimester, patients with PE had lower 6-keto-prostaglandin F(1)(alpha) levels than did control subjects. The prostacyclin/thromboxane ratio favored vasoconstriction early in gestation in women in whom PE developed. A 6-keto-prostaglandin F(1)(alpha)/thromboxane B2 ratio of less than or equal to 3.0 at 22–26 weeks of gestation had a high predictive value for the development of PE.[51]

In the rat, long term NO deficiency induces clinical and biological features of PE.[48] Suppression of arginine intake in the pregnant rat leads to an increase in perinatal mortality and low birth weight.[52] In 1994, Molnar et al. caused a PE like syndrome in the pregnant rat by a prolonged inhibition of NO production.[48,53] This PE like syndrome comprised hypertension, proteinuria, intrauterine growth retardation, thrombocytopenia and hypovolemia. Akar et al.[54] showed that basal NO activity was increased in the umbilical vessels of preeclamptic women, but stimulated NO release was decreased. Pinto et al.[55] reported an 80–90% reduction in the stimulation of NO activity in response to bradykinin in the umbilical vessels of placentas in preeclamptic women. Yet another study[56] found that NO synthase activity was decreased in placentas from women with PE and fetal growth restriction but not in those from normal pregnancies. Nakatsuka et al.[57]

applied transdermal isosorbide dinitrate to four preeclamptic women with fetal growth restriction and high resistance in the uterine arteries on Doppler, and the average pulsatility index was reduced to 67% of that before treatment. Similarly, Thaler et al.[58] in a double-blind randomized study of 23 women with pregnancy induced hypertension, found that a sublingual tablet of isosorbide dinitrate produced a significant fall of resistance in both umbilical arteries and uterine arteries, while mean blood pressure fell from 103 mm Hg to 90 mm Hg. But conflicting results exist and overall, due to methodological limitations, human studies have not reached a consensus on how NO activity is altered during PE.

Plasma asymmetric dimethylarginine (ADMA) levels are significantly higher in women with PE than gestationally matched normotensive controls. ADMA is the endogenous inhibitor of endothelial NO synthase (eNOS). A study[59] tested the hypothesis that endothelial dysfunction and raised plasma concentrations of ADMA, precede and contribute to the development of PE. Investigators assessed the uterine artery Doppler waveforms in 86 women at 23–25 weeks gestation. Endothelial function in all women was tested using flow mediated dilation of the brachial artery at 23–25 weeks gestation. Plasma concentrations of ADMA were also measured. Forty-three women had normal uterine artery Doppler waveforms and subsequently had a normal outcome. The second group of 43 had evidence of impaired placental perfusion and of these, 19 (44%) had normal outcome, 14 (33%) developed intrauterine growth restriction of the fetus, and PE arose in 10 (23%). Women who developed PE had significantly lower flow mediated dilation than did women who had normal outcome [3.58%, standard deviation (SD), 2.76 vs 8.59%, SD, 2.76; p < 0.0001]. Irrespective of pregnancy outcome, women with evidence of impaired placental perfusion had significantly higher levels of ADMA than did women with normal Doppler waveforms. There was a strong inverse correlation between ADMA and flow mediated dilation but only in the group of women who eventually developed PE. The authors concluded that maternal endothelial function is impaired in women who eventually develop PE and it occurs before the development of the clinical syndrome.[59] Another study[60] analyzed the association between the Glu298Asp eNOS gene variant and PE. Investigators identified a variant within exon 7 of the eNOS gene—G to T conversion at nucleotide position 894 resulting in replacement of glutamic acid with aspartic acid at codon 298 (Glu298Asp). The study included 152 PE patients (35 mild, 80 severe and 37 superimposed) and 170 control subjects. Screening for the Glu298Asp eNOS gene variant was carried out by analysis of polymerase chain reaction-restriction fragment length polymorphism. The frequency of the Glu298Asp variant was significantly higher in the severe PE group (28.8%) than in the control (14.1%; $p < 0.01$), superimposed PE (8.1%; $p < 0.01$), and mild PE (11.4%; $p < 0.01$) groups. The authors concluded that the presence of the Glu298Asp eNOS gene could be a marker of increased risk of developing severe PE.[60]

◼ CHANGES IN CIRCULATING ANGIOGENIC FACTORS IN PREECLAMPSIA

Preeclampsia is characterized by a change in the balance of a range of circulating bioactive factors. Placental hypoxia due to inadequate spiral artery remodeling is thought to induce the release of various bioactive factors. An increase has been shown in the release of antiangiogenic factors and apoptotic material from the syncytium of the trophoblast.[42] Increased plasma and vascular tissue levels of such factors during pregnancy cause endothelial dysfunction, severe vasoconstriction and end organ changes of PE. Changes in the renin-angiotensin-aldosterone axis are also observed in PE. Vascular sensitivity to angiotensin II levels is increased and plasma renin or aldosterone is suppressed. Angiotensin II hypersensitivity may result from auto antibodies that activate the angiotensin II (ATII) receptor.[61]

In normal pregnancy, placental growth factor (PlGF) and VEGF are both potent angiogenic agents. They play a crucial role in normal vasculogenesis in early pregnancy and later in normal maternal endothelial function. In PE, there is increased placental release of soluble antiangiogenic factors such as soluble Flt-1 (sFlt-1) and soluble endoglin (sEng).[62-64] These antagonize the actions of VEGF-A, PlGF and transforming growth factor beta

(TGF-β) leading to inhibition of angiogenesis and systemic endothelial dysfunction.

Soluble Flt-1 is a circulating antiangiogenic protein that adheres to the receptor binding domains of PlGF and VEGF, thus preventing interaction with endothelial cell receptors and leading to endothelial dysfunction. Endoglin is a cell surface co receptor for the TGF-β1 and β3. Its soluble form is a novel potent antiangiogenic factor and acts in synergy with sFlt-1. In PE, levels of PlGF and VEGF are lower and serum sFlt-1 and sEng levels are raised.[62-64]

Neutrophil gelatinase-associated lipocalin is a glycoprotein found in the granules of human neutrophils and serves as marker of endothelial damage. It has previously been shown to be elevated in the second trimester in women who subsequently develop preeclampsia.[65] P-selectin is yet another cell adhesion molecule expressed in platelets and a marker of platelet activation and endothelial dysfunction. Increased levels of P-selectin have been reported in the first trimester in women who subsequently develop PE.[66] Research continues using above factors to device a test (possibly a combination of serum factors with Doppler) which could be used in future for accurate prediction of risk of PE.

◼ CONCLUSION

Preeclampsia remains an important cause of maternal and perinatal mortality. The present understanding of the disorder suggests two different facets of pathophysiology. First is characterized by inadequate trophoblast invasion and defective development of the placenta and appears to be the primary event leading to placental ischemia/hypoxia and second is brought about by release of bioactive factors in the circulation. These bioactive factors in turn decrease the vasodilator mediators and increase the production of vasoconstrictors leading to severe vasoconstriction, increased vascular resistance and endothelial dysfunction. Vascular changes, such as capillary rarefaction, and changes in the NO/prostaglandin pathways appear to play an important role and need further research. The disorder appears to be a spectrum of pathology with variation in gestation of onset and severity of phenotype. Predisposing cardiovascular and metabolic risks for endothelial dysfunction increases the risk of development of PE. However, PE itself is associated with increased rates of cardiovascular and metabolic diseases later in life. It is unlikely that a single predictive test or treatment will be effective for all presentations of PE but a deeper understanding of the pathophysiology and vascular endothelial changes of PE could provide more specific and efficient measures for its prevention, diagnosis and treatment in future.

■ REFERENCES

1. Brosens I, Dixon HG. The anatomy of the maternal side of the placenta. J Obstet Gynaecol Br Commonw. 1966;73(3):357-63.

2. Khong TY, De Wolf F, Robertson WB, et al. Inadequate maternal vascular response to placentation in pregnancies complicated by pre-eclampsia and by small-for-gestational age infants. Br J Obstet Gynaecol. 1986;93(10):1049-59.

3. Brosens I, Robertson WB, Dixon HG. The physiological response of the vessels of the placental bed to normal pregnancy. J Pathol Bacteriol. 1967;93(2):569-79.

4. Lash GE, Schiessl B, Kirkley M, et al. Expression of angiogenic growth factors by uterine natural killer cells during early pregnancy. J Leukoc Biol. 2006;80(3):572-80.

5. Plaisier M, Rodrigues S, Willems F, et al. Different degrees of vascularization and their relationship to the expression of vascular endothelial growth factor, placental growth factor, angiopoietins, and their receptors in first-trimester decidual tissues. Fertil Steril. 2007;88(1):176-87.

6. Charnock-Jones DS. Soluble flt-1 and the angiopoietins in the development and regulation of placental vasculature. J Anat. 2002;200(6):607-15.

7. Huppertz B, Peeters LL. Vascular biology in implantation and placentation. Angiogenesis. 2005;8(2):157-67.

8. Burton GJ, Jauniaux E, Watson AL. Maternal arterial connections to the placental intervillous space during the first trimester of human pregnancy: the Boyd collection revisited. Am J Obstet Gynecol. 1999;181(3):718-24.

9. Jauniaux E, Watson AL, Hempstock J, et al. Onset of maternal arterial blood flow and placental oxidative stress. A possible factor in human early pregnancy failure. Am J Pathol. 2000;157(6):2111-22.

10. Kingdom JC, Kaufmann P. Oxygen and placental villous development: origins of fetal hypoxia. Placenta. 1997;18(8):613-21.

11. Brosens I, Robertson WB, Dixon HG. The role of the spiral arteries in the pathogenesis of pre-eclampsia. Obstet Gynecol Annu. 1972;1:177-91.

12. Pijnenborg R, Vercruysse L, Brosens I. Deep placentation. Best Pract Res Clin Obstet Gynaecol. 2011;25(3):273-85.

13. Dunk C, Smith S, Hazan A, et al. Promotion of angiogenesis by human endometrial lymphocytes. Immunol Invest. 2008;37(5):583-610.

14. Quenby S, Nik H, Innes B, et al. Uterine natural killer cells and angiogenesis in recurrent reproductive failure. Hum Reprod. 2009;24(1):45-54.

15. Kadyrov M, Kingdom JC, Huppertz B. Divergent trophoblast invasion and apoptosis in placental bed spiral arteries from pregnancies complicated by maternal anemia and early-onset preeclampsia/intrauterine growth restriction. Am J Obstet Gynecol. 2006;194(2):557-63.

16. Burton GJ, Jauniaux E. Placental oxidative stress: from miscarriage to preeclampsia. J Soc Gynecol Investig. 2004;11(6):342-52.

17. Pijnenborg R, Vercruysse L, Carter AM. Deep trophoblast invasion and spiral artery remodelling in the placental bed of the chimpanzee. Placenta. 2011;32(5):400-8.

18. Leslie K, Thilaganathan B, Papageorghiou A. Early prediction and prevention of pre-eclampsia. Best Pract Res Clin Obstet Gynaecol. 2011;25(3):343-54.

19. Prefumo F, Sebire NJ, Thilaganathan B. Decreased endovascular trophoblast invasion in first trimester pregnancies with high-resistance uterine artery Doppler indices. Hum Reprod. 2004;19(1):206-09.

20. Plasencia W, Maiz N, Bonino S, et al. Uterine artery Doppler at 11 + 0 to 13 + 6 weeks in the prediction of pre-eclampsia. Ultrasound Obstet Gynecol. 2007;30(5):742-9.

21. Papageorghiou AT, Yu CK, Bindra R, et al. Multicenter screening for pre-eclampsia and fetal growth restriction by transvaginal uterine artery Doppler at 23 weeks of gestation. Ultrasound Obstet Gynecol. 2001;18(5):441-9.

22. Abularrage CJ, Sidawy AN, Aidinian G, et al. Evaluation of macrocirculatory endothelium-dependent and endothelium-independent vaso-reactivity in vascular disease. Perspect Vasc Surg Endovasc Ther. 2005;17(3):245-53.

23. Carmeliet P. Angiogenesis in health and disease. Nat Med. 2003;9(6):653-60.

24. Smith SK. Angiogenesis and implantation. Hum Reprod. 2000;15 Suppl 6:59-66.

25. Rossi M, Fabbri A, Vagheggini G, et al. Endothelial function of dermal microcirculation in patients with essential arterial hypertension. Minerva Cardioangiol. 1999;47(12):617-8.

26. Farkas K, Nemcsik J, Kolossváry E, et al. Impairment of skin microvascular reactivity in hypertension and uraemia. Nephrol Dial Transplant. 2005;20(9):1821-7.

27. Lindstedt IH, Edvinsson ML, Edvinsson L. Reduced responsiveness of cutaneous microcirculation in essential hypertension—a pilot study. Blood Press. 2006;15(5):275-80.

28. Korner PI, Angus JA. Structural determinants of vascular resistance properties in hypertension. Haemodynamic and model analysis. J Vasc Res. 1992;29(4):293-312.

29. Savvidou MD, Kametas NA, Donald AE, et al. Non-invasive assessment of endothelial function in normal pregnancy. Ultrasound Obstet Gynecol. 2000;15(6):502-7.

30. Bowyer L, Brown MA, Jones M. Forearm blood flow in pre-eclampsia. BJOG. 2003;110:383-91.

31. Lampinen KH, Rönnback M, Kaaja RJ, et al. Impaired vascular dilatation in women with a history of pre-eclampsia. J Hypertens. 2006;24(4):751-6.

32. Vollebregt KC, Boer K, Mathura KR, et al. Impaired vascular function in women with pre-eclampsia observed with orthogonal polarisation spectral imaging. BJOG. 2001;108(11):1148-53.

33. Feihl F, Liaudet L, Waeber B, et al. Hypertension: a disease of the microcirculation? Hypertension. 2006;48(6):1012-7.

34. Greene AS, Tonellato PJ, Lui J, et al. Microvascular rarefaction and tissue vascular resistance in hypertension. Am J Physiol. 1989;256(1 Pt 2): H126-31.

35. Prewitt RL. Autoregulation of blood flow, endothelial nitric oxide synthase and microvascular rarefaction. J Hypertens. 2002;20(2):177-8.

36. Hasan KM, Manyonda IT, Ng FS, et al. Skin capillary density changes in normal pregnancy and pre-eclampsia. J Hypertens. 2002;20(12):2439-43.

37. Nama V, Manyonda IT, Onwude J, et al. Structural capillary rarefaction and the onset of preeclampsia. Obstet Gynecol. 2012;119(5):967-74.

38. Petty RG, Pearson JD. Endothelium--the axis of vascular health and disease. J R Coll Physicians Lond. 1989;23(2):92-102.

39. Poston L, Williams DJ. The endothelium in human pregnancy. In: Vallance PJ and Webb DJ (Eds). Vascular Endothelium in Human Physiology and Pathophysiology. Harwood Academic Publishers, 2000. pp. 247-81.

40. Conrad KP, Joffe GM, Kruszyna H, et al. Identification of increased nitric oxide biosynthesis during pregnancy in rats. FASEB J. 1993;7(6):566-71.

41. Roberts JM, Redman CW. Pre-eclampsia: more than pregnancy-induced hypertension. Lancet. 1993;341(8858):1447-51.

42. Sheppard SJ, Khalil RA. Risk factors and mediators of the vascular dysfunction associated with hypertension in pregnancy. Cardiovasc Hematol Disord Drug Targets. 2010;10(1):33-52.

43. Pober JS, Cotran RS. Cytokines and endothelial cell biology. Physiol Rev. 1990;70(2):427-51.

44. Benyo DF, Miles TM, Conrad KP. Hypoxia stimulates cytokine production by villous explants from the human placenta. J Clin Endocrinol Metab. 1997; 82(5):1582-8.

45. Faas MM, Schuiling GA, Baller JF, et al. A new animal model for human preeclampsia: ultra-low-dose endotoxin infusion in pregnant rats. Am J Obstet Gynecol. 1994;171(1):158-64.

46. Kraayenbrink AA, Dekker GA, van Kamp GJ, et al. Endothelial vasoactive mediators in preeclampsia. Am J Obstet Gynecol. 1993;169(1):160-5.

47. Greer IA, Leask R, Hodson BA, et al. Endothelin, elastase, and endothelial dysfunction in pre-eclampsia. Lancet. 1991;337(8740):558.

48. Carbillon L, Uzan M, Uzan S. Pregnancy, vascular tone, and maternal hemodynamics: a crucial adaptation. Obstet Gynecol Surv. 2000;55(9):574-81.

49. Greenberg SG, Baker RS, Yang D, et al. Effects of continuous infusion of endothelin-1 in pregnant sheep. Hypertension. 1997;30(6):1585-90.

50. Fitzgerald DJ, Rocki W, Murray R, et al. Thromboxane A2 synthesis in pregnancy-induced hypertension. Lancet. 1990;335(8692):751-4.

51. Chavarría ME, Lara-González L, González-Gleason A, et al. Prostacyclin/thromboxane early changes in pregnancies that are complicated by preeclampsia. Am J Obstet Gynecol. 2003;188(4):986-92.

52. Pau MY, Milner JA. Arginine deficiency during gestation and lactation in the rat. J Nutr. 1981; 111(1):184-93.

53. Molnár M, Sütö T, Tóth T, et al. Prolonged blockade of nitric oxide synthesis in gravid rats produces sustained hypertension, proteinuria, thrombocytopenia, and intrauterine growth retardation. Am J Obstet Gynecol. 1994;170(5 Pt 1):1458-66.

54. Akar F, Ark M, Uydeë BS, et al. Nitric oxide production by human umbilical vessels in severe pre-eclampsia. J Hypertens. 1994;12(11):1235-41.

55. Pinto A, Sorrentino R, Sorrentino P, et al. Endothelial-derived relaxing factor released by endothelial cells of human umbilical vessels and its impairment in pregnancy-induced hypertension. Am J Obst Gynecol. 1991;164(2):507-13.

56. Morris NH, Sooranna SR, Learmont JG, et al. Nitric oxide synthase activities in placental tissue from normotensive, pre-eclamptic, and growth retarded pregnancies. Br J Obstet Gynaecol. 1995;102(9): 711-4.

57. Nakatsuka M, Tada K, Kimura Y, et al. Clinical experience of long-term transdermal treatment with nitric oxide donor for women with preeclampsia. Gynecol Obstet Invest. 1999;47(1):13-9.

58. Thaler I, Amit A, Kamil D, et al. The effect of isosorbide dinitrate on placental blood flow and maternal blood pressure in women with pregnancy induced hypertension. Am J Hypertens. 1999;12(4 Pt 1): 341-7.

59. Savvidou MD, Hingorani AD, Tsikas D, et al. Endothelial dysfunction and raised plasma concentrations of asymmetric dimethylarginine in pregnant women who subsequently develop pre-eclampsia. Lancet. 2003;361(9368):1511-7.

60. Yoshimura T, Yoshimura M, Tabata A, et al. Association of the missense Glu298Asp variant of the endothelial nitric oxide synthase gene with severe preeclampsia. J Soc Gynecol Investig. 2000;7(4):238-41.

61. Plaisier M. Decidualisation and angiogenesis. Best Pract Res Clin Obstet Gynaecol. 2011;25(3):259-71.

62. Maynard SE, Min JY, Merchan J, et al. Excess placental soluble fms-like tyrosine kinase 1 (sFlt1) may contribute to endothelial dysfunction, hypertension, and proteinuria in preeclampsia. J Clin Invest. 2003;111(5):649-58.

63. Woolcock J, Hennessy A, Xu B, et al. Soluble Flt-1 as a diagnostic marker of pre-eclampsia. Aust N Z J Obstet Gynaecol. 2008;48(1):64-70.

64. ten Dijke P, Goumans MJ, Pardali E. Endoglin in angiogenesis and vascular diseases. Angiogenesis. 2008;11(1):79-89.

65. D'Anna R, Baviera G, Giordano D, et al. Second trimester neutrophil gelatinase-associated lipocalin as a potential prediagnostic marker of preeclampsia. Acta Obstet Gynecol Scand. 2008;87(12):1370-3.

66. Banzola I, Farina A, Concu M, et al. Performance of a panel of maternal serum markers in predicting preeclampsia at 11-15 weeks' gestation. Prenat Diagn. 2007;27(11):1005-10.

6 Antihypertensive Therapy in Hypertension

Evita Fernandez, Sirisha Rao Gundabattula

▪ INTRODUCTION

According to the National High Blood Pressure Education Program (NHBPEP) working group on high blood pressure in pregnancy, hypertension complicates 6–8% of pregnancies and contributes significantly to stillbirths and neonatal morbidity and mortality.[1] Despite years of research, there is a lack of consensus on classification/definition of hypertensive disorders, the blood pressure (BP) at which antihypertensive therapy needs to be initiated, appropriate therapy and maternofetal risk-benefit ratio of treatment.

▪ SEVERITY OF HYPERTENSION

The National Institute for Health and Clinical Excellence (NICE) clinical guideline in 2010[2] has classified the degrees of hypertension in pregnancy as:

*   *Mild*: Diastolic blood pressure (DBP) 90–99 mm Hg, systolic blood pressure (SBP) 140–149 mm Hg
*   *Moderate*: DBP 100–109 mm Hg, SBP 150–159 mm Hg
*   *Severe*: DBP greater than or equal to 110 mm Hg, SBP greater than or equal to 160 mm Hg.

Hypertensive emergency and urgency have been defined by the NHBPEP Joint National Committee (JNC) VII[3] report as:

*   *Hypertensive emergency (crisis)*: DBP greater than or equal to 120 mm Hg, SBP greater than or equal to 180 mm Hg complicated by evidence of impending or progressive target organ dysfunction
*   *Hypertensive urgency*: Severe elevation in BP without progressive target organ dysfunction.

The American College of Obstetricians and Gynecologists (ACOG) has stated that acute-onset, persistent (lasting 15 min or more) severe systolic (≥ 160 mm Hg) or diastolic (≥ 110 mm Hg) hypertension or both in pregnant or postpartum women with preeclampsia or eclampsia constitutes a hypertensive emergency.[4]

▪ GOAL OF TREATMENT

Antihypertensive agents are mainly used to treat severe hypertension to prolong pregnancy for as long as safely possible in order to maximize the gestational age and prevent neonatal complications of extreme prematurity such as cerebral hemorrhage. The goal of therapy is to maintain BP at a level that prevents cardiovascular and central nervous system consequences of severe and rapid elevation in BP in the mother without compromising uteroplacental blood flow and fetal perfusion. Ultimately, this protects the mother from the extremes of hypertension and potential morbidity, thereby allowing the pregnancy to continue and the fetus to grow and mature.

Medications used to reduce BP target the physiologic control systems that regulate BP which include vascular tone, vascular volume and the sympathetic system. They do not prevent preeclampsia nor do they reverse the primary pathogenic process of placental underperfusion and severe preeclampsia. Uncontrolled hypertension is a frequent trigger for delivery and control of hypertension may allow prolongation of pregnancy.

ANTIHYPERTENSIVE RATIONALE—HOW DOES IT DIFFER FROM NONPREGNANT ADULTS?

It is important to make the correct diagnosis, i.e. to distinguish between pre-existing (chronic hypertension) and pregnancy-induced (gestational hypertension and preeclampsia) hypertensive disease.[5]

The focus, during pregnancy has been on DBP rather than SBP. A DBP greater than 90 mm Hg identifies a level above which perinatal morbidity is increased in nonproteinuric hypertension and DBP is a better predictor of adverse pregnancy outcomes than is SBP.[6] However, the degree of systolic hypertension (as opposed to the level of diastolic hypertension or relative increase or rate of increase of mean arterial pressure from baseline levels) may be the most important predictor of cerebral injury and infarction.[7] Severe hypertension of greater than or equal to 170/110 mm Hg represents a level of BP above which cerebral autoregulation is overcome in normotensive individuals, with the risk of cerebral hemorrhage and hypertensive encephalopathy.

CHRONIC HYPERTENSION

Preconception Counseling

Women with chronic hypertension who are taking angiotensin-converting enzyme (ACE) inhibitors, angiotensin receptor blockers and chlorothiazide should be informed about the increased risk of congenital abnormalities if these drugs are taken during pregnancy. They should be switched over to alternative antihypertensive medication suitable for pregnancy such as amlodipine or methyldopa prior to planning conception. In those who inadvertently become pregnant while taking ACE inhibitors or angiotensin receptor blocking agents, the risk of birth defects rises from 3% to 7%.[8] In some cases, medications of any type may be unnecessary, and can be stopped while maintaining close surveillance.

Antenatal Period

Many of these women will experience a physiological lowering of BP due to gestational vascular relaxation. Hence, reducing or even discontinuing medication and monitoring is possible in women with mild or moderate hypertension. Therapy can be initiated if the BP again rises to more than 150/100 mm Hg. In women with underlying renal dysfunction, it may be reasonable to choose a slightly lower threshold for treatment.[9]

Postnatal Period

The antenatal antihypertensive is continued to maintain BP less than 140/90 mm Hg. If methyldopa was used in the antenatal period, it is stopped after delivery and prepregnancy antihypertensive therapy is restarted.

GESTATIONAL HYPERTENSION AND PREECLAMPSIA

Antenatal Period

The aim is to maintain BP less than 150/80–100 mm Hg.

Postnatal Period

Antenatal antihypertensive therapy is continued or commenced if BP rises above 150/100 mm Hg. The dose is reduced once the BP falls to less than 130/80 mm Hg. If antihypertensive needs to be continued, medical review is to be scheduled at 2 weeks and 6 weeks postpartum. The persistence or refractoriness of hypertension in the postpartum state is likely due to underlying chronic hypertension and/or mobilization of edema fluid with redistribution into the intravascular compartment.

ANTIHYPERTENSIVE AGENTS IN PREGNANCY

Not all the drugs used in the nonpregnant state can be used during pregnancy as many antihypertensive agents exert an adverse effect on the growing fetus and often reduce the uteroplacental circulation causing fetal growth restriction (FGR) and even death. Most antihypertensive agents used in pregnancy are designated as "category C", which states that human studies are lacking, animal studies are either positive for fetal risk or are lacking and the drug should be given only if potential benefits justify potential risks to the fetus.

Angiotensin-converting Enzyme Inhibitors

Angiotensin-converting enzyme inhibitors are to be avoided in all trimesters of pregnancy. First trimester exposure has been associated with a greater incidence of congenital malformations of the cardiovascular and central nervous systems with a risk ratio of 2.71 when compared with no antihypertensive medication or other types of antihypertensive medication.[8] Reported complications when used during second and third trimesters include oligohydramnios, FGR, bony malformations, hypocalvaria, limb contractures, persistent patent ductus arteriosus, pulmonary hypoplasia, respiratory distress syndrome, prolonged neonatal hypotension and neonatal death.[10]

Some of the commonly used drugs are discussed in Table 6.1.

Methyldopa

Undoubtedly, methyldopa remains one of the most widely used drugs for the treatment of hypertension in pregnancy. Treatment with methyldopa has been reported to prevent subsequent progression to severe hypertension in pregnancy and does not seem to have adverse effects on uteroplacental or fetal hemodynamics[11] or on fetal well-being.[12] Many years of use attest to its safety including

Table 6.1: Antihypertensive agents in pregnant women

Drug	FDA Category	Mechanism of Action	Maternal Effects	Fetal Effects	Contraindications
Methyldopa	B	Central sympatholytic—α_2 agonist inhibiting impulses from medulla and hypothalamus	Hypotension, sedation, depression, hemolytic anemia, dryness of mouth, blurred vision, elevated liver enzymes		Hepatitis, depression, congestive cardiac failure
Propranolol	C	$\beta_1 + \beta_2$ blocker	Fatigue, severe hypotension, bradycardia, bronchospasm, cardiac failure	Neonatal hypoglycemia	Asthma, renal insufficiency, diabetes mellitus
Atenolol	C	β_1 blocker		FGR	
Labetalol	C	$\alpha_1 + \beta_1 + \beta_2$ blocker	Bradycardia, headache, nausea	FGR	Asthma
Nifedipine	C	Calcium channel blocker causing arteriolar dilatation	Flushing, hypotension, headache, tachycardia, inhibition of labor, peripheral edema, constipation		Aortic stenosis
Hydralazine	C	Arteriolar vasodilator (tachyphylaxis on prolonged use)	Hypotension, tachycardia, arrhythmia, lupus like syndrome	Neonatal thrombocytopenia	
Nitroprusside	C	Vasodilator (nitric oxide donor)	Nausea, vomiting, severe hypotension	Cyanide toxicity may occur after 4 hours of use	

Abbreviations: FDA, Food and Drug Administration; FGR, fetal growth restriction

7 years of follow-up of offspring in which the children exhibited intelligence and neurocognitive development similar to controls.[13] It has a slow onset of action over 24 hours and BP control is gradual because of the indirect mechanism of action. Patients become tolerant to the sedative effect of this drug. Depression or liver function abnormalities which persist or are severe and hemolytic anemia necessitate change to a second-line drug.

Beta-Blockers

Beta (β)-blockers have been used extensively in pregnancy. None of them have been associated with teratogenicity. Atenolol resulted in clinically significant FGR and decreased placental weight compared with placebo.[14] Oral β-blockade was reportedly associated with nonclinically significant neonatal bradycardia and parenteral therapy was found to increase the risk of neonatal bradycardia, requiring intervention in one of six newborns.[15] In a Cochrane systematic review in 2003,[16] oral β-blockers were reported to decrease the risk of severe hypertension and the need for additional antihypertensives in women with mild to moderate hypertension. They seemed to be associated with an increase in small-for-gestational-age (SGA) infants. They appeared to be as safe as and more effective in lowering BP than methyldopa.

Nifedipine

Orally administered nifedipine does not pose teratogenic risks to fetuses exposed in the first trimester. Short-acting calcium antagonists, particularly when administered sublingually, are not recommended for the treatment of hypertension in nonpregnant patients because of reports of myocardial infarction and death in hypertensive patients with coronary artery disease.[17] A concern with the use of calcium channel blockers was the concomitant use of magnesium sulfate due to the possible risk of neuromuscular blockade and myocardial depression. However, there seems to be no increased risk when the two are used together.[18]

Hydralazine

Hydralazine selectively relaxes arteriolar smooth muscle. Its greatest use is in the urgent control of severe hypertension or as a third-line agent for multidrug control of refractory hypertension. Effects on uteroplacental blood flow are unclear because of variation in the degree of reflex sympathetic activation and fetal distress may result due to a precipitous drop in maternal pressure. In a meta-analysis of 21 trials comprising 1,085 women, parenteral hydralazine, compared with other short-acting antihypertensives, was found to be associated with more adverse effects including maternal hypotension, Cesarean sections and adverse fetal heart rate effects.[19] Vasodilators (hydralazine and nifedipine) cause headache and tachycardia in many patients. These side effects simulate features of impending eclampsia, and are lessened if the sympathetic nervous system is already inhibited by methyldopa.

Sodium Nitroprusside

Sodium nitroprusside is seldom used in pregnancy, usually only in cases of life-threatening refractory hypertension as a last resort in the critical care unit. An indwelling arterial line to obtain BPs is desirable. Administered only by continuous intravenous (IV) infusion, it is easily titrated because it has a near-immediate onset of action and duration of effect of 3 minutes. Adverse effects include excessive vasodilation and syncope in volume-depleted preeclamptic women. Cyanide poisoning of the fetus can occur when infusion rates exceed 5 µg/kg/min.

Diuretics

Diuretics to treat hypertension are normally avoided in pregnancy, as in preeclampsia they cause further depletion of a reduced intravascular volume. Although volume contraction might be expected to limit fetal growth, outcome data have not supported these concerns and the NHBPEP Working Group on High Blood Pressure in Pregnancy concluded that diuretics may be continued during pregnancy at a lower dose if possible, especially for women likely to have salt-sensitive hypertension.[1] However, mild volume contraction with diuretic therapy may lead to hyperuricemia and in doing so invalidate serum uric acid levels as a laboratory marker in the diagnosis of superimposed preeclampsia. The use of low doses (12.5–25 mg daily) of hydrochlorothiazide may minimize untoward metabolic effects such as impaired glucose tolerance and hypokalemia.[20] Spironolactone is not recommended because of its antiandrogenic effects during fetal development. The use of diuretics should be reserved for the treatment of heart failure, pulmonary edema and idiopathic intracranial hypertension.[21]

Ketanserin

Ketanserin is a selective S2-receptor-blocking drug that decreases SBP and DBP in nonpregnant patients with acute or chronic hypertension. It has been studied in small trials, which suggest that it may be safe and useful in the treatment of chronic hypertension in pregnancy, preeclampsia, and hemolysis, elevated liver enzymes and low platelet count (HELLP) syndrome.[22] However, there are reports of more persistent high BP than hydralazine and it is probably best avoided as per the Cochrane review in 2006.[23]

■ WHEN TO START ANTIHYPERTENSIVE THERAPY?

Severe Hypertension

Severe hypertension, i.e. BP greater than or equal to 160/110 mm Hg requires treatment because of the risk of a cardiovascular accident or target organ damage. There is consensus that women with severe hypertension in pregnancy are at an increased risk of intracerebral hemorrhage, and that treatment decreases the risk of maternal death. It is important to control severe hypertension at any gestation and postpartum. Induction of labor or Cesarean section does not control hypertension even though delivery begins the process of resolution of preeclampsia. Thus, antihypertensive medication will usually be required even when delivery has been arranged. Maternal stabilization is a must before delivery, even in urgent circumstances.[4]

Mild to Moderate Hypertension

The issue of efficacy of antihypertensive agents in mild to moderate hypertension was addressed in a Cochrane review.[24] The results of this review showed that antihypertensive agents halved the risk of developing severe hypertension, but there was no overall significant difference in risk of preeclampsia development, preterm births, SGA babies and fetal/neonatal deaths. Calcium antagonists and β-blockers versus no drug yielded altered risks of preeclampsia [relative risk (RR),

1.68; 95% confidence interval (CI), 1.17–2.41 and RR, 0.76; 95% CI, 0.59–0.98 respectively]. Beta-blockers demonstrated a statistically significant risk of SGA (RR, 1.56; 95% CI, 1.10–2.22). The authors concluded that it is unclear whether antihypertensive drug therapy for mild to moderate hypertension during pregnancy is worthwhile.

International guidelines for the treatment of hypertension in pregnancy vary with respect to thresholds for starting treatment:

- *Canadian Hypertension Society*:[25] 140–150/90–95 mm Hg
- *NHBPEP Working Group*:[1] Greater than or equal to 160/100 mm Hg
- *SOMANZ*:[26] 140–160/90–100 mm Hg

It seems reasonable to conclude that a DBP of greater than or equal to 100 mm Hg warrants therapy.

■ WHAT IS THE TARGET BLOOD PRESSURE TO BE ACHIEVED?

Target BP is disputed; overzealous control runs the risk of jeopardizing the uteroplacental circulation. There are no studies addressing safe BP treatment targets for pregnant women, and guidelines and reviews generally recommend treating to BP levels that are likely to be protective against acute adverse cerebrovascular or cardiovascular events, which is usually in the range of 140–155/90–105 mm Hg.

The Society of Obstetricians and Gynaecologists of Canada (SOGC)[27] recommends that for women without comorbid conditions, antihypertensive drug therapy should be used to maintain SBP at 130–155 mm Hg and DBP at 80–105 mm Hg. For women with comorbid conditions, the recommended targets are SBP of 130–139 mm Hg and DBP of 80–89 mm Hg. This goal reflects a concern that DBP less than 80 mm Hg may limit uteroplacental perfusion.

Those with hypertensive encephalopathy, hemorrhage or eclampsia require treatment with parenteral agents to lower mean arterial pressure by 25% over minutes to hours and then to further lower BP to 160/100 mm Hg over subsequent hours.[1] In treating severe hypertension, it is important to avoid hypotension, because aggressive lowering may cause fetal distress. As hypotension may result with any short-acting antihypertensive agent administered to women with preeclampsia, because they are intravascularly volume depleted, it may be prudent to continuously monitor fetal heart rate until BP stabilizes.[4]

■ WHICH ANTIHYPERTENSIVE MEDICATION IS PREFERRED?

The most important consideration in choice of antihypertensive agent is that the unit has experience and familiarity with that agent. It is recommended that protocols for the management of severe hypertension should be readily accessible in all obstetric units.[26]

Nonsevere Hypertension

The first-line agents for nonsevere hypertension are methyldopa and labetalol, with nifedipine as second line, followed by others in third line. The second-line medications should be used in conjunction with methyldopa in women who fail to respond to monotherapy, or be used to replace it in those who are unable to tolerate it. Alpha (α)-adrenergic blockers, e.g. doxazosin are also safe and well tolerated, and can be used as second- or third-line therapy.[21] A Cochrane review did not demonstrate any clear difference in the risk of developing severe hypertension or preeclampsia when different antihypertensive agents were compared. There was a 51% reduction in the risk of fetal/neonatal deaths when any agent was compared with methyldopa. But many outcomes were assessed on data from a small number of studies and hence they concluded that the choice

of the agent should depend on the obstetrician's experience and the patient.[24]

Severe Hypertension

A meta-analysis of the use of IV hydralazine in severe hypertension in pregnancy concluded that parenteral labetalol or oral nifedipine were preferable first-line agents, with hydralazine as a suitable second-line agent as IV hydralazine has been associated with more maternal and perinatal adverse effects than IV labetalol or oral nifedipine.[19] The ACOG considers both IV labetalol and hydralazine as first-line medications for the management of acute-onset severe hypertension in pregnant and postpartum women.[4]

Very High Blood Pressure

Drugs for the treatment of very high BP were the subject of a Cochrane review of 24 randomized trials comprising 2,949 women.[23] Women who received calcium channel blockers were less likely to have persistent high BP than hydralazine. Labetalol was associated with a lower risk of hypotension and Cesarean section than diazoxide. The reviewers concluded that no good evidence exists that any short-acting antihypertensive is better than another.

■ HOW TO ADMINISTER THERAPY?

The dosages of the antihypertensive medications for long-term and immediate control of BP are detailed in Table 6.2.

Table 6.2: Dose and route of administration of antihypertensive agents

Drug	Oral	Parenteral
Methyldopa	250 mg BD to 1 g TID	—
Labetalol	100 mg BD to 500 mg QID (2,400 mg/day maximum)	20 mg IV, then 20–80 mg every 20 min up to 300 mg maximum Infusion 1–2 mg/min
Nifedipine slow-release	10 mg BD to 40 mg BD (120 mg/day maximum) For acute severe hypertension: 10–30 mg PO which can be repeated after 45 min	—
Hydralazine	25 mg TID to 75 mg QID	5–10 mg IV, then 10 mg after 20 min Consider another drug if no response with 20 mg IV
Nitroprusside	—	Infusion 0.25—5 µg/kg/min
Hydrochlorothiazide	12.5–25 mg/day	—

Abbreviations: BD, twice a day; TID, thrice a day; QID, four times a day; IV, intravenous; PO, per orally

◼ ANTIHYPERTENSIVES IN THE POSTPARTUM PERIOD

Postpartum hypertension occurs most commonly 3–6 days after delivery.[21] The maximum increase in BP usually occurs toward the end of the 1st postpartum week (when, in most settings, women have been already discharged from facility care). There are no reliable data to guide management of women who are hypertensive postpartum and any antihypertensive agent used should be based on a clinician's familiarity with the drug.

Beta-blockers [e.g. atenolol 50–100 mg once daily (OD)] with addition of a calcium antagonist (e.g. slow-release nifedipine 10–20 mg OD) and/or an ACE inhibitor [e.g. enalapril 5–10 mg twice a day (BD)], if required, are appropriate for the treatment of postpartum hypertension.[21]

Labetalol, nifedipine, enalapril, captopril, atenolol and metoprolol have no known adverse effects on babies receiving breast milk. There is insufficient evidence on the safety of other drugs such as amlodipine, angiotensin receptor blockers and ACE inhibitors other than enalapril and captopril.[2]

Diuretics should be generally avoided as they may reduce milk production. Methyldopa should be avoided because of its tendency to cause depression.[21] In select cases of women with severe preeclampsia, there seems to be some benefit to a brief course of furosemide diuresis in the postpartum period, particularly for patients with hypertension accompanied by symptomatic pulmonary or peripheral edema.[28] A Cochrane review of three trials which compared furosemide or nifedipine capsules with no therapy or placebo concluded that postnatal furosemide may decrease the need for postnatal antihypertensive therapy in hospital. Based on a few case reports of elevated BP in the postpartum period with the use of nonsteroidal anti-inflammatory drugs, in women who are already hypertensive, these drugs should be used cautiously or should perhaps be avoided.[29]

Clinical practice often depends on capacity for postpartum clinical monitoring of changes in BP. Locally available resources to follow-up postpartum patients vary widely between settings. Initiating antihypertensive drug treatment where follow-up is not guaranteed carries both potential benefits and harms. Continued antihypertensive drug use is more resource intensive than interrupting the use of antihypertensive drugs. It is unclear whether the continued use of antihypertensive drugs will reduce adverse outcomes and, thereby, reduce the use of resources.[30]

◼ CONCLUSION

- There is no conclusive evidence to support the concept that BP control in pregnant women with chronic hypertension will prevent the subsequent occurrence of preeclampsia, itself the cause for most adverse outcomes in these patients.
- As BP falls in early pregnancy, decreasing or even discontinuing medication and monitoring is often possible in women with mild or moderate hypertension.
- An acceptable threshold for treatment would be 150 mm Hg SBP and/or 100 mm Hg DBP.
- Acceptable agents include methyldopa, labetalol and nifedipine in standard doses. Atenolol use should probably be avoided in pregnancy because it has been associated with slightly lower birth weights.
- Intravenous labetalol or oral nifedipine is as effective as IV hydralazine, with fewer adverse effects for the treatment of acute-onset severe hypertension.
- Good control of BP is important, but it should not preclude the definitive treatment of delivery if this is indicated for maternal or fetal reasons.

Future research should include multicentered, randomized controlled trials of sufficient sample size to assess maternal-perinatal benefits and adverse effects of antihypertensive therapy including long-term follow-up of children who entered trials as fetuses. Better surveillance systems to monitor adverse events are required to assess drug safety and guide treatment.

◼ REFERENCES

1. Report of the National High Blood Pressure Education Program Working Group on High Blood Pressure in Pregnancy. Am J Obstet Gynecol. 2000; 183(1):S1-22.
2. National Institute for Health and Clinical Excellence. (2010). Hypertension in pregnancy: The management of hypertensive disorders during pregnancy. NICE clinical guideline 107. [online]

Available from www.nice.org.uk/nicemedia/
live/13098/50418/50418.pdf. [Accessed May 2013].

3. US Department of Health and Human Services,
National Institutes of Health, National Heart, Lung,
and Blood Institute. (2004). National High Blood
Pressure Education Program. The Seventh Report
of the Joint National Committee on Prevention,
Detection, Evaluation, and Treatment of High Blood
Pressure. NIH Publication No. 04-5230. [online]
Available from www.nhlbi.nih.gov/guidelines/
hypertension/jnc7full.pdf. [Accessed May 2013].

4. Committee on Obstetric Practice. Committee
Opinion no. 514: emergent therapy for acute-
onset, severe hypertension with preeclampsia or
eclampsia. Obstet Gynecol. 2011;118(6):1465-8.

5. Podymow T, August P. Update on the use of
antihypertensive drugs in pregnancy. Hypertension.
2008;51(4):960-9.

6. Peek M, Shennan A, Halligan A, et al. Hypertension
in pregnancy: which method of blood pressure
measurement is most predictive of outcome? Obstet
Gynecol. 1996;88(6):1030-3.

7. Martin JN, Thigpen BD, Moore RC, et al. Stroke and
severe preeclampsia and eclampsia: a paradigm
shift focusing on systolic blood pressure. Obstet
Gynecol. 2005;105(2):246-54.

8. Cooper WO, Hernandez-Diaz S, Arbogast PG,
et al. Major congenital malformations after first-
trimester exposure to ACE inhibitors. N Engl J Med.
2006;354(23):2443-51.

9. Sibai BM. Chronic hypertension in pregnancy.
Obstet Gynecol. 2002;100(2):369-77.

10. Buttar HS. An overview of the influence of ACE
inhibitors on fetal-placental circulation and
perinatal development. Mol Cell Biochem. 1997;
176(1-2):61-71.

11. Montan S, Anandakumar C, Arulkumaran S,
et al. Effects of methyldopa on uteroplacental
and fetal hemodynamics in pregnancy-induced
hypertension. Am J Obstet Gynecol. 1993;168
(1 Pt 1):152-6.

12. Sibai BM, Mabie WC, Shamsa F, et al. A comparison
of no medication versus methyldopa or labetalol
in chronic hypertension during pregnancy. Am J
Obstet Gynecol. 1990;162(4):960-6.

13. Cockburn J, Moar VA, Ounsted M, et al. Final report of
study on hypertension during pregnancy: the effects
of specific treatment on the growth and development
of the children. Lancet. 1982;1(8273):647-9.

14. Butters L, Kennedy S, Rubin PC. Atenolol in essential hypertension during pregnancy. BMJ. 1990;
301(6752):587-9.

15. Magee LA, Ornstein MP, von Dadelszen P. Fort-
nightly review: management of hypertension in
pregnancy. BMJ. 1999;318(7194):1332-6.

16. Magee L, Duley L. Oral beta-blockers for mild
to moderate hypertension during pregnancy.
Cochrane Database Syst Rev. 2003;(3):CD002863.

17. Furberg CD, Psaty BM, Meyer JV. Nifedipine. Dose-
related increase in mortality in patients with coronary
heart disease. Circulation. 1995;92(5):1326-31.

18. Magee LA, Miremadi S, Li J, et al. Therapy with both
magnesium sulfate and nifedipine does not increase
the risk of serious magnesium-related maternal side
effects in women with preeclampsia. Am J Obstet
Gynecol. 2005;193(1):153-63.

19. Magee LA, Cham C, Waterman EJ, et al. Hydralazine
for treatment of severe hypertension in pregnancy:
meta-analysis. BMJ. 2003;327(7421):955-60.

20. Magee LA. Drugs in pregnancy. Antihypertensives.
Best Pract Res Clin Obstet Gynaecol. 2001;15(6):
827-45.

21. Nelson-Piercy C. Hypertension and pre-eclampsia.
In: Handbook of Obstetric Medicine, 4th edition.
London, UK: Informa Healthcare; 2010. pp. 1-18.

22. Steyn DW, Odendaal HJ. Serotonin antagonism
and serotonin antagonists in pregnancy: role of
ketanserin. Obstet Gynecol Surv. 2000;55(9):582-9.

23. Duley L, Henderson-Smart DJ, Meher S. Drugs
for treatment of very high blood pressure
during pregnancy. Cochrane Database Syst Rev.
2006;(3):CD001449.

24. Abalos E, Duley L, Steyn DW, et al. Antihypertensive
drug therapy for mild to moderate hypertension
during pregnancy. Cochrane Database Syst Rev.
2007;(2):CD002252.

25. Rey E, LeLorier J, Burgess E, et al. Report of
the Canadian Hypertension Society Consensus
Conference:3. Pharmacological treatment of
hypertensive disorders in pregnancy. Can Med
Assoc J 1997;157:1245-54.

26. SOMANZ. (2008). Guidelines for the Management
of Hypertensive Disorders of Pregnancy. [online]
Available from www.somanz.org/guidelines.asp.
[Accessed May 2013].

27. Magee LA, Helewa M, Moutquin JM, et al. (2008).
Diagnosis, Evaluation, and Management of the
Hypertensive Disorders of Pregnancy. SOGC
Clinical Practice Guideline No. 206. [online]
Available from www.preeclampsia.org/pdf/
gui206CPG0803_001.pdf. [Accessed May 2013].

28. Ascarelli MH, Johnson V, McCreary H, et al.
Postpartum preeclampsia management with
furosemide: a randomized clinical trial. Obstet
Gynecol. 2005;105(1):29-33.

29. Magee L, Sadeghi S. Prevention and treatment of
postpartum hypertension. Cochrane Database Syst
Rev. 2005;(1):CD004351.

30. World Health Organization. (2011). WHO recommendations for prevention and treatment of preeclampsia or eclampsia: Evidence base. WHO/
RHR/11.25. [online] Available from whqlibdoc.who.
int/hq/2011/WHO_RHR_11.25_eng.pdf. [Accessed
May 2013].

7

Fetal Assessment in Hypertensive Diseases in Pregnancy

PK Shah, Parikshit D Tank

◼ INTRODUCTION

Hypertensive disease is probably the most common medical disorder arising in pregnancy. Hypertensive disorders and their complications are also a leading cause of maternal and perinatal mortality and morbidity worldwide. In the Indian population, perinatal mortality rate in severe preeclampsia has been reported to be 4.76%.[1] A common feature of hypertensive disease in pregnancy (HDP) irrespective of whether it is chronic hypertension, early or late onset preeclampsia or preeclampsia superimposed on chronic hypertension, is vascular damage. The vascular damage is seen in every vessel of the maternal and fetal circulation but is more pronounced in the placental vessels. Vascular damage along with oxidative stress and endothelial damage are the origins of the fetal complications of HDP and possibly of the etiology of HDP itself.

◼ RATIONALE FOR FETAL ASSESSMENT IN HYPERTENSIVE DISEASE IN PREGNANCY

Nearly one-third of pregnancies with HDP are affected by growth restriction as a result of chronic hypoxia.[2] The chronic hypoxia also leads to poor fetal reserves and high chances of abnormal fetal heart rate pattern, meconium stained amniotic fluid and other poor outcomes in labor. Two other events that need to be predicted are less common but have more severe implications i.e. abruption and fetal death. The earlier the onset of HDP, the more common and more severe the impact and outcomes related to perinatal health. An onset

before 28 weeks of pregnancy is associated with a 27% risk of growth restriction, while the risk falls to 9% if the onset is after 32 weeks of pregnancy.[3]

The rationale of fetal assessment is to predict poor perinatal outcomes and allow obstetric intervention before irreversible damage occurs. The obstetric intervention in such situations is usually delivery. If the period of gestation is remote from term, the fetus is faced with the risks of prematurity. This could be a significant burden depending on the period of gestation. An earlier period of gestation indicates a higher risk of all prematurity related complications such as respiratory distress, intraventricular hemorrhage, necrotizing enterocolitis, metabolic disturbances and sepsis. A balance has to be maintained between intervention and conservation that may arise from the fetal assessment. Fetal assessment should therefore be sensitive to diagnose fetal compromise and specific to prevent unnecessary delivery of a healthy fetus before term.

◼ EVIDENCE FOR FETAL ASSESSMENT IN HYPERTENSIVE DISEASE IN PREGNANCY

On the basis of the rationale presented above, it would make intuitive sense to believe that fetal assessment should be conducted on a routine basis in HDP and it would reduce perinatal morbidity and mortality. However, much of the knowledge and literature has been shaped from the prevailing clinical practice and available tests at a particular point in time and place. The usefulness of fetal assessment tests is yet to be examined in randomized trials. It should also be borne in mind that such randomized trials are unlikely to be undertaken as there would be grave concern about not monitoring the fetus at all in HDP. There have been numerous studies comparing various modalities of testing. Due to the plethora of available tests, differences in the methodology of studies, varying period of gestation and frequency of testing, there is no consensus as to the ideal protocol for fetal assessment in HDP. A brief summary of recommendations from various authorities is presented in Table 7.1.

FETAL ASSESSMENT IN EARLY PREGNANCY

Standard tests for fetal assessment include first and second trimester ultrasounds for biometry, early assessment for chromosomal abnormality risk and structural evaluation. These tests are not affected in HDP. Biochemical screening tests have been used since the past three decades for identifying pregnancies at risk for chromosomal anomalies, particularly Trisomy 21. Observations from large series have shown that women with false-positive screening tests for chromosomal anomalies are at risk for a number of adverse perinatal outcomes including HDP.[8] Pregnancies which are destined to develop HDP usually have decreased first trimester maternal serum pregnancy-associated plasma protein A (PAPP-A), and in the second trimester decreased unconjugated oestriol (uE3), increased serum alpha fetoprotein (AFP), or increased total human chorionic gonadotrophin (hCG). Extrapolating from this, a number of workers are involved in using these and other markers to predict HDP.[9] Similarly, abnormal color Doppler

Table 7.1: Recommendations from world authorities on fetal assessment in hypertensive disease in pregnancy

Authority	Guideline Title	Recommendation	Evidence Level
RCOG	The management of severe preeclampsia/eclampsia[4]	Cardiotocography should be used in acute settings	Level III
		If conservative management is planned then further assessment of the fetus with ultrasound measurements of fetal size, umbilical artery Doppler and liquor volume should be undertaken. Serial assessment will allow timing of delivery to be optimized.	Level II, Level I A
SOGC	Diagnosis, evaluation, and management of the hypertensive disorders of pregnancy[5]	Umbilical artery Doppler velocimetry may be useful to support a placental origin for intrauterine fetal growth restriction.	Level II 2B
NHBPEP	NHBPEP report on high BP in pregnancy[6]	Daily fetal movement counts and periodic fetal NST and BPP. Weekly or biweekly testing is appropriate in most women, but daily testing is indicated in women with severe disease.	Level III
SOMANZ	Guidelines for the management of hypertensive disorders in pregnancy 2008[7]	Ultrasound for fetal growth, amniotic fluid volume and umbilical artery Doppler at the onset of disease and repeated every 2–3 weeks with the addition of cardiotocographs twice weekly. If fetal growth restriction is also present, ultrasound for amniotic fluid volume or umbilical artery Doppler twice weekly.	Level II, III

Abbreviations: RCOG, Royal College of Obstetricians and Gynaecologists; SOGC, Society of Obstetricians and Gynaecologists of Canada; NHBPEP, National High Blood Pressure Education Program; SOMANZ, Society of Obstetric Medicine of Australia and New Zealand

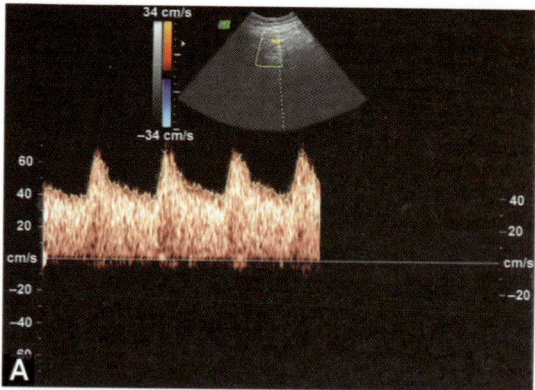 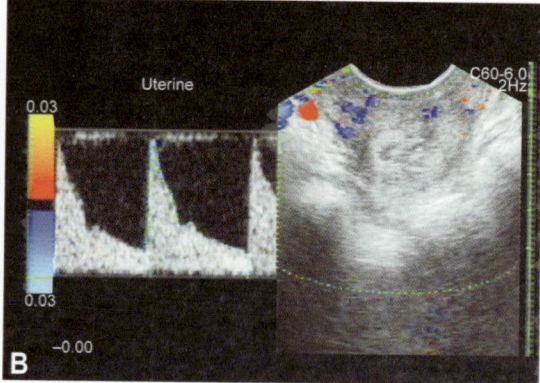

Figs 7.1A and B: (A) Uterine artery waveform without notching indicates a low risk pattern; (B) Uterine artery waveform with persistent notch after 20–22 weeks gestation suggests a higher risk of developing hypertensive disease in pregnancy

of the uterine artery (Figs 7.1A and B) is associated with a number of abnormal perinatal outcomes. Uterine artery notching has been studied from 14 to 22 weeks. A positive correlation with the risk of developing HDP has been seen in most of these studies. The positive predictive value has been variable in different studies.[10]

GENERAL PRINCIPLES FOR FETAL ASSESSMENT IN LATE PREGNANCY

For clinical practice, fetal assessment becomes relevant in the third trimester. Since abnormal fetal assessment results could indicate a need for delivering the fetus, testing should be initiated only at a period of gestation when an obstetric unit can offer a reasonable chance of survival to the neonate in terms of outcomes of prematurity. Initiation of fetal wellbeing tests at very early gestational ages is usually academic and could lead to anxiety for the patient and the caregiver. It is also relevant that care for the mother with HDP when she is at risk for preterm delivery with a viable fetus should be undertaken in a unit where neonatal care facilities are available. In utero transfer of the fetus with the mother is ideal and it would obviate the need for neonatal transport and delays in neonatal care.

As in other clinical situations, one should bear in mind the availability; cost and feasibility of performing tests. Below authors present a review of fetal assessment tests including present state of evidence for each of the tests.

Fetal Movement Counting

The perception of fetal movements by the mother is highly subjective. In an effort to make this more objective, there are various techniques described to quantify fetal movement.[11] Decreased fetal movements are regarded as a marker for suboptimal intrauterine conditions. The fetus responds to chronic hypoxia by conserving energy and the subsequent reduction of fetal movements is an adaptive mechanism to reduce oxygen consumption. At present, there is no specific study or data that addresses the effectiveness of fetal movement counting specifically in HDP. Inferences can be drawn from general populations. The largest review in the Cochrane database involves four trials with over 70,000 women studied. The reviewers could not conclude if fetal movement count was an effective method of fetal surveillance. As such, every pregnant woman who presents with reduced fetal movement on her own accord or on routine enquiry at an antenatal visit should be assessed for fetal growth and fetal wellbeing status with further testing. Although this is a simple, inexpensive and low-resource modality, there is good quality data to suggest that the use of formal counting or kick charts increases the possibility of hospital admissions, interventions and Cesarean section.[12]

Electronic Fetal Heart Rate Monitoring

The earliest electronic fetal heart rate monitoring (EFHRM) method was the contraction stress test.

This is no longer practiced due to the inherent risks of hyperstimulation and starting labor and the numerous contraindications. The contraction stress test is replaced today by the nonstress test (NST) in most obstetric units as the mainstay of fetal assessment. Definitions and classification of NST patterns are now standardized.[13] A reactive NST has a high negative predictive value and is of great assurance to the obstetrician. The converse is not true. The NST may be nonreactive due to a number of other reasons besides fetal compromise and could initiate unnecessary obstetric intervention.[14] NST is used in women with HDP with the thought that this is a high-risk population and the number of false-positive results would be lower. This has not been borne out in clinical practice or in literature. In fact, in women with HDP, the use of alphamethyldopa (a centrally acting antihypertensive agent) is likely to reduce fetal heart rate variability and produce a nonreactive NST in a healthy fetus.[15] The same is true if sedation or anxiolytics have been used. At present, most authorities recommend a weekly NST for women with HDP and twice weekly for women with severe disease or evidence of fetal compromise (growth restriction or oligohydramnios). These recommendations are opinion based. At present, the use of NST in women with HDP and especially those with fetal growth restriction represents an area where research is needed urgently.

Fetal Biometry

Fetal growth is the single most important aspect of fetal assessment that needs to be accurately estimated. This generally outlines the further course of fetal assessment, perinatal outcomes and often obstetric decisions. Growth restriction is more likely to occur when disease onset is remote from term and growth restricted fetuses are more likely to have greater perinatal morbidity and mortality.[2,3,16] Therefore, it is of primary importance to identify growth restriction in HDP. Abdominal palpation and symphysiofundal height measurement have limited accuracy and value in diagnosing growth restriction. Abdominal circumference (AC) (Figs 7.2A to C) and estimated fetal weight (EFW) are the most accurate diagnostic measurements to predict growth restriction. In high-risk women, AC at less than the 10th centile

has sensitivities of 72.9–94.5% and specificities of 50.6–83.8% in the prediction of fetuses with birth weight at less than the 10th centile. The respective figures for EFW are sensitivities of 33.3–89.2% and specificities of 53.7–90.9%.[17] Ideally, fetal biometry should be performed serially over intervals of 3–4 weeks and customized growth charts and growth velocity should be used to make the final diagnosis (Fig. 7.3). However, this may not always be possible in settings of HDP, where delivery may be indicated due to deteriorating maternal condition before the next biometry assessment can be made.

Amniotic Fluid Index and Biophysical Profile

The fetal biophysical profile is a multiparameter test that assesses various aspects of fetal behavior that may be affected by fetal hypoxia and involves ultrasound based criteria (fetal tone, breathing, movements and amniotic fluid) and NST. The standard method of assessing amniotic fluid volume is either measuring the deepest pocket of liquor or calculating the amniotic fluid index (AFI) based on the four quadrant technique. Amniotic fluid levels vary according to the gestation and are depicted in Figure 7.4. Amniotic fluid index and continuous cardiotocography (CTG) together constitute the modified biophysical profile (BPP). Biophysical testing is comprehensive and duration of testing is longer as compared to other fetal assessment tests. Though it has been introduced in clinical practice in the 1980s and is included in various recommendations and guidelines, the BPP or its variants have never been subjected to a single randomized trial in HDP. A Cochrane review of the use of BPP in high-risk pregnancies in general concluded that there is currently insufficient evidence from randomized control trials to support the use of BPP as a test of fetal well-being in high-risk pregnancies.[18] However, there is evidence from uncontrolled observational studies that biophysical profile in high-risk women has good negative predictive value, i.e. fetal death is rare in women with a normal biophysical profile.[19] The BPP, therefore cannot be recommended as the primary surveillance tool in high-risk HDP with growth restriction but can be a useful test in fetuses where the umbilical artery Doppler shows abnormal results.

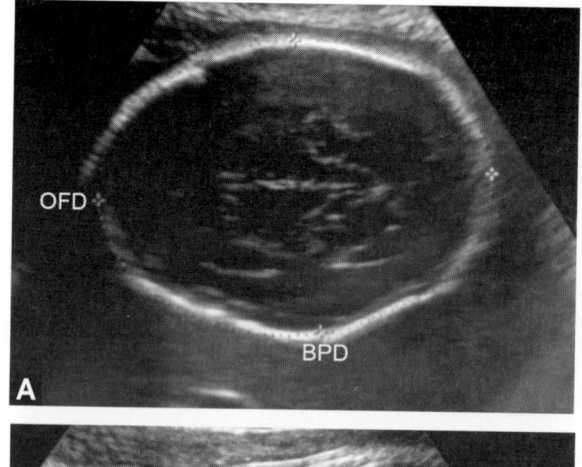

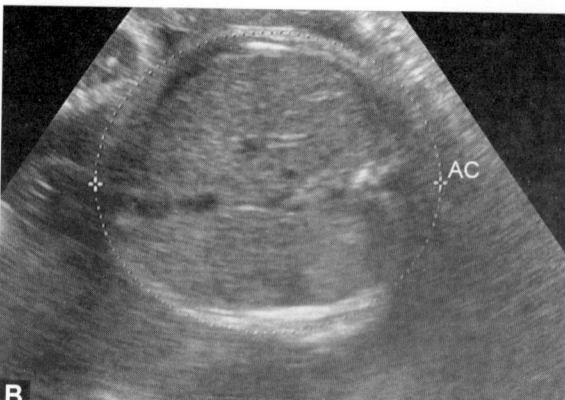

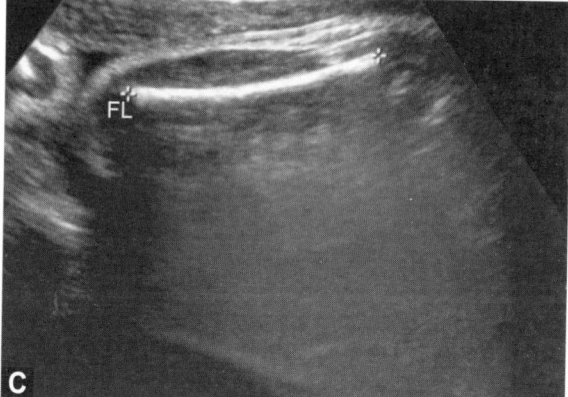

Figs 7.2A to C: Fetal biometry. (A) Measurement of the fetal biparietal diameter (BPD), occipitofrontal diameter (OFD) and head circumference (HC) represented by the dotted line; (B) Measurement of the abdominal circumference (AC); (C) Measurement of the femur length (FL)

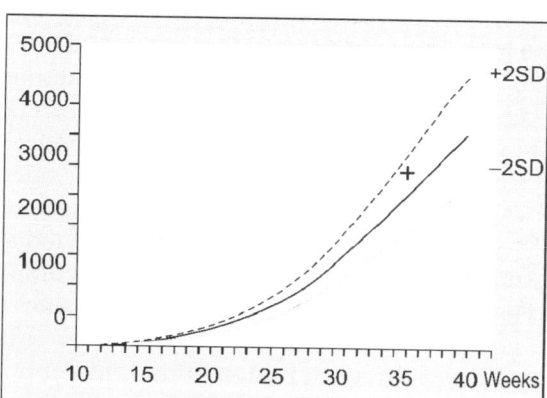

Fig. 7.3: Individual growth chart

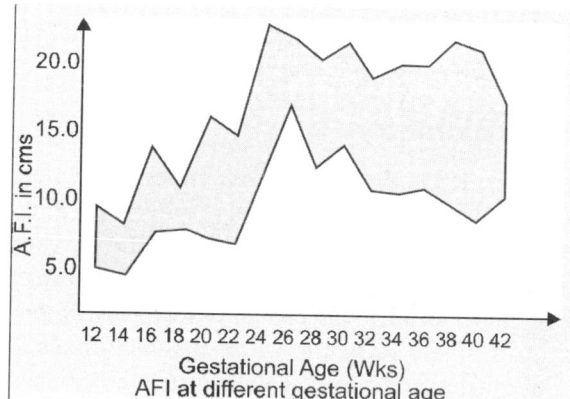

Fig. 7.4: Amniotic fluid index and gestational age

Color Doppler Velocimetry— Umbilical Artery

The vascular basis of fetal compromise is the common link between HDP etiopathogenesis and the morbidity of the growth-restricted fetus. Color Doppler velocimetry of the uteroplacental and fetoplacental circulation gives us a quantitative noninvasive analysis. Data from growth restricted fetuses of normotensive and hypertensive pregnancies show a great degree of correlation in the patterns of umbilical artery, middle cerebral artery (MCA), ductus venosus and cardiac performance indices.[20] Therefore, it is reasonable to extrapolate the literature from studies on growth restriction of other causes to HDP. Every vessel of these circulations has been studied. The most important one is the umbilical artery Doppler velocimetry. Of all indices used clinically to evaluate the umbilical arterial flow, the systolic–diastolic (S/D) ratio has been the most widely studied. In recent studies, umbilical artery pulsatility index (PI) is being used as a measurement of choice rather than S/D ratio. A PI greater than 1.2 was associated with a higher risk of fetal growth restriction and Cesarean deliveries even in low-risk populations.[21] With decreasing uteroplacental circulation, the forward flow in the umbilical artery, which is seen in all phases of the cardiac cycle gradually starts diminishing with an increasing S/D ratio. This continues till there is no flow in the diastolic phase absent end diastolic flow (AEDF) and further till there is a reversal in the blood flow in the diastole reverse end-diastolic flow (REDF). The gradual changes in umbilical artery Doppler flows are depicted in Figures 7.5A to C. It is estimated that abnormally high S/D ratios are seen when about 60–70% of the placental vascular tree is no longer functional.

A recent systematic review of the use of umbilical Doppler in high-risk pregnancies, including preeclampsia and fetal growth restriction, examined a total of 18 studies, which included 10,156 women.[22] Results indicated that umbilical artery Doppler assessment was associated with a significant decrease in perinatal mortality (RR 0.71, 95% CI 0.52 to 0.98). The rate of Cesarean section was decreased in the Doppler group (RR 0.90, 95% CI 0.84 to 0.97), as was the number of inductions of labor (average RR 0.89, 95% CI 0.80 to 0.99). Taken together, these data suggested that Doppler interrogation of the umbilical artery contributed to the accurate identification of the fetus at risk. These results apply to women with severe, early onset disease, or both, particularly with fetal growth restriction, as the underlying pathology of interest is uteroplacental insufficiency. Doppler studies of the umbilical artery should be incorporated into protocols for fetal monitoring in high-risk pregnancies thought to be at risk of placental insufficiency.

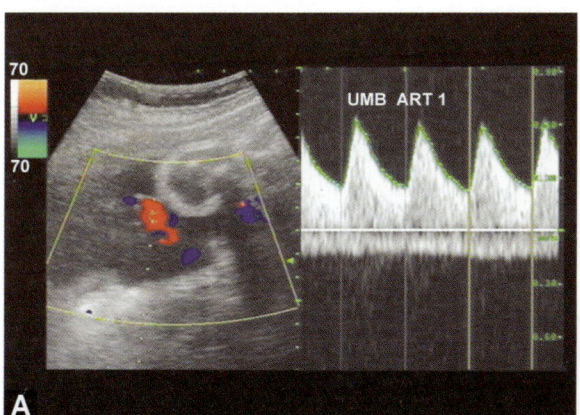

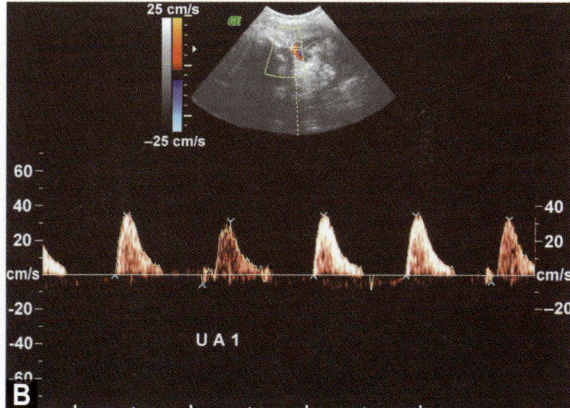

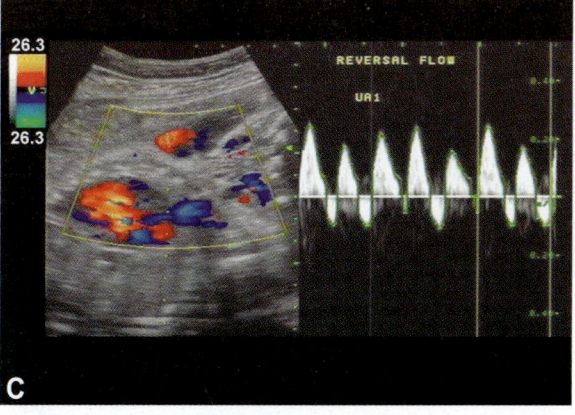

Figs 7.5A to C: Sequence of changes in umbilical artery Doppler velocimetry with worsening fetal hypoxia in hypertensive disease in pregnancy. (A) Increasing resistance in umbilical artery with high systolic/diastolic (S/D) ratio; (B) Absent end diastolic flow (AEDF) in the umbilical artery; (C) Reversal of end-diastolic flow (REDF) in umbilical artery

Color Doppler Velocimetry— Other Vessels

With progressively poor uteroplacental circulation, there is a "brain sparing" effect that the fetus uses as an adaptive mechanism to maintain circulation to the brain, heart and shunt blood away from the kidneys and gut. This results in autoregulation of the cerebral circulation with the changes evident in the MCA. The pulsatility index (PI) and peak systolic flows are increased (Figs 7.6A and B). This was found to be predictive of perinatal mortality, especially when used in conjunction with venous Doppler parameters.[23]

As the uteroplacental and fetoplacental circulations get further compromised, there is an increased shunting of blood from the umbilical vein through the ductus venosus and reduced liver perfusion. This supports fetal survival until there is cardiac decompensation in the form of stiffening of the fetal myocardium and valvular regurgitation. At this point, there is increase in the central venous pressure and it is reflected as reduced or negative flow during atrial contraction (A-wave) in the ductus venosus and pulsatility in the umbilical vein. These are shown in Figures 7.7A to C. These changes indicate a very high-risk of perinatal morbidity and mortality and are considered a late finding along the spectrum of fetal compromise. In a cohort of 74 fetuses with growth restriction and AEDF/REDF, umbilical vein pulsations, followed by waveform abnormalities in the ductus venosus were the most sensitive Doppler parameters for identifying fetuses at risk for stillbirth, perinatal or neonatal death.[24]

■ CONCLUSION

From the published literature on each of these modalities, it is clear that the first step in the assessment should be to identify the small fetus in HDP. Surveillance and monitoring should be then undertaken by umbilical artery Doppler. There is a steady deterioration of the uteroplacental circulation and it can be evaluated by a predictable series of Doppler changes that precede abnormalities in the biophysical evaluation and heart rate changes. Further evaluation can be done with Doppler velocimetry of other vessels or one or more components of the biophysical profile (Flow charts 7.1 and 7.2). The protocols should be followed until such time that the fetus is mature or the obstetric unit is confident of fetal salvage based on the gestational age. It is not necessary or desirable to wait for all the Doppler parameters to be abnormal before taking a decision to deliver the fetus if gestational age is favorable. Multiparameter testing would be of greater value rather than relying on a single testing modality. The goal of assessment and monitoring is to optimize the time and route

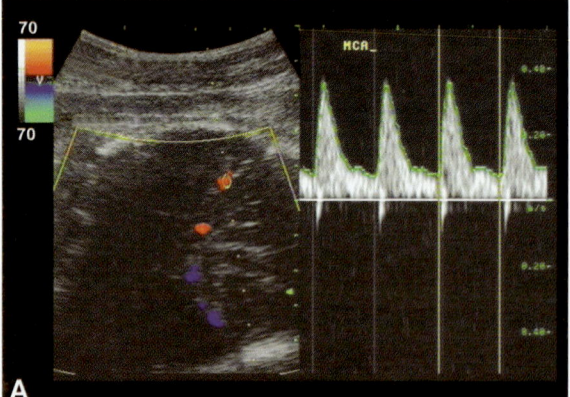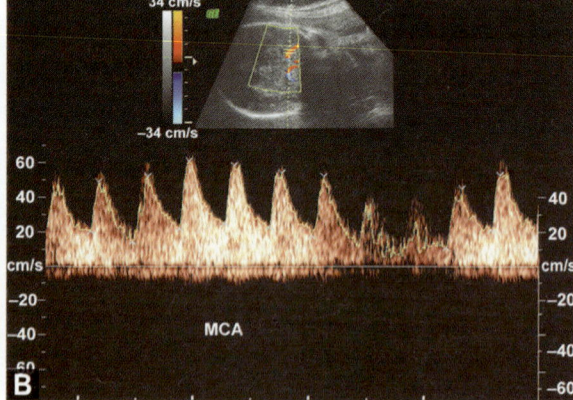

Figs 7.6A and B: Doppler velocimetry waveforms of the middle cerebral artery. (A) Middle cerebral artery waveform showing a high pulsatility index indicating a normal circulation; (B) Middle cerebral artery waveform showing a greater diastolic component and low pulsatility index suggesting redistribution of fetal blood flow and due to growth restriction or hypoxia

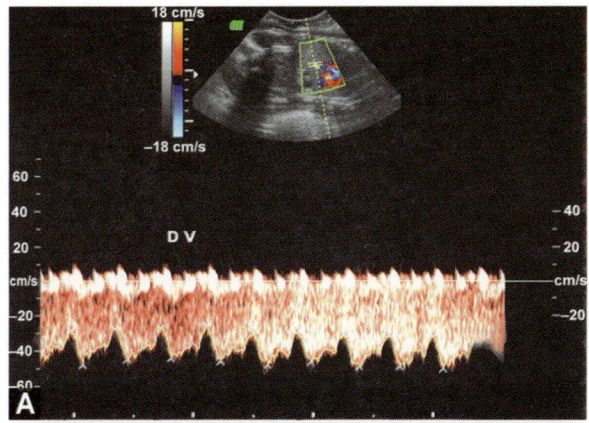

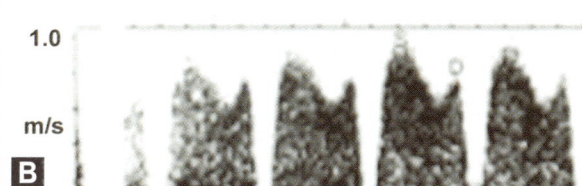

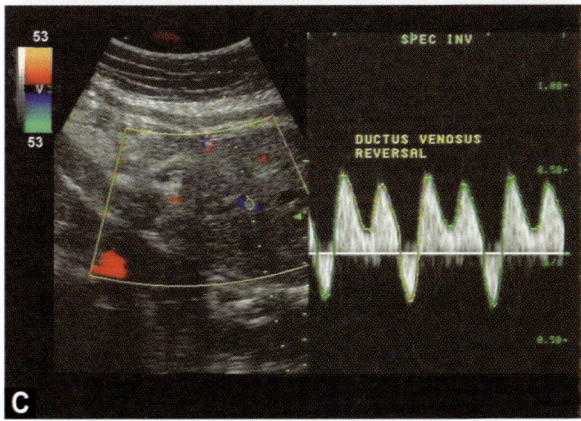

Figs 7.7A to C: Sequence of changes in the ductus venosus showing progressing fetal hypoxia and fetal cardiac failure. (A) Normal ductus venosus (DV) waveform; (B) Ductus venosus waveform with high pulsatility due to decrease of early diastolic forward flow and low velocity during atrial contraction; (C) Ductus venosus–increased reverse flow

Flow chart 7.1: Fetal assessment in hypertensive disease in pregnancy with normal biometry

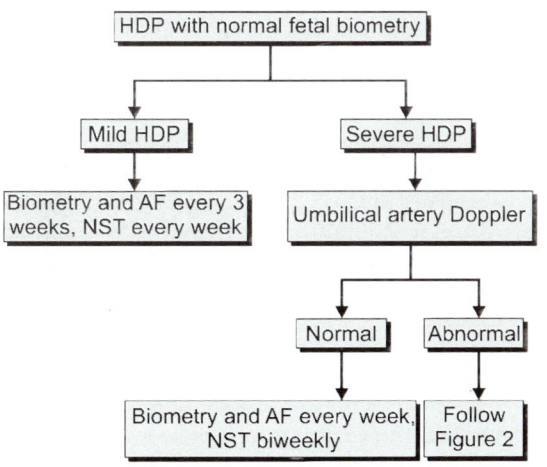

Flow chart 7.2: Fetal assessment in hypertensive disease in pregnancy with growth restriction (small-for-dates fetus)

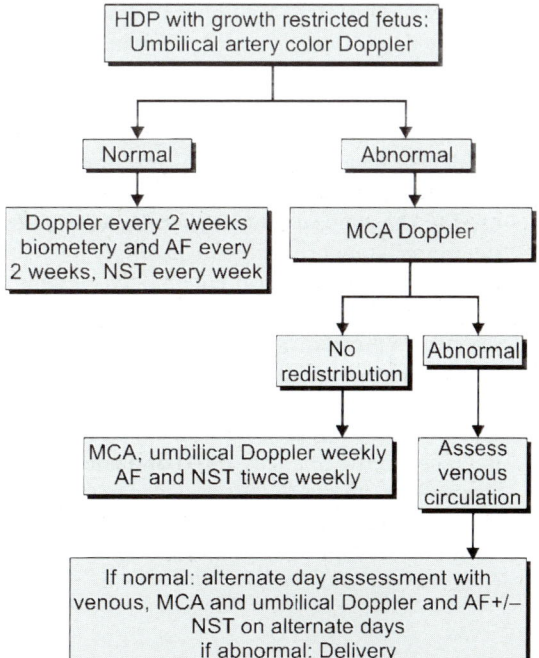

of delivery so that there is a balance between the risks of growth restriction and hypoxia versus the risks of prematurity.

74

■ REFERENCES

1. Shah D, Shroff S, Ganla K. Factors affecting perinatal mortality in India–the FOGSI Perinatal Mortality Study. Int J Gynecol Obstet. 2000;5:288-302.
2. Yücesoy G, Ozkan S, Bodur H, et al. Maternal and perinatal outcome in pregnancies complicated with hypertensive disorder of pregnancy: a seven year experience of a tertiary care center. Arch Gynecol Obstet. 2005;273:43-9.
3. Haddad B, Deis S, Goffinet F, et al. Maternal and perinatal outcomes during expectant management of 239 severe preeclamptic women between 24 and 33 weeks' gestation. Am J Obstet Gynecol. 2004;190:1590-5.
4. Royal College of Obstetricians and Gynecologists. The management of severe preeclampsia and eclampsia. Green Top Guidleine No.10A. London: RCOG Press; 2006.
5. The Society of Obstetricians and Gynecologists of Canada. Diagnosis, Evaluation and Management of the Hypertensive Disorders of Pregnancy. J Obstet Gynecol Canada. 2008;30:S9-S16.
6. Report of the National High Blood Pressure Education Program Working Group on High Blood Pressure in Pregnancy. National high blood pressure education program working group on high blood pressure in pregnancy. Am J Obstet Gynecol. 2000;183(Suppl. 1): S1-22.
7. Society of Obstetric Medicine of Australia and New Zealand. Guidelines for the management of hypertensive disorders of pregnancy 2008. SOMANZ Endorsed Guideline 1. 2008.
8. Huang T, Hoffman B, Meschino W, et al. Prediction of adverse pregnancy outcomes by combinations of first and second trimester biochemistry markers used in the routine prenatal screening of Down syndrome. Prenat Diagn. 2010;30:471-7.
9. Kolla V, Jenö P, Moes S, et al. Quantitative proteomic (iTRAQ) analysis of 1st trimester maternal plasma samples in pregnancies at risk for preeclampsia. J Biomed Biotechnol. 2012;2012:305964.
10. Myatt L, Clifton RG, Roberts JM, et al. The Utility of Uterine artery Doppler Velocimetry in Prediction of Preeclampsia in a Low-Risk Population. Obstet Gynecol. 2012;120:815-22.
11. Unterscheider J, Horgan R, O'Donoghue K, et al. Reduced fetal movements. The Obstetrician & Gynecologist. 2009;11:245-51.
12. Sinha D, Sharma A, Nallaswamy V, et al. Obstetric outcome in women complaining of reduced fetal movements. J Obstet Gynaecol. 2007;27:41-3.
13. Electronic fetal heart rate monitoring: research guidelines for interpretation. National Institute of Child Health and Human Development Research Planning Workshop. Am J Obstet Gynecol. 1997; 177:1385-90.
14. Pattison N, McCowan L. Cardiotocography for antepartum fetal assessment. Cochrane Database Syst Rev. 2010;1:CD001068.
15. Rayburn WF, Motley ME, Zuspan FP. Conditions affecting nonstress test results. Obstet Gynecol. 1982;59:490-3.
16. Sibai BM, Barton JR. Expectant management of severe preeclampsia remote from term: patient selection, treatment, and delivery indications. Am J Obstet Gynecol. 2007;196:514-9.
17. Chang TC, Robson SC, Boys RJ, et al. Prediction of the small for gestational age infant: which ultrasonic measurement is best? Obstet Gynecol. 1992;80:1030-8.
18. Lalor JG, Fawole B, Alfirevic Z, et al. Biophysical profile for fetal assessment in high risk pregnancies. Cochrane Database Syst Rev. 2008;1:CD000038.
19. Dayal AK, Manning FA, Berck DJ, et al. Fetal death after normal biophysical profile score: An eighteen-year experience. Am J Obstet Gynecol. 1999; 181:1231-6.
20. Crispi F, Comas M, Hernández-Andrade E, et al. Does preeclampsia influence fetal cardiovascular function in early-onset intrauterine growth restriction? Ultrasound Obstet Gynecol. 2009;34:660-5.
21. Bolz N, Kalache KD, Fotopoulu C, et al. Value of Doppler sonography near term: can umbilical and uterine artery indices in low-risk pregnancies predict perinatal outcome? J Perinat Med. 2012 Sep 10. doi:pii: /j/jpme.ahead-of-print/jpm-2012-0042/jpm-2012-0042.xml. 10.1515/jpm-2012-0042. [Epub ahead of print]
22. Alfirevic Z, Stampalija T, Gyte GM. Fetal and umbilical Doppler ultrasound in high-risk pregnancies. Cochrane Database Syst Rev. 2010;1: CD007529.
23. Mari G, Hanif F, Kruger M, et al. Middle cerebral artery peak systolic velocity: a new Doppler parameter in the assessment of growth-restricted fetuses. Ultrasound Obstet Gynecol. 2007;29:310-6.
24. Schwarze A, Gembruch U, Krapp M, et al. Qualitative venous Doppler flow waveform analysis in preterm intrauterine growth-restricted fetuses with ARED flow in the umbilical artery–correlation with short-term outcome. Ultrasound Obstet Gynecol. 2005;25:573-9.

8 Maternal Assessment in Hypertensive Disease of Pregnancy

Suchitra N Pandit, Gorakh G Mandrupkar, Rana Choudhary

INTRODUCTION

Hypertension in pregnancy is one of the major causes of maternal and perinatal morbidity and mortality. The challenge lies in early diagnosis which facilitates appropriate maternal and fetal assessment by various methods, correct management and timely intervention to get an optimal outcome. Treating clinicians must detect the cases as early as possible, so utmost care can be offered anticipating good maternal and fetal outcome.

Current chapter attempts to give recent data regarding maternal screening and assessment on hypertensive disease in pregnancy.

Hypertensive disorders of pregnancy (HDP) comprise of chronic hypertension, gestational hypertension, preeclampsia, superimposed pre-eclampsia in chronic hypertensive and eclampsia. These conditions range from mild disease to multiorgan failure causing significant harm. Society of Obstetricians and Gynaecologists of Canada (SOGC) Clinical Practice Guideline No. 206 states that despite extensive research, the onset of hypertension during pregnancy has proven difficult to predict.[1]

Hypertension in pregnancy is defined by South Australian Perinatal Practice Guidelines, 28 June 2004, as:[2]

- Systolic blood pressure greater than or equal to 140 mm Hg, and/or
- Diastolic blood pressure greater than or equal to 90 mm Hg.

These measurements should be confirmed by repeated readings. S Seligman S in the British Journal of Obstetrics and Gynaecology (June 1987) states that elevations of both systolic and diastolic blood pressures have been associated with an adverse fetal outcome and therefore both are important.[3] There is supporting evidence also as:

- Perinatal mortality rises with diastolic blood pressures above 90 mm Hg[4]
- Readings above these levels were beyond two standard deviations of mean blood pressure.[5]

Previously, a rise in blood pressure from pre-conception or first visit by more than 30/15 mm Hg was considered as one of the criteria for diagnosis of preeclampsia.

Available evidence does not support increased incidence of adverse outcomes.[6,7]

SEVERITY OF HYPERTENSION

Brown et al. (2001) mentioned hypertension in pregnancy is considered to be severe when systolic blood pressure is greater than or equal to 160 mm Hg and/or diastolic blood pressure greater than or equal to 100 mm Hg. These levels represent cut off levels of overcoming cerebral autoregulation. Severe hypertension should be lowered promptly and carefully to prevent cerebral hemorrhage and hypertensive encephalopathy.[8]

CLASSIFICATION

Accurate classification of women having either pre-existing hypertension or preeclampsia or gestational hypertension is very important. The management and prognosis are very different in each condition as well as the impact on maternal and perinatal outcomes is also different. It facilitates the action plan, vigilant care and early detection of complications thereby reducing maternal and perinatal morbidity and mortality.

Gestational Hypertension

It is the new onset of hypertension after 20 weeks gestation without proteinuria. It returns to normal within 3 months postpartum.

Preeclampsia

Preeclampsia is hypertension after 20 weeks gestation with proteinuria.[9] It is a multisystem disorder. It is considered severe with one of the following:

- Significant proteinuria (more than 2+): Renal involvement
- Thrombocytopenia, hemolysis, disseminated intravascular coagulation: Hematological involvement
- Epigastric pain, elevated liver enzymes: Liver involvement
- Hyperreflexia, headache, visual disturbances: Neurological involvement
- Pulmonary edema: Cardiorespiratory involvement
- Abruption, intrauterine growth restriction, oligohydramnios: Placental involvement.

Chronic Hypertension

It is defined as a blood pressure more than 140/90 mm Hg confirmed before pregnancy or before 20 weeks of pregnancy. These women are at high risk of superimposed preeclampsia than with normotensive women.

Preeclampsia Superimposed on Chronic Hypertension

It is diagnosed when preeclampsia develops in a woman with chronic hypertension after 20 weeks. In such women significant increases in blood pressure, proteinuria and other systemic features will help in making diagnosis.

Eclampsia

It is characterized by generalized tonic, clonic convulsions in patients with preeclampsia.

◼ MEASUREMENT OF BLOOD PRESSURE

- It is measured with arm at heart level with woman seated at 45°.
- It is better to avoid supine position.

- First Korotkoff sound (K1) is systolic and disappearance of sound (K5) is diastolic reading.[10,11]
- The correct method as well as correct cuff size of apparatus minimizes overdiagnosis.[12]

Measurement Devices

- Mercury manometers are the gold standards.
- Newly designed automated devices may give similar mean blood pressure.
- Calibration of devices must be done regularly. There is a wide intraindividual error and their accuracy may be further compromised in women with preeclampsia.

Twenty-four Hour Ambulatory Blood Pressure Monitoring

- Normal blood pressure values by ambulatory blood pressure monitoring (ABPM) are established for pregnancy.
- It is useful in evaluation of early (< 20 weeks gestation) hypertension.
- It is less useful in screening in the second half of pregnancy.[13]
- It has also been helpful in prediction of hypertension in high risk women but its sensitivity and specificity is low.[9]

◼ INVESTIGATION OF NEW ONSET HYPERTENSION IN PREGNANCY

Any pregnant woman with hypertension should be thoroughly investigated for assessment of type of HDP, etiology, severity and fetal well-being. Investigations may be carried out on outpatient basis but if there are premonitory symptoms like vomiting, headache, epigastric pain or established complications, admission becomes necessary.

The following investigations should be performed in all patients:

- Urine dipstick testing for proteinuria
- Complete blood count (CBC)
- Urea, creatinine, electrolytes
- Liver function tests (LFTs)
- Ultrasound assessment of fetal growth, amniotic fluid volume and umbilical artery flow.

Normal values of blood investigations are given in Table 8.1.

Measurement of Proteinuria

All pregnant women should be assessed for proteinuria testing by dipstick method. It is done for screening.

Table 8.1: Normal values of blood investigations

Test	Normal Values	Test	Normal Values
Creatinine	0.4–1.2 mg/dL	SGOT	Up to 40 IU/L
Blood urea	20–40 mg/dL	SGPT	Up to 40 IU/L
Serum Na+	135–145 mmol/L	Albumin	3.8–5 g/dL
Serum K+	3.5–5.0 mmol/L	Globulin	2.3–3.5 g/dL
Uric acid	3–6.5 mg/dL	LDH	80–460 U/L

• Frequency of any investigations is individualized as per need in that case.
• There are no strict guidelines for the same.
(Abbreviations: SGOT, serum glutamic oxaloacetic transaminase; SGPT, serum glutamic pyruvate transaminase; LDH, lactate dehydrogenase)

Though it is not an accurate method, approximate measurements are done as:
• 1+ corresponds to 0.3 g/L
• 2+ corresponds to 1 g/L
• 3+ corresponds to 3 g/L

More definitive testing is advocated when preeclampsia is suspected. A protein creatinine ratio more than 30 mg/mmol corresponds with a 24 hour urine excretion of more than 300 mg. This is used to check for significant proteinuria.

One Canadian study measured many parameters including CBC, uric acid and creatinine levels along with coagulation profile, LFTs and urinary dipstick proteinuria, and 24 hour urinary protein.[14]

Higher levels of proteinuria were not always associated with increased maternal or perinatal morbidity/mortality[15,16] and have not predicted short-term maternal renal failure.[16]

Complete Blood Count

It gives an idea about anemia status and thrombocytopenia, which is one of the worsening signs of preeclampsia. Total leukocyte count will identify current infections which may aggravate the condition.

Liver Function Tests

Elevated liver enzymes—serum glutamic oxaloacetic transaminase (SGOT), serum glutamic pyruvate transaminase (SGPT) and lactate dehydrogenase (LDH)—are the markers for severity of underlying HDP. Approximately 12% women with severe preeclampsia may develop HELLP syndrome consisting of hemolysis, elevated liver enzymes and low platelets.

Renal Function Tests

Though acute renal failure is a rare complication in preeclampsia these tests not only indicate the severity but also help in diagnosis of causes of chronic hypertension during pregnancy. One must not forget the following causes of chronic hypertension—chronic kidney disease, e.g. glomerulonephritis, reflux nephropathy, and adult polycystic kidney disease. Serum electrolytes help in fluid management.

Special Investigations

• Patients with severe early onset preeclampsia warrant investigation for associated conditions, e.g. systemic lupus erythematosus, underlying renal disease, antiphospholipid syndrome or thrombophilias.
• Undiagnosed pheochromocytoma, though rare, in pregnancy is potentially fatal and may present as preeclampsia.[17]
• Twenty-four hour urinary catecholamines should be undertaken in the presence of very labile or severe hypertension.
• If there is thrombocytopenia or falling hemoglobin, investigations for DIC (coagulation studies, peripheral blood smear, LDH, fibrinogen, D-Dimer) should be done.

▮ MONITORING

Monitoring is individualized depending upon the situation of the case. In severe preeclampsia:
• Blood pressure is best measured every 15 minutes initially and then half hourly.
• Foley's catheter should be inserted.
• Detailed input and output records are kept.
• Oxygen saturation, respiratory rate and temperature should be measured.
• Neurological assessment should be performed hourly.
• Fetal well-being should be assessed carefully.

The Research Need of the Hour

Uterine artery Doppler study is a poor predictor of preeclampsia as it has limited test accuracy.

The trials should compare a policy of revealed versus unrevealed uterine artery Doppler group of patients. The study outcomes should be consequences of preeclampsia including need for high dependency units, perinatal mortality and morbidity.

Fetal Surveillance

Perinatal outcome is compromised in many cases of hypertensive disease in pregnancy as compared to normotensive women.

Fetal surveillance is commonly recommended and performed in women with hypertensive disease in pregnancy.[8] There are no definitive guidelines on how it should be performed.[18]

Frequency, intensity, and modality of evaluation will differ in each case. Details of monitoring for fetal well-being is provided in another chapter.

▇ REFERENCES

1. Magee LA, Helewa M, Moutquin JM, et al. (2008). Clinical Practice Guideline No. 206: Diagnosis, Evaluation and Management of the Hypertensive Disorders of Pregnancy. [online] Available from sogc.org/wp-content/uploads/2013/01/gui206CPG0803hypertensioncorrection.pdf. [Accessed July, 2013].

2. Government of South Australia. (2004). Hypertensive disorders in pregnancy; South Australian Perinatal Practice Guidelines. [online] Available from www.health.sa.gov.au/ppg/Default.aspx?PageContentMode=1&tabid=103. [Accessed July, 2013].

3. Seligman S. Which blood pressure? Br J Obstet Gynaecol. 1987; 94(6):497-8.

4. MacGillivray I. Pre-eclampsia. The hypertensive diseases of pregnancy. Toronto, Canada: Harcourt Canada Limited; 1983. pp. 174-90.

5. Stone P, Cook D, Hutton J, et al. Measurements of blood pressure, oedema and proteinuria in a pregnant population of New Zealand. Australian N Z J Obstet Gynaecol. 1995;35(1):32-7.

6. North RA, Taylor RS, Schellenberg JC. Evaluation of a definition of pre-eclampsia. Br J Obstet Gynaecol. 1999;106(8):767-73.

7. Levine RJ, Ewell MG, Hauth JC, et al. Should the definition of preeclampsia include a rise in diastolic blood pressure >/=15 mm Hg to a level < 90 mm Hg in association with proteinuria? Am J Obstet Gynecol. 2000;183(4):787-92.

8. Brown MA, Lindheimer MD, de Swiet M, et al. The classification and diagnosis of the hypertensive disorders of pregnancy: statement from the International Society for the Study of Hypertension in Pregnancy (ISSHP). Hypertens Pregnancy. 2001; 20(1):9-14.

9. Report of the National High Blood Pressure Education Program Working Group on High Blood Pressure in Pregnancy. Am J Obstet Gynecol. 2000; 183(1):S1-S22.

10. Brown MA, Mangos G, Davis G, Homer C. The natural history of white coat hypertension during pregnancy. BJOG. 2005;112(5):601-6.

11. Shennan A, Gupta M, Halligan A, et al. Lack of reproducibility in pregnancy of Korotkoff phase IV as measured by mercury sphygmomanometry. Lancet. 1996;347(8995):139-42.

12. Brown MA, Reiter L, Smith B, et al. Measuring blood pressure in pregnant women: a comparison of direct and indirect methods. Am J Obstet Gynecol. 1994;171(3):661-7.

13. Brown MA, Davis GK, McHugh L. The prevalence and clinical significance of nocturnal hyper-tension in pregnancy. J Hypertens. 2001;19(8):1437-44.

14. Caetano M, Ornstein MP, von Dadelszen P, et al. A survey of Canadian practitioners regarding diagnosis and evaluation of the hypertensive disorders of pregnancy. Hypertens Pregnancy. 2004;23(2):197-209.

15. Newman MG, Robichaux AG, Stedman CM, et al. Perinatal outcomes in preeclampsia that is complicated by massive proteinuria. Am J Obstet Gynecol. 2003;188(1):264-8.

16. Hall DR, Odendaal HJ, Steyn DW, et al. Urinary protein excretion and expectant management of early onset, severe pre-eclampsia. Int J Gynaecol Obstet. 2002;77(1):1-6.

17. Hudsmith JG, Thomas CE, Browne DA. Undiagnosed phaeochromocytoma mimicking severe preeclampsia in a pregnant woman at term. Int J Obstet Anesth. 2006;15(3):240-5.

18. Sibai BM. Diagnosis and management of gestational hypertension and preeclampsia. Obstet Gynecol. 2003;102(1):181-92.

9

Medical Disorders Presenting with Hypertension in Pregnancy—Renal, Vascular, Connective Tissue and Endocrine Disease: Diagnosis and Management

Vikram Sinai Talaulikar, Sabaratnam Arulkumaran

INTRODUCTION

Hypertension in pregnancy can be a result of chronic disease or a new onset hypertension (gestational hypertension or preeclampsia) in the second half of pregnancy. In either situation there is an increased risk of maternal and perinatal morbidity and mortality. Hypertensive disorders of pregnancy (HDP) affect about 10% of all pregnant women around the world.[1] While preeclampsia predominantly affects women in their first pregnancy (2–8%), prevalence of chronic hypertension in pregnancy is estimated to be about 3%.[2,3] Due to their unpredictable nature and potential for poor outcomes, patients with HDP need a multidisciplinary care with senior obstetric, neonatal and anesthetic input to optimize both maternal and fetal outcomes. This chapter discusses the etiology, diagnosis and management of medical disorders resulting in chronic hypertension in pregnancy.

DEFINITION AND MAGNITUDE OF THE PROBLEM

Chronic hypertension in pregnancy is defined as a blood pressure (BP) of at least 140 mm Hg systolic or 90 mm Hg diastolic before pregnancy, or before 20 weeks of gestation. In a normal pregnancy, BP levels tend to fall in the first and second trimesters. Therefore, women with high BP before the 20th week are assumed to have pre-existing hypertension.

Some women may have been diagnosed as hypertensive prior to pregnancy but it is common for other women, especially in under-resourced parts of the world, to only seek healthcare when they are pregnant. Thus, for many women of reproductive age, chronic hypertension is diagnosed for the first time in the first half of pregnancy. Occasionally, diagnosis of chronic hypertension may only be made retrospectively up to 3–6 months after delivery, when the BP fails to return to normal.

The estimated prevalence of chronic hypertension is about 3% however it is expected to rise in future because of growing epidemic of obesity, diabetes and older obstetric population.[3]

RISKS TO MOTHER AND FETUS

Most women with chronic hypertension have good pregnancy outcomes, but they are at an increased risk for pregnancy complications in comparison to the general population.

Major maternal and fetal risks include:

- Increased frequency of preeclampsia (17–25%)
- Placental abruption
- Stillbirth
- Intrauterine growth restriction (IUGR) (10–20%)
- Preterm birth
- Increased rate of Cesarean delivery

These risks increase with severity of hypertension[4] and the risk of superimposed preeclampsia increases with an increasing duration of hypertension.[5] In addition to those women with chronic hypertension who develop superimposed preeclampsia, 7–20% of women experience worsening of hypertension during pregnancy without the development of preeclampsia.[4,6]

ETIOLOGY OF CHRONIC HYPERTENSION IN PREGNANCY

Ninty to ninty-five percent of cases of chronic hypertension are considered to be essential.

Box 9.1: Medical conditions presenting with chronic hypertension in pregnancy

Idiopathic essential hypertension

Vascular Disorders
- Renovascular hypertension
- Aortic coarctation

Endocrine Disorders
- Diabetes mellitus
- Hyperthyroidism
- Pheochromocytoma
- Acromegaly
- Cushing's syndrome
- Conn's syndrome

Renal Disorders
- Diabetic nephropathy
- Reflux nephropathy
- Chronic glomerulonephritis
- Nephritic and nephrotic syndrome
- Polycystic kidney

Connective Tissue Disorders
- Systemic lupus erythematosus
- Systemic sclerosis
- Polyarteritis nodosa
- Rheumatoid disease

Secondary causes that account for approximately 5–10% cases are listed in Box 9.1.

◼ DIAGNOSIS AND INVESTIGATION OF MEDICAL CONDITIONS PRESENTING WITH HYPERTENSION IN PREGNANCY

History

Women may remain asymptomatic until their BP is significantly high. Therefore, hypertension can progress undetected until the maternal condition has deteriorated to the point of severe organ failure and/or fetal demise. Besides obstetric history, a detailed history of underlying medical condition should be obtained wherever possible. Any treatment received in the past as well as ongoing medications should be discussed. Symptoms pertaining to hypertensive end organ disease should be specifically sought for.

Clinical Examination

A thorough system-wise clinical examination should be performed in addition to the obstetric examination. Mercury sphygmomanometry remains the gold standard for measurement of BP. If other electronic devices are used they need to be regularly validated and calibrated. Correct size of cuff is very important to avoid erroneous measurements (if the mid-arm circumference is more than 33 cm, a large cuff should be used). Blood pressure should be measured with the woman rested and seated with a slight lateral tilt at a 45°, with the arm at the level of the heart. At least two high readings should be obtained minimum 4–6 hours apart before a diagnosis is confirmed. A single BP of 140/90 mm Hg or above is not uncommon in pregnancy and has been reported in nearly 40% of pregnant women in a study.[7] Femoral pulses should be examined to look for radio-femoral delay suggesting coarctation of aorta and renal bruits may be heard in case of renal artery stenosis.

Other condition specific symptoms and signs are discussed in individual sections below.

Blood, Urine and Imaging Investigations

In women presenting with chronic hypertension in pregnancy, it is important to look for an underlying cause. Although the type and frequency of investigations depends on the etiology, commonly performed tests include:
- Urine analysis (for blood, protein and glucose)
- Serum urea and creatinine (for renal impairment)
- Serum electrolytes (for hypokalemia–Conn's syndrome and renal impairment)
- Electrocardiography (ECG)
- Serum lipoproteins
- Renal tract ultrasound
- Urinary catecholamines in cases suggestive of pheochromocytoma
- Adrenal/Pituitary imaging by USG/MRI if tumor is suspected
- Assessment of fetus after 26 weeks—ultrasound assessment of fetal growth and the volume of amniotic fluid, Doppler velocimetry of umbilical arteries and cardiotocography (CTG)
- Fundoscopy—to look for changes in retinal vasculature/papilloedema
- Other condition specific tests (discussed below)

Identifying superimposed preeclampsia in women with chronic hypertension can be challenging; however, it should be considered when the BP increases in pregnancy or when there is a new onset of or an increase in baseline proteinuria. An elevated uric acid level, presence of thrombocytopenia or abnormal liver function tests (LFT) favor the diagnosis of preeclampsia.

■ MANAGEMENT OF CHRONIC HYPERTENSION IN PREGNANCY

Rationale Behind Treatment

Management of women with hypertensive disease in pregnancy aims at preventing further complications, avoiding unnecessary prematurity and optimizing maternal and infant outcomes. To ensure patient safety and the optimal clinical outcomes, management should be multidisciplinary and evidence based.

Prepregnancy Care and Counseling

The care of women with chronic hypertension should begin before pregnancy. Appropriate preconception counseling and preparations are necessary for optimal control of BP. Medications may need to be changed before conception to reduce the risk of fetal anomalies. In very high-risk situations, pregnancy may need to be discouraged or postponed until maternal condition has improved.

Evaluation of renal functions, 24 hour urine for total protein and creatinine clearance, ECG and fundoscopy are recommended to establish baseline profiles and end organ status. Restriction of dietary sodium intake to more than 2.4 g sodium daily should be advised. Lifestyle modifications, including weight reduction and increased physical activity, should be encouraged. Should medical therapy become necessary, antihypertensives should be started preconceptionally and continued in pregnancy at the lowest effective dose. Due to risk of fetal anomalies, angiotensin converting enzyme (ACE) inhibitors and angiotensin-II (ATII) receptor antagonists are contraindicated and should be discontinued with substitution by suitable alternatives. Folic acid supplementation and Rubella immunization (if seronegative) should be recommended to all women.

Antenatal Care and Antihypertensive Therapy

Depending of the nature and severity of underlying medical condition, women should be seen with increased frequency in the antenatal clinic and cared for by a multidisciplinary team. The use of antihypertensive drugs in hypertensive women without renal impairment is considered to be beneficial in preventing sudden increases in BP, cerebrovascular accident or hypertensive encephalopathy. A Cochrane systematic review[6] with meta-analysis of 28 randomized trials comparing antihypertensive treatment either with placebo or with no treatment showed that antihypertensive treatment significantly reduced the risk of severe hypertension. However, treatment did not reduce the risks of superimposed preeclampsia, placental abruption, or growth restriction, nor did it improve neonatal outcomes.[6] There is still lack of robust evidence for benefit of antihypertensive agents in treatment of mild to moderate chronic hypertension as the treatment. In fact some obstetricians have expressed concerns that, too tight control of BP may impair uteroplacental perfusion and fetal growth leading to adverse perinatal outcomes. The ongoing Control of Hypertension in Pregnancy Study (CHIPS)[8] is a multicenter randomized controlled trial (RCT) looking at nonsevere, nonproteinuric hypertension which may clarify this issue. It aims to answer whether "less tight" control (target diastolic BP 100 mm Hg) versus "tight" control (target diastolic BP 85 mm Hg) increases or decreases the likelihood of pregnancy loss, high level neonatal care and serious maternal outcomes.

Timing of Initiation and Goals of Therapy

Opinions also differ regarding the timing of initiation of treatment in pregnancy. Until recently, the focus remained on treating elevated BP based on the diastolic readings with treatment generally recommended for sustained diastolic BP more than 100 mm Hg. There is now however increasing awareness on the importance of systolic BP values.

Both Center for Maternal and Child Enquiries (CMACE)[9] and National Institute for Health and Clinical Excellence (NICE)[10] clinical guidelines in the United Kingdom on hypertension in pregnancy recommend that all pregnant women with a systolic BP of 150 mm Hg or more require antihypertensive treatment. Antihypertensive therapy may be considered at lower pressures if the overall clinical picture suggests rapid deterioration or if development of severe hypertension can be anticipated. A systolic BP more than 180 mm Hg should be considered a medical emergency and quick effective treatment is advocated to prevent hemorrhagic stroke.

The goal of antihypertensive therapy in women with essential hypertension is to keep the systolic BP between 130–155 mm Hg and diastolic BP between 80–105 mm Hg. The diastolic BP should not be allowed to drop below 80 mm Hg due to concerns of diminishing uteroplacental blood flow. For pregnant women with end organ damage secondary to hypertension, the aim should be to keep the BP lower than 140/90 mm Hg. For women whose antihypertensive therapy is continued, aggressive lowering of BP should be avoided. Occasionally, prepregnancy

dose of antihypertensive agents may need to be reduced, particularly in the second trimester, when BP tend to fall in comparison to the levels before pregnancy or during the first trimester.

Choice of Antihypertensive Agent

A Cochrane review concluded that there is no clear evidence to recommend one antihypertensive over another for improving outcome for women with very high BP during pregnancy.[11] Choice of drug depends on the experience of physician, costs and local availability. Table 9.1 lists the commonly used antihypertensive agents in pregnancy. Labetalol is a popular first line antihypertensive of choice. It is a combined beta (β) and alpha (α) adrenoceptor blocker. Labetalol is contraindicated in women with history of asthma. At intravenous doses of 50–100 mg or oral doses of 200–800 mg, a BP drop of approximately 20% is observed in nonpregnant subjects.[12,13] Although data exist suggesting an association between atenolol and fetal growth restriction, this finding has not been reported with

Table 9.1: Commonly used antihypertensive agents in pregnancy

Drug	Action-mechanism and Timing	Main Adverse Effects	Additional Features
Methyl dopa (Oral 250–500 mg QDS)	Central action, Onset 6–10 hours after oral administration and lasts up to 24 hours	Drowsiness, tiredness in 75%, depression	Slow onset of action, preferred for mild hypertension, avoid postpartum due to depression
Labetalol (Oral 200–400 mg TDS and IV 50 mg over 2 min and repeat every 5 min until BP controlled followed by 20 mg/hr infusion)	Alpha and beta sympathetic blocker, Onset 2 hours after oral administration and lasts 8–12 hours	Postural hypotension, tiredness, nightmares, bradycardia	Drug most commonly used in modern settings–oral for mild cases and IV for crisis
Nifedipine (Oral 10 mg QDS)	Calcium channel blocker Onset 10–15 min after oral administration and lasts 3 hours Modified Release: 1–2 hours after oral administration and lasts 24 hours	Hypotension, flushing, headache, tachycardia, palpitations due to rapid onset of vasodilation, ankle edema	Commonly used orally in low-resourced settings
Hydralazine (IV–5–10 mg over 15–30 min followed by infusion 3–5 mg/hr)	Direct acting vasodilator	Hypotension, headache	Used IV for severe hypertension

Abbreviations: TDS, ter die sumendus (three times a day); QDS, quater die sumendus (four times a day).

the use of other labetalol.[13] Nifedipine a calcium channel blocker is a common alternative used in the treatment of chronic hypertension in pregnancy. The principal side effect is headache however use of the long-acting, once daily preparation improves compliance.[13] Sublingual administration of nifedipine may cause profound drop in BP and should be avoided. Alpha methyldopa (a centrally acting α adrenergic agonist) has been the most commonly used and studied agent for the control of BP during pregnancy.[13] Its safety is well established both in pregnancy and in the long-term follow-up of the infants. However, it is slow acting and one of the most frequent side effects is sedation, which can be profound.

Traditionally, diuretics have been contra-indicated in pregnancy because of concern about volume depletion leading to reduced uteroplacental perfusion. However, a review of nine randomized trials showed no significant difference in pregnancy outcomes among women with hypertension who took diuretics and those without antihypertensive medication.[14]

Some authorities therefore support the continuation of diuretic therapy during pregnancy in women with chronic hypertension who were previously treated with these agents.[4,15,16]

Women taking ACE inhibitors or ATII receptor blockers should be counseled that there is an increased risk of congenital abnormalities if these drugs are taken during pregnancy.[13,17-20] Second and third trimester exposure to ACE inhibitors appears to be fetotoxic, producing fetal hypocalvaria, renal defects, oligohydramnios, fetal limb contractures, craniofacial deformations and pulmonary hypoplasia.[4] Intrauterine growth restriction, prematurity, persistence of a patent ductus arteriosus, severe neonatal hypotension, neonatal anuria and neonatal or fetal death have all been observed with use of these drugs and they should therefore be discontinued pre-conceptionally or as early in the first trimester as possible.[4]

Fetal Surveillance

Hypertension in pregnancy can have a significant impact on fetal well-being.[21] Chronic uteroplacental insufficiency may result in IUGR and oligohydramnios. Oligohydramnios in turn may result in loss of protection of the umbilical cord from mechanical compression. Such a fetus is prone to abnormal fetal heart rate patterns during labor as well as hypoxia and in extreme cases antepartum or intrapartum fetal demise.

The highest risk patients are those with severe hypertension, IUGR, associated medical complications such as diabetes, systemic lupus erythematosus (SLE), chronic renal disease or history of a prior stillbirth. Most authorities believe that well controlled mild hypertension without superimposed preeclampsia does not constitute an indication for fetal surveillance. Unfortunately, no RCTs have been carried out to indicate which testing modality and at what frequency should be used to achieve the best results. A combination of fetal movement counting, nonstress test, bio-physical profile and umbilical artery Doppler weekly for women with mild disease and twice weekly or more frequently for those with severe disease is recommended.[21] Evidence suggests that in cases of severe IUGR, integrating Doppler of the fetal venous circulation may help further define the risk of perinatal death and assist in determining the optimal timing of delivery.[21] Testing should begin when intervention for fetal indication is considered to be appropriate, usually 26–28 weeks gestation. Management of preterm pregnancies with signs of fetal growth restriction and hypertension is complex, especially before 32 weeks gestation. The risk of prolonged hypoxia and acidemia leading to stillbirth or neonatal death if the pregnancy is allowed to progress must be balanced against the risks of neonatal morbidity and mortality associated with prematurity if early delivery is chosen. Doppler umbilical arterial velocimetry appears to have its maximum use as secondary surveillance in such pregnancies early in the third trimester.

Intrapartum and Postpartum Care

In women with chronic hypertension without additional complications, delivery should be planned around the estimated date of delivery (EDD).

Early delivery may become necessary in cases of maternal complications such as worsening hypertension or disease, nonreassuring fetal testing or severe fetal growth restriction. Continuous intrapartum electronic fetal monitoring is recommended. Vaginal delivery is desired in most cases except in specific situations however rates of Cesarean delivery are higher in this group of women. Syntometrine should be avoided for the active management of the third stage to avoid its pressor effects.

All women should be offered a medical review at the postnatal clinic (6–8 weeks after the birth) to check status of their BP, medical condition and review antihypertensive medication. Breast-feeding should be encouraged in women with chronic hypertension, including those requiring medication. Atenolol and ACE inhibitors should be avoided where possible. Although most antihypertensive agents can pass into the breast milk, their levels are generally lower than those in maternal plasma.[4,22]

SPECIFIC MEDICAL CONDITIONS IN PREGNANCY

Renal Disorders in Pregnancy

Women with underlying renal disease (glomerulo-nephritis, diabetic or reflux nephropathy) are at significantly increased risk of poor pregnancy outcomes and require multidisciplinary care involving a renal physician.[23] The outcomes of pregnancies with renal problems depend on the nature of underlying condition, degree of renal impairment, control of hypertension and amount of proteinuria. The presence of proteinuria at baseline increases the risks of superimposed preeclampsia and growth restriction.[5]

Prepregnancy counseling is very important in this group of women. Baseline investigations including creatinine clearance should be performed. ACE inhibitors should be stopped as soon as pregnancy is confirmed and medications altered accordingly. Diabetic women with creatinine clearance less than 50 mL/min, proteinuria more than 2 gm/24 hours, creatinine more than 2 mg/dL or uncontrolled hypertension should be discouraged from pregnancy before the above conditions can be improved. With chronic renal disease in pregnancy, the fetal prognosis is best if maternal renal function and BP are optimized. If the plasma creatinine is less than 125 µmol/L, the maternal and perinatal outcome is usually good. If prepregnancy creatinine is more than 250 µmol/L,

there is high-risk of renal function deterioration in pregnancy. Fifty percent of such women will experience long-term worsening of renal function and at least 50% of babies will have IUGR and prematurity. Other risks include thromboembolism and urinary tract infections. With intermediate levels of creatinine there are both maternal (renal deterioration and preeclampsia) and fetal risks such as preterm birth, IUGR or intrauterine death. A successful outcome may be achieved in 60–90% of cases.

Prophylactic low-dose aspirin is recommended to reduce the risk of preeclampsia. Regular and frequent antenatal visits should be planned especially for fetal surveillance (growth and Doppler) and BP monitoring in latter half of pregnancy. Urea, creatinine, electrolytes, serum proteins, urine proteins, midstream specimen urine (MSU) should be checked at each visit and monthly quantification of proteinuria should be undertaken by either 24 hour urine collection or protein-creatinine ratio. Hemoglobin levels should be closely monitored and anemia promptly treated. Hypertension should be treated aggressively. If renal function deteriorates underlying cause should be sought such as infection, dehydration, obstruction, superimposed preeclampsia or renal vein thrombosis. Vaginal delivery is the preferred mode of delivery.

Pregnancies in women who have had a success-ful renal transplant are becoming increasingly common. Women should be advised to avoid pregnancy for 2 years after transplant as good renal function at that stage predicts very good long-term survival. Such pregnancies usually have a good outcome if renal function is normal prior to conception and immunosuppressive therapy is continued throughout pregnancy. Commonly used drugs include prednisolone, azathioprine, cyclosporine and tacrolimus. Maternal risks include ectopic pregnancy as a result of pelvic adhesions secondary to surgery, peritoneal dialysis and pelvic infection. Up to 15% may develop permanent renal deterioration. Pregnancy generally has no effect on graft survival or function. LFTs, calcium, phosphate, CMV titres and immunosuppressant drug levels are additional investigations every 6–8 weeks. Delivery should be managed according to obstetric indications, with the addition of antibiotic and steroid cover. Breastfeeding should be avoided with cyclosporine and tacrolimus use.

Pregnancy should generally be discouraged in women on dialysis as the fetal prognosis is poor. Live birth rates approximate 40–50% and management in tertiary unit is required often needing extreme preterm delivery.[23] Besides other management strategies as described above for other renal conditions, specific measures include correction of anemia with erythropoietin and/ or blood, nutritional support and continuation of hemo or peritoneal dialysis. Fetal monitoring should be undertaken during dialysis, when it is performed after 28 weeks of gestation.

Coarctation of the Aorta

Coarctation of the aorta has usually been corrected before pregnancy and is generally well tolerated if corrected. The condition is a moderate risk heart disease with mortality up to 15%. The main risk with the condition is aortic dissection. Hypertension increases the risk of this complication and beta blockers are commonly used antihypertensives in such cases.

If coarctation is uncorrected or recurrent, BP must be well controlled. Angina, hypertension, heart failure and pulmonary edema are the major risks. Cardiology team should be involved throughout the care. Balloon angioplasty should be avoided in pregnancy for fear of dissection and Cesarean section is indicated if there is associated aortic dilatation.

Connective Tissue Disorders

Systemic Lupus Erythematosus

Systemic lupus erythematosus is ten times more common in women than men. It has an estimated an incidence of 1:1,000. Criteria for diagnosis of SLE based on American rheumatology[24] are summarized in Box 9.2. Pregnancy does not affect the long-term prognosis of SLE. There is probably an increased chance of an exacerbation of the disease (flare-up) occurring in pregnancy and during the postnatal period. Diagnosis of exacerbation in pregnancy can be tricky as symptoms such as joint pains, fatigue, anemia are nonspecific and erythrocyte sedimentation rate (ESR) is raised in a normal pregnancy. Low C3

Box 9.2: Diagnostic criteria for systemic lupus erythematosus (1997 update on 1982 American College of Rheumatology classification criteria for systemic lupus erythematosus)

Any combination of 4 or more of 11 criteria, well documented at any time during a woman's history, makes it likely that she has SLE (specificity 95% and sensitivity 75%)

- Malar rash
- Discoid rash
- Serositis—pleurisy or pericarditis
- Oral ulcers or nasopharyngeal ulcers
- Arthritis—nonerosive arthritis of two or more peripheral joints
- Photosensitivity
- Neurologic disorder—seizures or psychosis
- Hematologic disorder—hemolytic anemia, leukopenia, lymphopenia or thrombocytopenia in the absence of offending drug
- Renal disorder—more than 0.5 g per day protein in urine or cellular casts
- Antinuclear antibody test positive
- Immunologic disorder—positive anti-Smith, anti-ds DNA, anti-phospholipid antibody and/or false-positive serological test for syphilis

or raised anti-DNA levels are useful. Long-term prognosis of the disease is generally not affected by the pregnancy.

Women should be discouraged from becoming pregnant when their disease is active to minimize problems. Active SLE nephritis during pregnancy is associated with significant risk of preeclampsia as well as maternal and perinatal morbidity and mortality.[25] SLE is associated with increased fetal loss from spontaneous miscarriage, preterm birth, IUGR and stillbirth. There is increased incidence of preeclampsia and its onset needs to be differentiated from disease flare-up carefully as both may cause hypertension and proteinuria. Although there is no increased rate of fetal anomalies, fetal congenital heart block can occur with the presence of anti-Ro (3%) and anti-La antibodies.[25] Rarely neonatal lupus can result in hemolytic anemia, leucopenia, thrombocytopenia, discoid skin lesions, pericarditis and congenital heart block.

Multidisciplinary management involving rheumatology team is important. If lupus anticoagulant or anti-cardiolipin antibodies are present, low-dose aspirin should be started and in women with previous thromboembolic disease or adverse pregnancy outcome low molecular weight heparin is indicated. Careful monitoring of renal functions and regular fetal growth scans should be performed and flare-ups managed with oral prednisolone therapy where possible (initiate or increase steroids).[25]

Rheumatoid Arthritis

Rheumatoid arthritis (RA) tends to improve in 75% of cases in pregnancy and may flare-up again postpartum. Generally it has no adverse effects on the pregnancy. Drugs such as nonsteroidal anti-inflammatory agents, gold, penicillamine, cyclophosphamide and methotrexate should be avoided in pregnancy.

Conn's Syndrome, Pheochromocytoma and Cushing's Syndrome

Conn's syndrome is rare in pregnancy. Primary hyperaldosteronism may be caused by adrenal adenoma or carcinoma or bilateral adrenal hyperplasia. It presents with hypokalemia and hypertension. Blood investigations reveal high aldosterone, low potassium and low rennin levels. Treatment consists of antihypertensives, potassium supplements or potassium sparing diuretics (avoid spironolactone) and surgery for adenoma, which may be deferred until after delivery.[26]

Pheochromocytoma is an adrenal medulla tumor which causes excessive secretion of catecholamines and labile hypertension. It is also rare in pregnancy, bilateral in 10% and malignant in 10% cases. It is associated with a high maternal and perinatal mortality if untreated. Symptoms (which may be episodic) include hypertension, headache, sweating, palpitations, anxiety and vomiting. Hypertensive crisis can lead to stroke or congestive cardiac failure. Raised 24 hour urinary catecholamines or their metabolites such as vanillylmandelic acid (VMA) confirm the diagnosis. Ultrasound and MRI are used to localize the tumor in pregnancy. Involvement of endocrine specialist, surgeon and senior anesthetist is vital. Treatment consists of commencement of α adrenoceptor blockers such as phenoxybenzamine to control BP then beta blockers to control the tachycardia. After pharmacological blockade has been achieved

surgery should be undertaken to excise the tumor. Surgery may be delayed until fetal maturity if diagnosis was made after 24 weeks of gestation. Cesarean is the preferred mode of delivery and tumor may be removed at the same time or later in some cases.[26]

Cushing's syndrome is very rare in pregnancy but causes may include excessive pituitary ACTH secretion and adrenal adenoma or carcinoma. Clinical features include tendency to bruising, myopathy, hypertension, striae, hirsuitism, excessive weight gain, headaches and acne. Investigations reveal increased 24 hour urinary free cortisol or plasma free cortisol which fails to suppress with high dose dexamethasone suppression test. Other investigations are plasma ACTH and CT/MRI for tumor imaging. Visual fields are plotted for a pituitary tumor. Complications of the condition include diabetes, hypertension, fetal prematurity and perinatal mortality as well as poor wound healing.[26] Generally, surgery is the treatment of choice for adrenal or pituitary tumors. Medical therapy (limited experience) may be used to either suppress cortisol production with metyrapone or ACTH activity with cyproheptadine.[26] Ketoconazole is teratogenic and should be avoided.

■ CONCLUSION

It is likely that obstetricians will encounter increasing number of women with medical disorders presenting with hypertension in pregnancy in the future. This may be attributable to the growing epidemics of obesity, diabetes, successful treatment of complex medical conditions in childhood and an older obstetric population. Prepregnancy counseling and preparation holds a key to preventing complications and optimizing outcomes in these women. Such evaluation should include assessment of end organ damage, evaluation for identifiable causes of hypertension, adjustment of antihypertensive therapy in addition to lifestyle modification and weight reduction advice. Labetalol and nifedipine are the current first line drugs of choice for hypertension in pregnancy. Depending on the nature and severity of the underlying condition, the mother and fetus should be closely followed during the pregnancy. The mother should be well informed regarding the potential risks of chronic hypertension in pregnancy. A multidisciplinary and evidence-based care should be offered to all women presenting with medical conditions and hypertension in pregnancy. Research and clinical trials are ongoing, which in future, are likely to shed light on some of the controversial areas in the management of such women and improve our understanding of underlying pathophysiology.

■ REFERENCES

1. WHO recommendations for Prevention and treatment of pre-eclampsia and eclampsia. World Health Organization. 2011.
2. Williams D, Craft N. Pre-eclampsia. BMJ. 2012; 345:e4437.
3. Sibai BM. Chronic hypertension in pregnancy. Obstet Gynecol. 2002;100:369-77.
4. Seely EW, Ecker J. Clinical practice. Chronic hypertension in pregnancy. N Engl J Med. 2011; 365(5):439-46.
5. Sibai BM, Lindheimer M, Hauth J, et al. Risk factors for preeclampsia, abruption placentae and adverse neonatal outcomes among women with chronic hypertension. N Engl J Med. 1998;339:667-71.
6. Abalos E, Duley L, Steyn DW, et al. Antihypertensive drug therapy for mild to moderate hypertension during pregnancy. Cochrane Database Syst Rev. 2007;(1):CD002252.
7. McCarthy F, Kenny L. Hypertension in pregnancy. Obstetrics, Gynecology and Reproductive Medicine. 2012;22(6):141-47.
8. Magee LA, von Dadelszen P, Chan S, et al. The control of hypertension in pregnancy study pilot trial. BJOG. 2007;114:770, e13-20.
9. Centre for Maternal and Child Enquiries (CMACE). Saving mothers' lives: reviewing maternal deaths to make motherhood safer: 2006-08. The eighth report on confidential enquiries into maternal deaths in the United Kingdom. BJOG. 2011;118(suppl 1): 1-203.
10. National institute for Health and Care Excellence. (2010). Hypertension in pregnancy. The management of hypertensive disorders during pregnancy. [online] Available from web address. www.nice.org. uk/guidance/CG107. [Accessed August 2010].
11. Duley L, Henderson-Smart DJ, Meher S. Drugs for treatment of very high blood pressure during pregnancy. Cochrane Database Syst Rev. 2006; 3:CD001449.
12. McInnes GT. Clinical Pharmacology and Therapeutics of Hypertension. Oxford: Elsevier; 2008.
13. Kernaghan D, Duncan A, McKay G. Hypertension in pregnancy: a review of therapeutic options. Obstetric Medicine. 2012;5:44-9.
14. Collins R, Yusuf S, Peto R. Overview of randomized trials of diuretics in pregnancy. Br Med J. 1985;290: 17-23.
15. Report of the National High Blood Pressure Education Program Working Group on High Blood Pressure in Pregnancy. Am J Obstet Gynecol. 2000; 183:S1-S22.
16. ACOG Committee on Practice Bulletins. Chronic hypertension in pregnancy. Obstet Gynecol. 2001; 98:Suppl:177-85.
17. Barr M Jr. Teratogen update: angiotensin-converting enzyme inhibitors. Teratology. 1994;50:399-409.
18. Brent RL, Beckman DA. Angiotensin converting enzyme inhibitors, an embryopathic class of drugs with unique properties: information for clinical teratology counselors. Teratology. 1991;43:543-6.
19. Gersak K, Cvijic M, Cerar LK. Angiotensin II receptor blockers in pregnancy: a report of five cases. Reprod Toxicol. 2009;28:109-12.
20. Serreau R, Luton D, Macher MA, et al. Developmental toxicity of the angiotensin II type 1 receptor antagonists during human pregnancy: a report of 10 cases. BJOG. 2005;112:710-2.
21. Gruslin A, Lemyre B. Pre-eclampsia: Fetal assessment and neonatal outcomes. Best Practice & Research Clinical Obstetrics and Gynecology. 2011; 25:491-507.
22. Beardmore KS, Morris JM, Gallery ED. Excretion of antihypertensive medication into human breast milk: a systematic review. Hypertens Pregnancy. 2002;21:85-95.
23. Williams D. Renal disease in pregnancy. Current Obstetrics & Gynecology. 2004;14(3):166-74.
24. American College of Rheumatology. Update of the American College of Rheumatology Revised Criteria for Classification of Systemic Lupus Erythematosus. Atlanta: ACR; 1997.
25. Cauldwell M, Nelson-Piercy C. Maternal and fetal complications of systemic lupus erythematosus. The Obstetrician & Gynecologist. 2012;14:167-74.
26. Nelson-Piercy C. Pituitary and adrenal disease. Handbook of Obstetric Medicine. 3rd edition. Informa UK Ltd. 2006. pp. 125-44.

10

HELLP Syndrome

Vikram Sinai Talaulikar, Sabaratnam Arulkumaran

INTRODUCTION

Over the last few decades it has been realized that preeclampsia is not a single disease entity but a spectrum of disorders ranging from clinically mild hypertension and proteinuria to severe life-threatening crisis with multiorgan failure. Progression of preeclampsia eventually results in placental insufficiency and maternal end organ dysfunction with increased risk of maternal and perinatal morbidity and mortality. Such end organ dysfunction may present with varied clinical features including eclampsia and hemolysis, elevated liver enzymes and low platelet count (HELLP) syndrome. The acronym HELLP syndrome was coined in 1982 by Weinstein and it is regarded as a complication or a variant of severe preeclampsia.[1]

DEFINITION

The definition, diagnosis and management of HELLP syndrome have been a subject of controversy over the years. The syndrome has been variously defined in several case studies and reports using varying criteria for platelet count and liver function test abnormalities, making comparison of data difficult and adding to confusion among clinicians. Although mild abnormalities of liver enzymes can occur in up to a third of women with preeclampsia, diagnosis of HELLP requires concomitant presence of additional abnormal laboratory findings.

Sibai et al.[2] established the diagnostic criteria for HELLP syndrome and defined the laboratory abnormalities sufficient for the diagnosis of each element of the syndrome as follows:

- *Hemolysis*: An abnormal peripheral smear, elevated bilirubin greater than 1.2 mg/dL, or elevated lactate dehydrogenase (LDH) greater than 600 U/L
- *Elevated liver enzymes*: Aspartate amino-transferase (AST) greater than 70 IU/L and LDH greater than 600 U/L
- *Low platelet count*: Less than 100,000/mm³

Laboratory evaluation of HELLP syndrome should include a full blood count with platelet count, a peripheral smear, coagulation profile, liver function tests (LFTs) including AST, creatinine, glucose, bilirubin, uric acid and LDH levels. Box 10.1 lists the clinical features and investigation

---

Box 10.1: Diagnosis of HELLP syndrome

Clinical features
- Malaise, nausea, vomiting, headache, epigastric/right upper quadrant abdominal pain
- Associated severe preeclampsia (hypertension, proteinuria)
- Right upper abdominal tenderness
- Abruption/DIC/renal failure/jaundice

Hemolysis
- Abnormal peripheral blood film
- Raised unconjugated bilirubin (>1.2 mg/dL)
- Elevated LDH (>600 U/L)

Elevated liver enzymes
- Raised ALT, AST (>70 U/L)
- Raised LDH (>600 U/L)

Low platelets (<100,000/mm³)

Ultrasound scan
- Liver scan
- Fetal growth, liquor volume and umbilical artery Doppler

Abbreviations: DIC, disseminated intravascular coagulopathy; ALT, alanine transaminase; AST, aspartate aminotransferase; LDH, lactate dehydrogenase

findings utilized in the diagnosis of HELLP syndrome.

The HELLP syndrome may be complete or incomplete. Diagnosis of the complete form requires the presence of all three components, while partial or incomplete HELLP syndrome consists of only one or two elements of the triad (H or EL or LP).

Women with partial HELLP have fewer symptoms, and may develop fewer complications than those with complete form but sometimes go on to develop the complete form of the syndrome.[3,4] Partial or total reversal of the syndrome is known to occur rarely.[5,6]

However, it is important to remember that despite its incomplete nature, a woman with partial HELLP is also at risk for significant fetal and maternal morbidity as the underlying pathophysiology remains the same.[7]

■ INCIDENCE

The HELLP syndrome occurs in 0.5–0.9% of all pregnancies and 10–20% of women with severe preeclampsia. Seventy percent of HELLP is diagnosed in the antenatal period with majority cases occurring between 27 weeks and 37 weeks. Thirty percent of cases occur in the postnatal stage, usually within 48 hours after delivery. Such postnatal cases tend to be missed or diagnosed with a delay, since they are often associated with no or uncomplicated preeclampsia before delivery. They are also associated with a high risk of pulmonary edema and renal failure.[8]

Maternal and Perinatal Risks

The HELLP syndrome is associated with increased maternal mortality (reported rates 1–24%) and perinatal mortality rates (7–60%). Serious risks include:
- Placental abruption
- Increased rates of wound hematomas and the need for blood transfusion
- Disseminated intravascular coagulopathy (DIC)
- Liver hematoma
- Liver rupture
- Pulmonary edema
- Acute renal failure
- Metabolic acidosis

- Adult respiratory distress syndrome (ARDS)
- Sepsis
- Cerebrovascular accident
- Maternal death
- Prematurity, fetal/neonatal death and neonatal thrombocytopenia

Hepatic hematoma and rupture remain the most dreaded complications of the HELLP syndrome. The conditions may be diagnosed by ultrasound, computerized tomography (CT) or magnetic resonance imaging (MRI) examination. Surgical repair has been traditionally recommended for hepatic hemorrhage without liver rupture; however, new evidence suggests that conservative management can be successful in patients who remain hemodynamically stable.[7,9,10] Management should include close monitoring of hemodynamic parameters and coagulation status. Serial assessment of the subcapsular hematoma with ultrasound or CT is required with immediate intervention for rupture or worsening of maternal status.[7]

Spontaneous rupture of a subcapsular liver hematoma is a rare but life-threatening complication (1 in 40,000 to 1 in 250,000 deliveries and in about 1% cases of HELLP).[11] The reported maternal and fetal mortality is over 50%. Rupture most often occurs in the right liver lobe.[12] The symptoms are sudden-onset severe pain in the epigastric and right upper abdominal quadrant radiating to the back, right shoulder pain, anemia and hypotension. Ruptured liver hematoma with shock is a surgical emergency requiring acute resuscitation in the form of massive transfusions of blood, correction of coagulopathy with fresh-frozen plasma (FFP) and platelets, and immediate laparotomy. Surgical techniques utilized at laparotomy may include: packing and drainage, ligation of the hemorrhaging hepatic segments, embolization of the hepatic artery to the involved segment, loosely suturing omentum or surgical mesh to the liver to improve integrity and even liver transplantation.[7] Recombinant factor VIIa is an effective adjunct in the treatment of preeclamptic patients with expanding or ruptured subcapsular liver hematoma.[12]

■ PATHOPHYSIOLOGY

The syndrome is a variant of severe preeclampsia and characterized by hepatic endothelial disruption, microangiopathic platelet activation and consumption leading to hepatocyte death. Research has suggested that HELLP syndrome represents a vasculopathy mediated by an abnormal concentration of vascular growth factors.[7,13]

The changes may be limited to a hepatic segment or occur diffusely throughout the liver. There is periportal or focal parenchymal necrosis in which hyaline deposits of fibrin-like material can be seen in the sinusoids.[5,14]

■ CLINICAL FEATURES AND LABORATORY FINDINGS

Symptoms and Signs

Symptoms of HELLP (present in 30–90% cases) are often nonspecific such as malaise, epigastric or right upper quadrant pain, headache, nausea and vomiting. Presentations may also include jaundice and hematuria (dark colored urine). Examination of abdomen may reveal tenderness in the right upper quadrant that is suggestive of liver capsule distension. Associated complications such as placental abruption with DIC/renal failure may be encountered in complicated cases.

Most women have accompanying preeclampsia and hypertension but blood pressures tend to be lower as compared to severe preeclampsia alone. A small number of cases do not demonstrate hypertension or proteinuria.[15]

Laboratory Findings

Hemolysis

Hemolysis occurs due to microangiopathic hemolytic anemia. It is characterized by presence of fragmented (schistocytes) red blood cells or contracted red blood cells with spicules (Burr cells) in the peripheral blood smear. Polychromatic red cells may also be seen in the smears along with increased reticulocyte count. Destruction of red blood cells causes increased serum LDH, indirect bilirubin levels and decreased hemoglobin concentrations. There are five different isoforms of LDH and only two of them, LDH1 and LDH2, are released from ruptured red blood cells. Low or undetectable haptoglobin concentration is a more specific indicator of extent of hemolysis.

Liver Enzymes

There is no consensus in the literature regarding what degree of abnormality of liver enzymes should be used to diagnose HELLP. Elevation of liver enzymes can occur due to both hemolysis as well as hepatic involvement. Alanine transaminase (ALT), AST and LDH are the most commonly utilized enzymes for diagnosis.

Platelets

Case reports vary in the use of cutoff values to diagnose thrombocytopenia in HELLP—ranging from 75,000/mm³ to 279,000/mm³. A value below 100,000/mm³ is used as a standard in most studies. In severe HELLP, platelet count may drop below 30,000/mm³ and DIC will develop in 20%. It is important to rule out low platelets due to severe preeclampsia with thrombocytopenia, gestational thrombocytopenia or immune thrombocytopenic purpura (ITP). Thrombocytopenia in HELLP syndrome is due to increased platelet consumption. Endothelial injury followed by platelet adhesion and activation leads to increased platelet turnover with shorter lifespan.

Ultrasonography

Ultrasound of abdomen and liver scan is useful to rule out other causes of right abdominal pain such as gallstones or cholecystitis and exclude liver hematoma. In antenatal patient, assessment of fetal growth, liquor volume and umbilical artery Doppler should be performed at the same time.

■ DIFFERENTIAL DIAGNOSIS

A diagnosis of HELLP syndrome should be suspected in any pregnant woman presenting in second or third trimester with epigastric/right upper quadrant pain and hepatic dysfunction. Reassessment of laboratory parameters in 4–6 hours after initial presentation may help confirm the diagnosis.

Common differential diagnosis of HELLP syndrome is listed in Box 10.2. Some of these conditions are associated with significant maternal morbidity and mortality and require a different treatment approach. Therefore, it is important to make careful use of laboratory and imaging investigations to reach the correct diagnosis.

Box 10.2: Differential diagnosis of HELLP syndrome

- Acute fatty liver of pregnancy (AFLP)
- Thrombotic thrombocytopenic purpura (TTP)
- Hemolytic uremic syndrome (HUS)
- Immune thrombocytopenic purpura (ITP)
- Systemic lupus erythematosus (SLE)
- Antiphospholipid syndrome (APS)
- Cholecystitis
- Fulminant viral hepatitis
- Acute pancreatitis
- Disseminated herpes simplex
- Hemorrhagic or septic shock
- Hyperemesis gravidarum
- Appendicitis
- Cholestasis of pregnancy
- Kidney stones
- Peptic ulcer
- Pyelonephritis
- Diabetes insipidus
- Gastroenteritis
- Hepatic encephalopathy

In severe cases, senior input and multidisciplinary approach including advice from liver physicians may be vital.

Acute Fatty Liver of Pregnancy

Distinguishing features include hypoglycemia, severe hyperuricemia and prolongation of prothrombin time. Hypertension and proteinuria are usually absent. Elevated ammonia levels and renal dysfunction are also typically associated with acute fatty liver of pregnancy (AFLP).

Thrombotic Thrombocytopenic Purpura

Cerebral dysfunction, fever, rash, abdominal pain and bleeding may be part of thrombotic thrombocytopenic purpura (TTP).[8] Profound thrombocytopenia is uncommon in HELLP syndrome. On the other hand, abnormal LFTs and coagulopathy favor a diagnosis of HELLP syndrome.

Hemolytic Uremic Syndrome

Most cases develop in the postpartum period with signs and symptoms of renal failure.[8] The mortality of hemolytic uremic syndrome (HUS) and TTP has decreased in modern times due to the use of plasma exchange and intensive care.

■ MANAGEMENT

Once a diagnosis of HELLP syndrome is made, the care of such women is based on principles similar to treatment of severe preeclampsia or eclampsia. As the syndrome can lead to sudden deterioration in maternal and fetal condition, women should be hospitalized immediately and monitored in high dependency unit (HDU) settings, where such facilities are not available (peripheral units), women should be immediately transferred to the nearest tertiary care center. The first priority is to assess and stabilize the maternal condition. Stabilization should begin with administration of intravenous magnesium sulfate as prophylaxis against seizures and antihypertensive medications to keep systolic blood pressure below 160 mm Hg and/or diastolic blood pressure below 105 mm Hg. Antenatal steroids should be administered for fetal lung maturity for women below 34 weeks gestation. Serial platelet counts, LFTs and coagulation profile monitoring are essential (every 6–8 hours) to monitor disease progression. Ultimate treatment is delivery of the fetus. Mode of delivery (induction of labor or Cesarean section) depends on the gestational age, fetal condition and cervical favorability with Cesarean more likely at earlier gestations. Martin et al.[16] have evaluated the effectiveness of the Mississippi Protocol (MP) to treat HELLP syndrome. Uniform early initiation of MP (corticosteroids, magnesium sulfate and systolic blood pressure control) was studied prospectively in patients admitted with severe preeclampsia/HELLP syndrome. One hundred and ninety patients between 2000 and 2007 received MP without suffering maternal death, stroke or liver rupture and early initiation of MP inhibited HELLP syndrome disease progression and severity.

In the management of women with severe preeclampsia and HELLP syndrome, following options may be considered:
- Immediate delivery which is the treatment of choice at or above 34 weeks gestation.
- Delivery within 48 hours after stabilization of the maternal clinical condition and steroids administration. This may be appropriate between 26 weeks and 34 weeks of gestation.

- Conservative management including steroids administration for more than 48–72 hours may be considered in select cases, especially those with partial HELLP syndrome. Possible advantages due to limited prolongation of pregnancy should be carefully weighed against the increased risks for maternal and fetal complications.

If the HELLP syndrome develops before 24 weeks gestation, termination of pregnancy should be strongly considered. Overall, the current best evidence does not demonstrate significant fetal benefits despite increasing maternal risks with expectant management of HELLP, and therefore, women with HELLP syndrome should not typically be managed expectantly and the delivery process initiated.[17,18] If delivery is delayed for antenatal steroid administration for fetal benefit, magnesium sulfate seizure prophylaxis should be continued and continuous fetal monitoring performed. Magnesium sulfate 4 g as one dose or 4 g followed by 1 g/hour for 24 hours prior to delivery appear to provide some neuroprotection to the newborn. Delivery should be pursued if the maternal or fetal condition worsens, or upon completion of steroid treatment. Conservative treatment is contraindicated in women with DIC. A suggested algorithm for management of HELLP syndrome is presented in Flow chart 10.1.

Intrapartum Management

The presence of HELLP syndrome alone is not an indication for immediate Cesarean delivery and vaginal delivery is preferable in most cases. The decision regarding mode of delivery should be based on fetal gestational age, fetal condition [cardiotocograph (CTG) and Doppler findings] and cervical score. There is a poor success rate for attempted induction of labor at preterm gestations with intrauterine growth restriction (IUGR) or abnormal Doppler studies. Many authors have suggested elective Cesarean delivery for all women with HELLP syndrome before 30 weeks of gestation who are not in labor and whose Bishop score is below 5.[15] Cesarean is also recommended for those with HELLP syndrome plus fetal growth restriction and/or oligohydramnios if the gestational age is below 32 weeks in the presence of an unfavorable cervical score.[15]

Flow chart 10.1: Suggested algorithm for management of antenatal HELLP syndrome

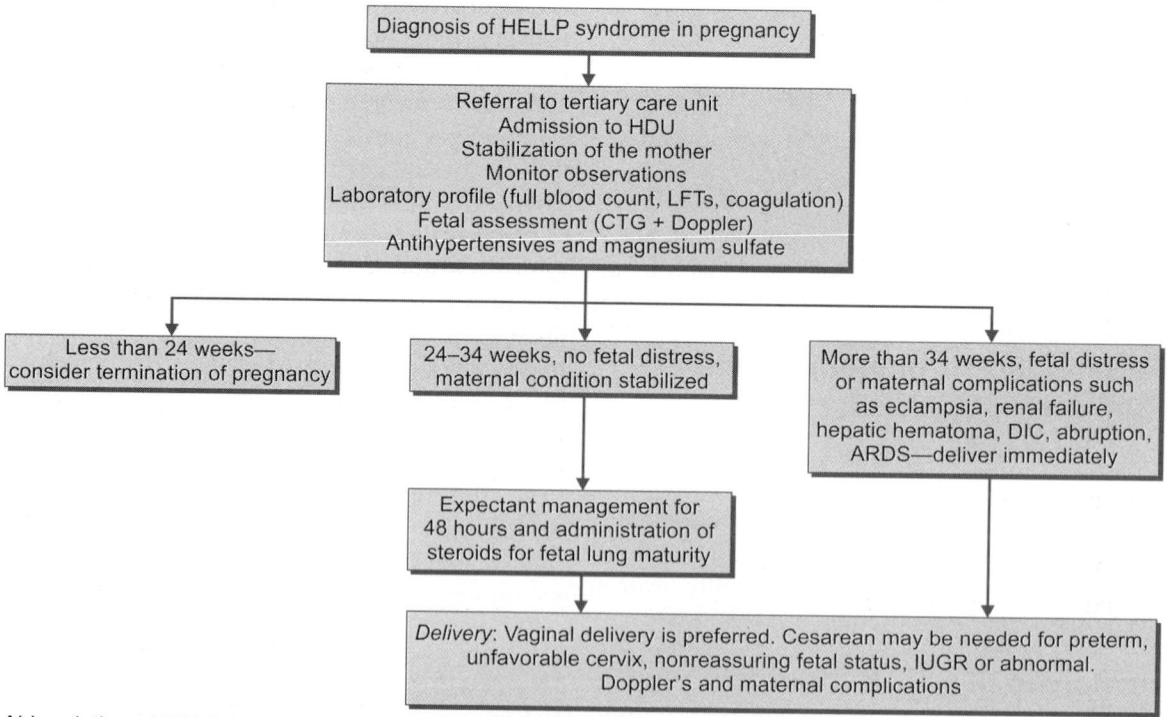

Abbreviations: HELLP, hemolysis, elevated liver enzymes and low platelet count; HDU, high dependency unit; LFTs, liver function tests; CTG, cardiotocograph; DIC, disseminated intravascular coagulopathy; ARDS, adult respiratory distress syndrome; IUGR, intrauterine growth restriction

In all other patient's induction of labor may be attempted with either prostaglandins or oxytocin infusion. Patients already in labor or with rupture of membranes may be allowed to deliver vaginally in the absence of obstetric complications.

Maternal pain relief during labor can be provided by intermittent use of small doses of systemic opioids. Local infiltration anesthesia can be used for episiotomy or laceration repair. The use of pudendal block is contraindicated because of the risk of bleeding and hematoma formation. Epidural anesthesia is contraindicated if the platelet count is less than 75,000/mm³. In patients with disordered coagulation or very low platelets, FFPs or platelet transfusions may be required perioperatively or peripartum. Platelets are transfused only if there is active bleeding or before operative intervention (if < 50,000/mm³), and are not usually required on a prophylactic basis. Transfusion is also indicated in all antepartum patients whose platelet count is less than 20,000/mm³.

CORTICOSTEROIDS FOR TREATMENT OF HELLP SYNDROME

It is well recognized that administration of corticosteroids may improve the hematological parameters of HELLP. A Cochrane review in 2010[19] which addressed this issue included 11 trials (550 women) which compared corticosteroids with placebo or no treatment for HELLP. There was no difference in the risk of maternal death [risk ratio (RR), 0.95; 95% confidence interval (CI), 0.28–3.21), maternal death or severe maternal morbidity (RR, 0.27; 95% CI, 0.03–2.12), or perinatal/infant death (RR, 0.64; 95% CI, 0.21–1.97). The only clear effect of treatment on individual outcomes was improved platelet count [standardized mean difference (SMD), 0.67; 95% CI, 0.24–1.10]. The effect on platelet count was strongest for women who commenced treatment antenatally (SMD, 0.80; 95% CI, 0.25–1.35). Two trials (76 women) compared dexamethasone with betamethasone. There was no clear evidence of a difference between groups in respect to perinatal/infant death (RR, 0.95; 95% CI, 0.15–6.17) or severe perinatal/infant morbidity or death (RR, 0.64; 95% CI, 0.27–1.48). In respect to platelet count, dexamethasone was superior to betamethasone. The authors concluded that there was no clear evidence of any effect of corticosteroids on substantive clinical outcomes.[19] Those receiving steroids showed significantly greater improvement in platelet counts which was greater for those receiving dexamethasone than those receiving betamethasone. Till date, there is insufficient evidence of benefits in terms of substantive clinical outcomes to support the routine use of steroids for the management of HELLP. Based on the current evidence, both Royal College of Obstetricians and Gynecologists/ National Institute for Health and Clinical Excellence (RCOG/NICE), United Kingdom (UK)[20] as well as World Health Organization (WHO) guidelines[21] do not recommend use of corticosteroids for the specific purpose of treating women with HELLP syndrome. High-dose corticosteroid treatment and repeated doses should be avoided for fear of long-term adverse effects on the fetal brain.

POSTPARTUM CARE AND COUNSELING FOR FUTURE PREGNANCIES

Following delivery, women should be placed in high dependency care with regular observations, blood, fluid balance and coagulation monitoring for at least 48 hours. There is a high risk of pulmonary edema and renal failure in these cases and maintenance of optimum fluid balance is critical. Most patients show evidence of resolution of the disease process within 48 hours. The maternal platelet count may continue to decrease immediately postpartum with an increasing trend on the 3rd day. The recovery is usually rapid and complete with no long-term hepatic sequelae. Some authors have considered corticosteroid treatment postpartum to hasten recovery but this remains controversial. Women with HELLP syndrome who show progressive elevation of bilirubin or creatinine for more than 72 hours after delivery may benefit from plasma exchange with FFP.[8,22-24]

Risk of recurrence of HELLP syndrome is 3–5% and there are also increased risks of preeclampsia (25%), preterm delivery and fetal growth restriction in future pregnancies. Most neonates born from a woman with HELLP will have a normal long-term development. Use of oral contraceptives is safe in women with a prior HELLP syndrome.[25]

▉ SUMMARY

The HELLP syndrome is a variant of severe preeclampsia, and is associated with significant maternal and perinatal morbidity and mortality. There is a need for a uniform definition and diagnostic evaluation of this syndrome. Clinical features can often be nonspecific and diagnosis is primarily laboratory based (evidence of HELLP). Once HELLP has been diagnosed, stabilization of maternal condition and serial monitoring of clinical and laboratory parameters is essential. To prevent complications and adverse outcomes, early delivery is indicated when the HELLP syndrome develops after 34 weeks of pregnancy. Expectant management for 48 hours with steroids for fetal lung maturity after stabilization of the maternal condition may be appropriate between 26 weeks and 34 weeks gestation, which is then followed by delivery.

Women with HELLP usually demonstrate a rapid and complete recovery after delivery; however, they remain at increased risk of preeclampsia in future pregnancies.

▉ REFERENCES

1. Weinstein L. Syndrome of hemolysis, elevated liver enzymes, and low platelet count: a severe consequence of hypertension in pregnancy. Am J Obstet Gynecol. 1982;142(2):159-67.
2. Sibai BM, Taslimi MM, el-Nazer A, et al. Maternal-perinatal outcome associated with the syndrome of hemolysis, elevated liver enzymes, and low platelets in severe preeclampsia-eclampsia. Am J Obstet Gynecol. 1986;155(3):501-9.
3. Audibert F, Friedman SA, Frangieh AY, et al. Clinical utility of strict diagnostic criteria for the HELLP (hemolysis, elevated liver enzymes, and low platelets) syndrome. Am J Obstet Gynecol. 1996;175(2):460-4.
4. Martin JN, Rose CH, Briery CM. Understanding and managing HELLP syndrome: the integral role of aggressive glucocorticoids for mother and child. Am J Obstet Gynecol. 2006;195(4):914-34.
5. Aarnoudse JG, Houthoff HJ, Weits J, et al. A syndrome of liver damage and intravascular coagulation in the last trimester of normotensive pregnancy. A clinical and histopathological study. Br J Obstet Gynaecol. 1986;93(2):145-55.
6. Visser W, Wallenburg HC. Temporising management of severe pre-eclampsia with and without the HELLP syndrome. Br J Obstet Gynaecol. 1995;102(2):111-7.
7. O'Brien J, Barton J. Controversies with the diagnosis and management of HELLP syndrome. Clin Obstet Gynaecol. 2005;48(2):460-77.
8. Haram K, Svendsen E, Abildgaard U. The HELLP syndrome: clinical issues and management. A Review. BMC Pregnancy Childbirth. 2009;9:8.
9. Goodlin RC, Anderson JC, Hodgson PE. Conservative treatment of liver hematoma in the postpartum period. A report of two cases. J Reprod Med. 1985;30(4):368-70.
10. Manas KJ, Welsh JD, Rankin RA, et al. Hepatic hemorrhage without rupture in preeclampsia. N Engl J Med. 1985;312(7):424-6.
11. Wicke C, Pereira PL, Neeser E, et al. Subcapsular liver hematoma in HELLP syndrome: Evaluation of diagnostic and therapeutic options—a unicenter study. Am J Obstet Gynecol. 2004;190(1):106-12.
12. Merchant SH, Mathew P, Vanderjagt TJ, et al. Recombinant factor VIIa in management of spontaneous subcapsular liver hematoma associated with pregnancy. Obstet Gynecol. 2004;103(5 Pt 2):1055-8.
13. Levine RJ, Maynard SE, Qian C, et al. Circulating angiogenic factors and the risk of preeclampsia. N Engl J Med. 2004;350(7):672-83.
14. Barton JR, Riely CA, Adamec TA, et al. Hepatic histopathologic condition does not correlate with laboratory abnormalities in HELLP syndrome (hemolysis, elevated liver enzymes, and low platelet count). Am J Obstet Gynecol. 1992;167(6):1538-43.
15. Sibai BM. Diagnosis, controversies, and management of the syndrome of hemolysis, elevated liver enzymes, and low platelet count. Obstet Gynecol. 2004;103(5 Pt 1):981-91.
16. Martin JN, Owens MY, Keiser SD, et al. Standardized Mississippi Protocol treatment of 190 patients with HELLP syndrome: slowing disease progression and preventing new major maternal morbidity. Hypertens Pregnancy. 2012;31(1):79-90.
17. Publications Committee, Society for Maternal-Fetal Medicine, Sibai BM. Evaluation and management of severe preeclampsia before 34 weeks' gestation. Am J Obstet Gynecol. 2011;205(3):191-8.
18. Magee LA, Yong PJ, Espinosa V, et al. Expectant management of severe preeclampsia remote from term: a structured systematic review. Hypertens Pregnancy. 2009;28(3):312-47.
19. Woudstra DM, Chandra S, Hofmeyr GJ, et al. Corticosteroids for HELLP (hemolysis, elevated liver enzymes, low platelets) syndrome in pregnancy. Cochrane Database Syst Rev. 2010;(9):CD008148.

94

20. National Institute for Health and Clinical Excellence. (2011). NICE clinical guideline 107. Hypertension in pregnancy: The management of hypertensive disorders during pregnancy. [online] Available from publications.nice.org.uk/hypertension-in-pregnancy-cg107/guidance. [Accessed May 2013].

21. World Health Organization, Department of Reproductive Health and Research, Department of Maternal, Newborn, Child and Adolescent Health, et al. (2011). WHO recommendations for Prevention and treatment of pre-eclampsia and eclampsia. [online] Available from www.who.int/reproductivehealth/publications/maternal_perinatal_health/9789241548335/en/. [Accessed May 2013].

22. Martin JN, Files JC, Blake PG, et al. Plasma exchange for preeclampsia. I. Postpartum use for persistently severe preeclampsia-eclampsia with HELLP syndrome. Am J Obstet Gynecol. 1990;162(1): 126-37.

23. Bayraktaroğlu Z, Demirci F, Balat O, et al. Plasma exchange therapy in HELLP syndrome: A single-center experience. Turk J Gastroenterol. 2006;17(2):99-102.

24. Eser B, Guven M, Unal A, et al. The role of plasma exchange in HELLP syndrome. Clin Appl Thromb Hemost. 2005;11(2):211-7.

25. Sibai BM. The HELLP syndrome (hemolysis, elevated liver enzymes, and low platelets): much ado about nothing? Am J Obstet Gynecol. 1990;162(2):311-6.

11

Atypical Presentations in Hypertensive Disease in Pregnancy

Alex C Vidaeff, Michael A Belfort

◼ INTRODUCTION

This chapter will review and challenge some current concepts surrounding the diagnosis of preeclampsia and will increase awareness of the nonclassical and atypical features of preeclampsia/eclampsia. Since, according to the World Health Organization (WHO), hypertensive disorders rank as the second leading cause of maternal death globally,[1] it is essential to be able to identify in a timely and correct manner those women with atypical preeclampsia.

◼ AREAS OF CONTENTION IN THE CONVENTIONAL DIAGNOSIS OF PREECLAMPSIA

The incidence of preeclampsia is the same (5–10% of pregnancies) throughout the world, indicating that the disorder is independent of environmental and ethnic influences. However, fetal and maternal morbidity and mortality related to preeclampsia, including the development of eclampsia, varies from country to country implying that the quality and accessibility of obstetrical care can influence the rate of complications derived from the same baseline condition. In developing countries, preeclampsia/eclampsia is responsible for 50,000 deaths annually.[2]

With the cause of preeclampsia still unknown, primary and even secondary prevention cannot be effectively achieved at present, other than avoiding pregnancy. Therefore, the first step in any successful approach to preeclampsia remains early recognition, allowing appropriate monitoring and intervention in order to reduce the risk of life-threatening or life-altering complications such as eclampsia or stroke. However, early diagnosis can be problematic because of the great variability in clinical presentation. Typically, preeclampsia used to be characterized by the triad of elevated blood pressure (BP), proteinuria and generalized edema. By the early 1990s, the presence of edema was no longer considered mandatory to establish the clinical diagnosis of preeclampsia/eclampsia by both the International Society for the Study of Hypertension in Pregnancy and the American College of Obstetricians and Gynecologists.[3,4] Indeed, edema is neither sufficient nor necessary to confirm the diagnosis of preeclampsia because edema is a common finding in normal pregnancy and, alternatively, significant edema can be absent in as much as 40% of preeclampsia cases progressing to eclampsia.[5] This does not mean that the clinical sign of edema should be ignored. Although no longer pathognomonic, significant peripheral edema usually signals the underlying capillary leak that may lead in many patients to important manifestations of the disease, such as generalized edema, excessive weight gain (> 5 lb/week), pulmonary edema, cerebral edema or ascites.

Hypertension, at least for typical cases, remains the hallmark for diagnosis in preeclampsia. The cutoff for abnormal BP in pregnancy has been arbitrarily established at 140/90 mm Hg. At least two BP readings at or above the cutoff, 6 hours apart (but not more than 1 week apart), are necessary to consider the BP level in abnormal range.[3,4] This threshold is low and subsequently may label as abnormal some borderline and possibly inconsequential cases of BP elevation. In a study of 6,790 pregnant women in the United Kingdom,

22% had a BP reading above 140/90 mm Hg at some point after 20 weeks' gestation—rate that is much higher than the universally reported rate of preeclampsia (5–10%).[6] Nevertheless, it is safer to err on the side of caution and use a more sensitive cutoff in order to prompt a careful examination for other features of preeclampsia. It has been suggested that the so called "white-coat" hypertension may contribute to the lower specificity. Although this may be the case especially early in pregnancy, "white-coat hypertension" cannot be considered entirely benign, since 40% of such cases will progress to gestational hypertension later in pregnancy, and even proteinuric preeclampsia in 8% cases.[7]

The cutoff for proteinuria, the third element in the conventional definition of preeclampsia, was also somewhat arbitrarily established at 300 mg in a 24 hour urine collection. It is recommended that the evaluation be based only on a 24 hour urine collection or, alternatively, spot protein/creatinine ratio because of the large discrepancies in results generated by other diagnostic modalities.[8] Although, largely used in routine clinical practice, dipstick urinalysis is inaccurate for diagnosis. A result of 1+ proteinuria is false-positive in 71% of cases compared to the 300 mg cutoff on 24 hour urine collection, and even 3+ results are false-positive in 7% of cases. Using the same 24 hour urine collection standard, the false-negative rate for dipstick urinalysis is 9%.[9] While detecting proteinuria is important, quantitative assessments for magnitude are less beneficial. Even though proteinuria levels of 5 g/day or more are considered definitive for severe preeclampsia, the degree of proteinuria by itself only rarely predicts adverse outcomes and should not be relied upon to dictate the timing of delivery. Even repeat testing at that point may be redundant. Once severe proteinuria has been identified, serum creatinine will suffice to monitor renal function and risk level.[10]

Most of the current literature considers proteinuria mandatory for the diagnosis of preeclampsia, implying that nonproteinuric hypertension (gestational hypertension) would be a less concerning entity than preeclampsia. However, the evidence has been accumulating indicating that nonproteinuric hypertension is not a benign disorder and may not represent a separate entity from preeclampsia.[6] It is important to note that even with mild range hypertension 25–50% of women with gestational hypertension will progress to preeclampsia. The rate of progression depends on gestational age at onset of hypertension, with rates approaching 50% when gestational hypertension develops before 32 weeks' gestation.[11] Moreover, when the level of hypertension is severe, the rate of adverse maternal or perinatal outcomes has been noted to be similar for women with nonproteinuric hypertension or preeclampsia.[11] Other investigators have reported a higher perinatal mortality rate in women with nonproteinuric hypertension compared with proteinuric preeclampsia.[12] In a cohort of 1,348 hypertensive pregnant women, Homer et al.[13] noted that while those cases with associated proteinuria had more frequently progressed to severe hypertension and had higher rates of preterm birth and perinatal mortality, those without proteinuria more commonly had thrombocytopenia or liver dysfunction.[13] These data suggest that the theoretical distinction between gestational hypertension and preeclampsia is unnecessary and unsupported by outcome. Furthermore, the conventional upper limit for normal 24 hour urinary protein excretion during pregnancy (< 300 mg) has little scientific basis and a lower cutoff (< 260 mg) has been recently proposed based on data derived from longitudinal studies of normal pregnancies.[14]

THE CHALLENGE OF SEVERE ATYPICAL PREECLAMPSIA

The classical signs of preeclampsia may not always be present (even in patients with established disease) and the condition may have an atypical presentation. In an analysis of all cases of eclampsia in the United Kingdom in 1992, it was noted that in 38% of cases the seizure occurred without any prior documentation of either hypertension or proteinuria. The authors concluded that "hypertension and proteinuria are neither the only nor necessarily the most important signs of preeclampsia".[15] It has also been reported that in high-order multifetal gestations the presentation of preeclampsia is frequently atypical, with only half of the patients having hypertension.[16] The clinical presentation of preeclampsia may be extremely vague and nonspecific, and at times, the only presenting element is the patient's statement that she does not feel well.

In the absence of the classical presentation, preeclampsia may assume presentations imitating nonobstetric disorders, potentially leading to misdiagnosis. Frequently, the patient will be seen by various medical or surgical subspecialists and the disease will be often misdiagnosed as viral hepatitis, cholangitis, lupus erythematosus, upper gastrointestinal ulceration, idiopathic thrombocytopenia, neurologic disorders, etc. In fact, Goodlin once called preeclampsia "the great imitator".[17] The opposite diagnostic pitfall is diagnosing preeclampsia where the condition does not exist, leading to potentially inappropriate management and possibly unnecessary early delivery. The presence of hypertension, proteinuria, or other laboratory test abnormalities may be due to lupus nephritis, antiphospholipid antibody syndrome, thrombotic thrombocytopenic purpura (TTP), hemolytic uremic syndrome (HUS), alpha-1-antitrypsin deficiency, severe folate deficiency, Wilson's disease, hemochromatosis, autoimmune hepatitis, or autoimmune hemolytic anemia, among other conditions unrelated to pregnancy.[18,19] Proteinuria may also occasionally be found as a reversible state transiently associated with high fever, strenuous exercise, stress, congestive heart failure, intracranial hemorrhage, status epilepticus and other acute medical illnesses.

In addition to such incomplete or equivocal clinical presentations, preeclampsia is also considered atypical when it develops before 20 weeks' gestation or beyond 48 hour postpartum (up to 4 weeks after delivery).[20] Preeclampsia/eclampsia before 20 weeks' gestation has been reported with molar or hydropic changes of the placenta with or without a coexistent fetus and with fetal diandric triploidy.[21]

Any woman with hypertension, proteinuria, headaches, blurred vision, or other symptoms suggestive of preeclampsia, with or without convulsions up to 4 weeks after delivery should be considered preeclamptic/eclamptic while other causes are being ruled out. Magnesium sulfate therapy for seizure prophylaxis should be initiated without delay and the BP should be stabilized at less than 160 mm Hg systolic and/or 100 mm Hg diastolic pressure. The most important intracranial complication of preeclampsia is that of hypertensive encephalopathy which, if left untreated, can cause cerebral infarction and bleeding. Hypertensive encephalopathy involves an overperfusion syndrome which stresses the cerebral autoregulation system and ultimately leads to breakthrough bleeding, vascular damage and cerebral vasospasm.[22] Hypertensive encephalopathy, also known as posterior reversible encephalopathy syndrome (PRES), is now believed to be the prime cause of convulsions (eclampsia) in preeclamptic patients and is best diagnosed using diffusion weighted imaging (DWI) magnetic resonance imaging (MRI). This modality allows the differentiation between vasogenic cerebral edema (free diffusion of water) which is reversible and does not result in permanent cerebral tissue loss (infarction) and cytotoxic edema (restricted diffusion) which indicates cell death and infarction. Zeeman et al.[23] and Loureiro et al.[24] have shown that eclampsia can be associated with long-term and permanent white matter loss, and for this reason hypertensive encephalopathy should be aggressively managed and prevented. In those cases where seizure activity is not associated with obvious vasogenic edema and hypertensive encephalopathy is not likely, the differential diagnosis may rely on CT scan and cerebrospinal fluid (CSF) investigation to rule out subarachnoid and intracerebral bleeding and magnetic resonance angiography to evaluate for possible dural sinus thrombosis, cerebral vasculitis, or benign postpartum angiopathy. The latter two conditions are characterized by segmental narrowing of cerebral arteries (the "chain of beads" sign), a finding usually absent in eclampsia. As opposed to cases with cerebral vasculitis, patients with benign postpartum angiopathy have normal CSF and recover without immunosuppressive treatment.[25] Benign postpartum angiopathy, also called Call-Fleming syndrome, was described in 1987 as a clinical syndrome characterized by reversible multifocal brain ischemia due to multilocular segmental narrowing of large- and medium-sized cerebral arteries.[26] Patients with this syndrome may develop severe generalized or occipital headaches with abrupt onset (similar to subarachnoid hemorrhage), seizures, cortical blindness, visual field deficits, confusion, aphasia, hemiparesis, or ataxia. Focal edema is revealed on MRI, similar to the PRES that can be detected in eclampsia, but the "chain of beads" sign is indicative of segmental vasospasm.

In a clinical context where the presentation may be atypical and the diagnosis based on elusive signs and symptoms, the clinician will be helped by a comprehensive assessment including biochemical and hematologic evaluation. Such a biochemical marker, first reported in the late 1800s, and still widely used, is the serum uric acid.[27] Plasma concentrations of uric acid normally increase in late pregnancy, and this is thought to be due to increased rates of fetal and/or placental production, decreased binding to albumin and a decline in uric acid clearance. The serum uric acid concentration increases to a greater extent in preeclampsia and may reflect the severity of the disease process.[28] The most commonly accepted explanation for hyperuricemia in preeclampsia, besides increased production, is the increased reabsorption and decreased excretion of uric acid in the proximal renal tubules. Although there is considerable variation among reports regarding the expected normal values in pregnancy or the discriminatory value for uric acid as a marker for preeclampsia, a uric acid value over 6 mg/dL is generally regarded as abnormal in pregnancy. Uric acid is the end product of purine metabolism and is synthesized by the enzyme xanthine oxidase. Hypoxia, placental ischemia and cytokines, all implicated in the pathogenic pathways of preeclampsia, induce the expression of xanthine oxidase and therefore increase the production of uric acid.[29] Several systematic reviews on the accuracy of serum uric acid as a predictor of pregnancy complications in preeclampsia have reached conflicting conclusions.[30,31] More recently however, hyperuricemia has been correlated with adverse maternal and perinatal outcome in preeclampsia, based on the observation that uric acid, which is a marker of oxidative stress, tissue injury and renal dysfunction may directly alter vascular endothelial function.[6,32] Through these known effects, uric acid may promote endothelial dysfunction, damage and inflammation, possibly playing a pathogenic role in preeclampsia.[33] Uric acid may also be reflective of the fetal state and an association between maternal hyperuricemia and poor pregnancy outcome has long been considered a "truism".[34] More recent data have reconfirmed the association between hyperuricemia and shorter gestation or reduced birth weight,[35,36] lending some support to the observation that uric acid may affect mechanisms relevant to fetal growth, such as placental amino acid uptake.[37]

Another valuable marker in the ancillary diagnosis of preeclampsia is the platelet count. It decreases by approximately 10% during pregnancy and counts slightly lower are encountered in multiple pregnancies.[38] A level less than 150,000/mm^3 is considered abnormal and 21% of all cases of thrombocytopenia in pregnancy are associated with preeclampsia, resulting from increased platelet activation, aggregation and consumption.[39] This diagnostic marker also reflects the severity of disease; however, reduced platelet counts are not found in all cases of preeclampsia or eclampsia.[40] Only about 20% of patients with preeclampsia have thrombocytopenia, varying from 7% in mild cases to 50% in severe cases.[41]

Pritchard et al. first noticed thrombocytopenia and hemolysis in severe preeclampsia in 1954.[42] Almost 30 years later, Weinstein reported a series of 29 patients with severe preeclampsia who all exhibited hemolysis, elevated liver enzymes and low platelets and he coined the mnemonic HELLP (Hemolysis, Elevated Liver enzymes, Low Platelets) for this form of severe preeclampsia.[43] While different classification systems have been proposed,[44] most clinicians now use the following criteria suggested by Sibai[45] to make the diagnosis: lactate dehydrogenase (LDH) should be elevated more than or equal to 600 IU/L, aspartate transaminase (AST) and alanine transaminase (ALT) should be equal to or exceed 70 IU/L, and the platelet count should be less than 100,000/mm^3. While it has been proposed that both HELLP syndrome and acute fatty liver of pregnancy represent advanced stages of severe preeclampsia,[46] there are some who feel that these conditions represent atypical forms of preeclampsia and perhaps even separate disease states.[47] Both HELLP syndrome and acute fatty liver of pregnancy may have an insidious and atypical onset, with up to 15% of the patients lacking either hypertension or proteinuria.[48] Because of this, authors suggest that liver function tests (LFT), markers of hemolysis (AST, ALT and LDH) and a platelet count should be routinely assessed in any case that is suggestive of atypical or severe preeclampsia, including women presenting with nonspecific symptoms such as nausea, vomiting, or malaise. Such nonspecific symptoms related to liver dysfunction may often be the only presenting features and may be the harbinger of significant illness. AST is the dominant transaminase released into the peripheral circulation in liver dysfunction due to preeclampsia and is related to periportal necrosis. The fact that AST is increased to a greater extent than ALT, at least initially, may help in distinguishing preeclampsia from other potential causes of parenchymal liver disease where ALT is usually higher than AST. However, both autoimmune hepatitis and alcoholic hepatitis may also present with AST as the predominant transaminase and these conditions should be excluded before diagnosing preeclampsia or HELLP syndrome based on AST level in an atypical presentation. Increased serum levels of LDH in preeclampsia are caused by both hepatic dysfunction with LDH derived from ischemic/necrotic tissues and hemolysis with LDH from red cell destruction. Increase in bilirubin secondary to significant hemolysis may develop only in the late stages of the disease. Similarly, alterations in PT, PTT and fibrinogen usually develop in advanced preeclampsia and evaluation of coagulation parameters is probably only useful when the platelet count is below 100,000/mm^3, there is significant liver dysfunction, or there is suspected abruption.[49] Abnormal LFT occur in 3–5% of pregnancies, from a wide variety of causes, and while it is reasonable to suspect preeclampsia, the total clinical picture should be used and the diagnosis should not be made purely on the basis of elevated liver enzymes.[50]

The belief that preeclampsia/eclampsia must be associated with high BP may cause unwarranted delays in diagnosis.[15] Not infrequently, atypical presentations of preeclampsia occur. In the pregnant woman meeting the laboratory diagnostic criteria for HELLP syndrome, preeclampsia should be considered as part of the differential diagnosis despite the absence of hypertension, proteinuria, or other clinical signs. Some patients may present with isolated elevated liver enzymes and/or low platelets. In some cases, the hematocrit may not appear decreased despite hemolysis because of baseline hemoconcentration. In such cases, if some diagnostic criteria are met, the safest approach is to consider the patient to have preeclampsia and treat accordingly.

◼ ATYPICAL ECLAMPSIA IN EPIDEMIOLOGIC AND CLINICAL CONTEXT

Maternal morbidity and mortality in preeclampsia are influenced, among other factors, by the occurrence, severity, type and number of seizures and therefore, preventing their occurrence and recurrence is essential. Seizures may lead to severe maternal hypoxia, trauma and aspiration pneumonia. Although residual neurologic damage is rare,[24] some women may have short-term and long-term consequences such as impaired memory and cognitive function, especially after recurrent seizures or uncorrected severe hypertension leading to cytotoxic edema or infarction.[51] Permanent white matter loss has been documented by Zeeman et al.[52] on MRI following eclampsia in up to one fourth of women; however, without clinical neurologic deficits. Perinatal mortality in preeclampsia is also particularly elevated following eclamptic seizures.[53]

From 1940 to 1970, there was a 90% reduction in both the rates of eclampsia and maternal death from eclampsia in high-income countries.[54] This reduction coincided with the widespread introduction of prenatal care and increased access to hospital care. Although the traditional view is that prenatal care improves pregnancy outcomes, the evidence suggests that the implementation of prenatal care based on a strategy of screening and incidental case finding demonstrates outcome improvements only in relation to preeclampsia detection and management. It has failed to significantly impact rates of preterm birth or fetal growth restriction.[55] Eclampsia rates in high-income countries have continued to decline and in Canada for example, the annual rate of eclampsia decreased by over 50% between 2003 and 2009.[56]

Eclampsia incidence and associated maternal mortality remain high in low-resource settings, primarily as a result of poor access to prenatal care and diminished hospital accessibility. Eclampsia occurs in 2–3 cases per 10,000 births in Europe,[57] while in low-and middle-income countries the incidence is about 16–69 cases per 10,000 births.[58] Similarly, eclampsia associated maternal mortality varies from 1.8% in the UK[15] or 4.9% in Canada[56] to as high as 15.6% in regional data from Africa.[59,60] The final expression of the disease (i.e. convulsions) may represent different degrees of severity, or even different pathology (reversible vasogenic edema versus permanent cytotoxic infarction) in high and low resource settings. It has been reported that where the incidence of eclampsia is high, a greater proportion of cases occur antepartum than postpartum[60] and status epilepticus with recurrent seizures is more common than isolated seizure episodes.[61]

There is no reliable way to predict eclampsia in women who have preeclampsia until late in the process when signs of cerebral irritation become apparent (severe headache, increased reflexes, visual disturbances) and even then the majority of women with these signs do not convulse. Although the traditional teaching is that eclamptic seizures (tonic-clonic, focal, or multifocal) are associated with hypertension, proteinuria (i.e. preeclampsia) and raised intracranial pressure,[62] in reality, a significant proportion of women (20–38%) do not demonstrate the signs of preeclampsia before the seizure episode.[15,61] Unheralded eclampsia is the term that has been used to describe this presentation. A symptomatic prodrome is however present in 78–83% of all eclampsia cases,[61,63] mainly characterized by refractory frontal or occipital headaches. Headache is believed to reflect the development of cerebral edema, elevated cerebral perfusion pressure and hypertensive encephalopathy.[64]

Research into the mechanisms of eclamptic seizures has offered insights into this apparent paradox—eclampsia without preeclampsia. Although some researchers have suggested that eclamptic seizures are caused by increased cerebral blood flow,[65] others considered cerebral perfusion pressure, with or without an increase in cerebral blood flow, to be the critical determinant.[66] In preeclamptic women with high cerebral perfusion pressure, protective cerebral vasoconstriction occurs as a function of cerebral autoregulation. The relationship between cerebral perfusion pressure and mean arterial pressure is not linear and cannot be reliably predicted because physiologic autoregulation is inconsistently affected in preeclampsia.[22] Some patients with low-range BP may have elevated cerebral perfusion pressure, while others with very high BP have normal cerebral perfusion pressure. These findings are consistent with the clinical observation that eclampsia may occur in the absence of established hypertension, with headaches being a more consistent prodromal clinical finding than the elevation in BP. It has also been shown that women with headaches are more likely to have elevated cerebral perfusion pressure than those without.[64]

Both unheralded eclampsia and eclampsia developing beyond 48 hour after delivery have been referred to as atypical eclampsia. Atypical eclampsia occurring beyond 48 hour postpartum appears to be increasing in incidence in high-income countries and more than 50% of patients affected with late postpartum eclampsia had no evidence of preeclampsia prior to delivery.[4] The recent trend toward early postpartum discharge from the hospital in these countries may contribute to the increased rate of undetected late preeclampsia.

The prevention of eclampsia is empirically based on the concept of prompt delivery once severe preeclampsia has been diagnosed. In general most would deliver a preeclamptic patient with severe preeclampsia after 32–33 weeks' gestation without consideration of prolongation of the pregnancy. Prompt diagnosis and delivery are essential because severe preeclampsia may progress within hours from a normal clinical evaluation to severe manifestations.[67] Once severe preeclampsia has been diagnosed, most would manage the condition using magnesium sulfate to prevent the development of eclampsia. Magnesium sulfate was introduced for care of women with eclampsia in 1925 and it was more readily accepted in North America than elsewhere.[68] In some European countries, as late as 1992, magnesium sulfate was still not considered standard treatment.[69] It was only after the Magpie study, a randomized placebo-controlled trial with 10,110 participants (two-thirds originating from developing countries), that the value of magnesium sulfate as prophylaxis for eclampsia in women diagnosed with preeclampsia was accepted globally.[70] In this study, the seizure rate was reduced overall by more than half with treatment, magnesium sulfate being effective in both mild and severe preeclampsia cases. It is interesting to note that the reduction in the rate of eclampsia was not statistically significant in the subset of women enrolled in high-resource countries in the Western world [Risk ratio (RR), 0.67; 95% confidence interval (CI), 0.19–2.37].

In a systematic review that included the Magpie study plus five others, magnesium sulfate compared to placebo more than halved the risk of eclampsia (RR, 0.41; 95% CI, 0.29–0.58), reduced the risk of placental abruption (RR, 0.64; 95% CI, 0.50–0.83), and reduced the risk of maternal mortality albeit nonsignificantly (RR, 0.54; 95% CI, 0.26–1.10). There were no differences in maternal morbidity or perinatal mortality. A quarter of women reported side effects with magnesium sulfate, primarily flushing and the rate of cesarean section was increased by 5% when magnesium sulfate was used.[71]

The question of whether magnesium sulfate is beneficial in the management of mild preeclampsia is still unanswered by conclusive randomized data. Only two randomized studies, totaling 357 enrolled subjects have evaluated the use of magnesium sulfate in mild preeclampsia.[72,73] The use of magnesium sulfate did not appear to reduce the rate of progression to severe preeclampsia and based on this limited data, the benefit-to-risk ratio of using magnesium sulfate as prophylaxis of seizures in patients with mild preeclampsia is not clear.[74]

In contrast, the use of magnesium sulfate prophylaxis in severe preeclampsia is supported by adequate data and now by general consensus. The rate of seizures in severe preeclampsia without magnesium prophylaxis is four times higher than in mild cases (2 in 100 vs 1 in 200), and the use of magnesium may reduce the risk of seizure by slightly more than 50%. It has been calculated that 129 women need to be treated to prevent one case of eclampsia in asymptomatic cases, whereas in symptomatic cases (severe headache, blurred vision, photophobia, hyperreflexia and epigastric pain), the number needed to treat is 36.[74] Although the benefit-to-risk ratio for routine prophylaxis is less compelling for patients in high-resource settings in the Western world, most experts agree that magnesium sulfate prophylaxis in severe preeclampsia is advisable.[74] Magnesium sulfate is more effective than phenytoin or nimodipine (calcium-channel blocker used in clinical neurology to reduce cerebral vasospasm) in reducing eclampsia and should be considered the drug of choice in the prevention of eclampsia intrapartum and immediately (24 hours) postpartum.[71,75]

The accumulated evidence is also compelling for the use of magnesium sulfate to prevent recurrent eclamptic seizures. Recent Cochrane reviews,[76-78] which include data from low-resource countries, show a significant reduction in recurrent seizures and eclampsia-related maternal mortality with the use of magnesium sulfate. Magnesium sulfate given intramuscularly or intravenously is superior to phenytoin, diazepam, or lytic cocktail (usually chlorpromazine, promethazine and pethidine) and is also associated with less maternal and neonatal morbidity.[76-78] Diazepam, one of the most frequently prescribed medications in the world, was first proposed for women with eclampsia in the 1960s.[79] The use of magnesium sulfate, rather than diazepam, reduces the relative risk of recurrent seizures by 57% and the relative risk of maternal death by 41%, and these risk reduction effects are noted both antepartum and postpartum. Not only are the mothers better off, but babies exposed to magnesium sulfate rather than diazepam had higher Apgar scores, needed less intubation immediately after birth and fewer stayed in the special care unit for more than 7 days. Benzodiazepines and phenytoin are now thought to be justified only in the context of epilepsy treatment or when magnesium sulfate is contraindicated (myasthenia gravis, hypocalcemia, moderate-to-severe renal failure, cardiac ischemia, heart block, or myocarditis).

The diagnosis of atypical eclampsia is also one that requires finesse given the multitude of differential diagnoses. Neuroimaging, when possible, usually forms the mainstay in this regard and is especially advisable in atypical eclampsia developing beyond 48 hours postpartum. It has been reported that 13% of late postpartum seizures (> 48 hour) may have cerebral pathology other than eclampsia.[80] The differential diagnosis includes eclampsia, intracranial hemorrhage, encephalopathy, vasculitis, thrombosis/embolus, epilepsy, meningitis and stroke. Given the fact that many signs may be common to a number of these conditions, neuroimaging becomes essential to determine the underlying pathology. Proteinuria and hypertension can occur as a result of intracranial bleeding, rather than as signs of a presumed cause (preeclampsia). Similarly, in epileptic seizures, proteinuria may occur,

BP may be labile, reflexes brisk and uric acid increased. A particularly vexing situation may occur in a pregnant epileptic patient who develops seizures. The differential diagnosis may not be straightforward; however, with control of seizures, proteinuria and hypertension tend to resolve. Contrary to the functional, transient proteinuria that can be present in status epilepticus, in women with preeclampsia the proteinuria is caused by glomerular endothelial damage and generally gets progressively worse until they are delivered. Hypertension related to preeclampsia also tends to be more resilient and even after delivery return to normal BP may take days if not weeks.

CONCLUSION

At this point we should reemphasize the particular challenges inherent to the diagnostic process in atypical eclampsia. An exhaustive discussion on the differential diagnosis of cerebrovascular disorders including seizures in their presentation in pregnancy and postpartum is beyond the scope of this review. Authors have tried to highlight the fact that seizures in pregnancy can be related to pregnancy, may be exacerbated by pregnancy, or may be purely incidental and unrelated to pregnancy, and that eclamptic convulsions are a sign and not a cause. Seizures in pregnancy need to be fully investigated and a diagnosis of the underlying cause must be made. There may be considerable overlap of clinical and neuroimaging features among different pathological states (i.e. PRES and cerebral edema from other causes and between pathologic cerebral vasospasm and Call-Fleming syndrome).[81] Hypertensive encephalopathy is an acute manifestation that can include seizures and coma, and can occur in pregnancy at diastolic BP levels lower than 130 mm Hg. Differentiating eclampsia caused by hypertensive encephalopathy from that associated with intracranial hemorrhage is difficult based on clinical signs and neuroimaging is paramount. Both hypertensive encephalopathy and eclampsia may be associated with an increasingly recognized brain disorder known as PRES, first described in 1996.[82] Posterior reversible encephalopathy syndrome is believed to be caused by vasogenic brain edema and typically presents with focal MRI features described as symmetric high-signal intensity lesions in the bilateral parietooccipital lobes. Any instance of abrupt hypertension or hypertensive encephalopathy may trigger the syndrome which has also been described in association with preeclampsia/eclampsia, renal failure and immunosuppressive treatment. The lesions generally disappear with appropriate treatment. From a practical point of view, the practitioner should always think of eclampsia first in a pregnant or recently pregnant woman who is unconscious or having seizures. Hypertensive encephalopathy (PRES), as an etiology of eclamptic convulsions should also be considered in a convulsing pregnant or recently pregnant woman.[83]

The diagnosis of eclampsia is by necessity a diagnosis of exclusion in the absence of other causative conditions such as cerebral arterial ischemia and infarction, intracranial hemorrhage, venooclusive disease, vasculitis, tumors, intracranial infection, acute hypoglycemia, acute intermittent porphyria, TTP, HUS, or drug use. It is helpful that in most cases of eclampsia focal neurologic deficits are absent, however, occasionally, such manifestations, including visual loss may be present. Moreover, preeclampsia and eclampsia are risk factors for ischemic and hemorrhagic stroke, and the work-up suggested in any atypical case (MRI and/or CT scan) should elicit the diagnosis, allowing appropriate medical and surgical management. Between 2000 and 2004 there were 14 deaths due to preeclampsia and eclampsia in the United Kingdom and of these, 9 had an associated intracranial hemorrhage.[81] Hemorrhage may be promoted and exacerbated by coexisting coagulopathy, such as thrombocytopenia or disseminated intravascular coagulopathy, both of which are not infrequently present in severe preeclampsia.

Thrombotic thrombocytopenic purpura and HUS must be differentiated from preeclampsia/eclampsia and this may on occasion be extremely difficult. Both are thrombotic microangiopathic syndromes, rare in pregnancy and in the postpartum period (less than one case in 100,000 pregnancies),[84] and TTP and HUS are often undistinguishable from each other. TTP may be precipitated by pregnancy, with 13% of all cases of TTP being associated with pregnancy.[85] In both, TTP and HUS, seizures occur and the differentiation from eclampsia is of outmost importance because of management implications. In TTP/HUS maternal condition is not expected to improve with delivery and administration of platelets and certain drugs (e.g. heparin) can result in a precipitous decline in clinical status due to an increase in microvascular thrombosis. Without adequate treatment (plasmapheresis and high-dose steroids in TTP, and a combination of plasma exchange and prednisone for HUS), maternal mortality in these conditions could exceed 80%.[86] Other conditions known to imitate preeclampsia/eclampsia include herpes encephalitis, lupus encephalitis and acute fatty liver of pregnancy.

Eclampsia remains one of the most common acute neurological events occurring during pregnancy and is still a significant cause of maternal death worldwide, particularly in low-resource settings. When the clinical presentation is atypical, difficulties in differential diagnosis may lead to improper management. Only an open minded, astute clinical diagnostic approach will favorably modify the life-threatening or life-altering potential of atypical preeclampsia/eclampsia.

■ REFERENCES

1. Paxton A, Wardlaw T. Are we making progress in maternal mortality? N Engl J Med. 2011;364:1990-3.
2. Roberts JM, Villar J, Arulkumaran S. Preventing and treating eclamptic seizures. BMJ. 2002;325:609-10.
3. Brown MA, Lindheimer MD, de Swiet M, et al. The classification and diagnosis of the hypertensive disorders of pregnancy: statement from the International Society for the Study of Hypertension in Pregnancy (ISSHP). Hypertens Pregnancy. 2001;20:IX-XIV.
4. Sibai BM. Diagnosis, differential diagnosis and management of eclampsia. Obstet Gynecol. 2005;105:402-10.
5. Mattar F, Sibai BM. Eclampsia: risk factors for maternal morbidity. Am J Obstet Gynecol. 2000; 182:307-12.
6. Pettit F, Brown MA. The management of pre-eclampsia: what we think we know. Eur J Obstet Gynecol Reprod Biol. 2012;160:6-12.
7. Brown MA, Mangos G, Davis G, et al. The natural history of white coat hypertension during pregnancy. BJOG. 2005;112:601-6.
8. Saudan PJ, Brown MA, Farrell T, et al. Improved methods of assessing proteinuria in hypertensive pregnancy. Br J Obstet Gynecol. 1997;104:1159-64.
9. Phelan LK, Brown MA, Davis GK, et al. A prospective study of the impact of automated dipstick urinalysis

on the diagnosis of preeclampsia. Hypertens Pregnancy. 2004;23:135-42.
10. Lindheimer MD, Kanter D. Interpreting abnormal proteinuria in pregnancy: the need for a more pathophysiological approach. Obstet Gynecol. 2010;115:365-75.
11. Magee LA, von Dadelszen P, Bohun CM, et al. Serious perinatal complications of non-proteinuric hypertension: an international, multicentre, retrospective cohort study. J Obstet Gynecol Can. 2003;2:372-82.
12. Thornton CE, Makris A, Ogle RF, et al. Role of proteinuria in defining pre-eclampsia: clinical outcomes for women and babies. Clin Exp Pharmacol Physiol. 2010;37:466-70.
13. Homer CS, Brown MA, Mangos G, et al. Non-proteinuric pre-eclampsia: a novel risk indicator in women with gestational hypertension. J Hypertens. 2008;26:295-302.
14. Espinoza J. The need to redefine preeclampsia. Expert Opin Med Diagn. 2012;6:347-57.
15. Douglas KA, Redman CW. Eclampsia in the United Kingdom. BMJ. 1994;309:1395-400.
16. Hardardottir H, Kelly K, Bork MD, et al. Atypical presentation of preeclampsia in high-order multifetal gestations. Obstet Gynecol. 1996;87: 370-4.
17. Goodlin RC. Severe preeclampsia: another great imitator. Am J Obstet Gynecol. 1976;125:747-53.
18. Goodlin RC. Preeclampsia as the great impostor. Am J Obstet Gynecol. 1991;164:1577.
19. Walker SP, Wein P, Ihle BU. Severe folate deficiency masquerading as the syndrome of hemolysis, elevated liver enzymes, and low platelets. Obstet Gynecol. 1997;90:655-7.
20. Stella CL, Sibai BM. Preeclampsia: diagnosis and management of the atypical presentation. J Matern Fetal Neonatal Med. 2006;19:381-6.
21. Stefos T, Plachouras N, Mari G, et al. A case of partial mole and atypical type I triploidy associated with severe HELLP syndrome at 18 weeks' gestation. Ultrasound Obstet Gynecol. 2002;20:403-4.
22. Belfort MA, Saade GR, Grunewald C, et al. Effect of blood pressure on orbital and middle cerebral artery resistance in healthy pregnant women and women with preeclampsia. Am J Obstet Gynecol. 1999;180:601-7.
23. Zeeman GG, Fleckenstein JL, Twickler DM, et al. Cerebral infarction in eclampsia. Am J Obstet Gynecol. 2004;190:714-20.
24. Loureiro R, Leite CC, Kahhale S, et al. Diffusion imaging may predict reversible brain lesions in eclampsia and severe preeclampsia: initial experience. Am J Obstet Gynecol. 2003;189:1350-5.

25. Neudecker S, Stock K, Krasnianski M. Call-Fleming postpartum angiopathy in the puerperium. Obstet Gynecol. 2006;107:446-9.

26. Call GK, Fleming MC, Sealfon S, et al. Reversible cerebral segmental vasoconstriction. Stroke. 1988; 19:1159-70.

27. Bainbridge SA, Roberts JM. Uric acid as a pathogenic factor in preeclampsia. Placenta. 2008;29(Suppl. A); S67-72.

28. Sagen H, Haram K, Nilsen ST. Serum urate as a predictor of fetal outcome in severe preeclampsia. Acta Obstet Gynecol Scand. 1984;63:71.

29. Martin AC, Brown MA. Could uric acid have a pathogenic role in pre-eclampsia? Nat Rev Nephrol. 2010;6:744-8.

30. Thangaratinam S, Ismail KM, Sharp S, et al. Accuracy of serum uric acid in predicting complications of pre-eclampsia: a systematic review. BJOG. 2006; 113:369-78.

31. Koopmans CM, van Pampus MG, Groen H, et al. Accuracy of serum uric acid as a predictive test for maternal complications in pre-eclampsia: bivariate meta-analysis and decision analysis. Eur J Obstet Gynecol Reprod Biol. 2009;146:8-14.

32. Parrish M, Griffin M, Morris R, et al. Hyperuricemia facilitates the prediction of maternal and perinatal adverse outcome in patients with severe/super-imposed preeclampsia. J Matern Fetal Neonatal Med. 2010;23:1451-5.

33. Martin AC, Brown MA. Could uric acid have a pathogenic role in pre-eclampsia? Nat Rev Nephrol. 2010;6:744-8.

34. Dunlop W, Furness C, Hill LM. Maternal hemoglobin concentration, hematocrit and renal handling of urate in pregnancies ending in the births of small-for-dates infants. Br J Obstet Gynecol. 1978;85: 938-40.

35. Roberts JM, Bodnar LM, Lain KY, et al. Uric acid is as important as proteinuria in identifying fetal risk in women with gestational hypertension. Hypertension. 2005;46:1263-9.

36. Hawkins TL-A, Roberts JM, Mangos GJ, et al. Plasma uric acid remains a marker of poor outcome in hypertensive pregnancy: a retrospective cohort study. BJOG. 2012;119:484-92.

37. Bainbridge SA, von Versen-Hoynck F, Roberts JM. Uric acid inhibits placental system amino acid uptake. Placenta. 2009;30:195-200.

38. Verdy E, Bessons V, Dreyfus M, et al. Longitudinal analysis of platelet count and volume in normal pregnancy. Thromb Hemost. 1997;77:806-7.

39. Burrows RF, Kelton JG. Thrombocytopenia at delivery: a prospective survey of 6,715 deliveries. Obstet Gynecol. 1990;162:731-4.

40. Sibai BM, Anderson GD, McCubbin JH. Eclampsia II clinical significance of laboratory findings. Obstet Gynecol. 1982;59:153-7.

41. Giles C, Inglis TC. Thrombocytopenia and macro-thrombocytosis in gestational hypertension. Br J Obstet Gynecol. 1981;88:1115-9.

42. Pritchard JA, Weisman R Jr, Ratnoff OD, et al. Intravascular hemolysis, thrombocytopenia and other hematologic abnormalities associated with severe toxemia of pregnancy. N Engl J Med. 1954; 250:89-98.

43. Weinstein L. Syndrome of hemolysis, elevated liver enzymes and low platelet count: a severe consequence of hypertension in pregnancy. Am J Obstet Gynecol. 1982;142:159-67.

44. Martin JN Jr, Blake PG, Perry KG Jr, et al. The natural history of HELLP syndrome: patterns of disease progression and regression. Am J Obstet Gynecol. 1991;164:1500-9.

45. Sibai BM. The HELLP syndrome (hemolysis, elevated liver enzymes, and low platelets): much ado about nothing? Am J Obstet Gynecol. 1990;162:311-6.

46. Minakami H, Oka N, Sato T, et al. Preeclampsia: a microvesicular fat disease of the liver? Am J Obstet Gynecol. 1988;159:1043-7.

47. Rigo J, Tanyi J, Varga I, et al. Atypical process of acute disturbance of liver function with severe thrombocytopenia in the third trimester. Zentralbl Gynakol. 2000;122:436-8.

48. Martin JN, Rinehart BK, May WL, et al. The spectrum of severe pre-eclampsia: comparative analysis by HELLP (hemolysis, elevated liver enzyme levels, and low platelet count) syndrome classification. Am J Obstet Gynecol. 1999;180:1373-84.

49. Leduc L, Wheeler JM, Kirshon B, et al. Coagulation profile in severe preeclampsia. Obstet Gynecol. 1992;79:14-8.

50. Hay JE. Liver disease in pregnancy. Hepatology. 2008;47:1067-76.

51. Zeeman GG. Neurologic complications of pre-eclampsia. Semin Perinatol. 2009;33:166-72.

52. Zeeman GG, Fleckenstein JL, Twickler DM, et al. Cerebral infarction in eclampsia. Am J Obstet Gynecol. 2004;190:714-20.

53. Eclampsia Trial Collaborative Group. Which anticonvulsant for women with eclampsia? Evidence from the collaborative eclampsia trial. Lancet. 1995;345:1455-63.

54. Goldenberg RL, McClure EM, MacGuire ER, et al. Lessons for low-income regions following the reduction in hypertension-related maternal mortality in high-income countries. Int J Gynecol Obstet. 2011;113:91-5.

55. Vidaeff AC, Franzini L, Low MD. The unrealized potential of prenatal care. A population health approach. J Reprod Med. 2003;48:837-42.

56. Liu S, Joseph KS, Liston RM, et al. Incidence, risk factors, and associated complications of eclampsia. Obstet Gynecol. 2011;118:987-94.

57. Knight M. Eclampsia in the United Kingdom. 2005. BJOG. 2007;114:1072-8.

58. Frias AE Jr., Belfort MA. Post Magpie: how should we be managing severe preeclampsia? Curr Opin Obstet Gynecol. 2003;15:489-95.

59. Ozumbia BC, Ibe AI. Eclampsia in Enugu, eastern Nigeria. Acta Obstet Gynecol Scand. 1993;72:189-92.

60. Igberase GO, Ebeigbe PN. Eclampsia: ten years of experience in a rural tertiary hospital in the Niger delta, Nigeria. J Obstet and Gynecol. 2006;26:414-7.

61. Noraihan MN, Sharda P, Jammal ABE. Report of 50 cases of eclampsia. J Obstet Gynecol Res. 2005;31:302-9.

62. Thomas SV. Neurological aspects of eclampsia. J Neurol Sci. 1998;144:37-43.

63. Cooray SD, Edmonds SM, Tong S, et al. Characterization of symptoms immediately preceding eclampsia. Obstet Gynecol. 2011;118:995-9.

64. Belfort MA, Saade GR, Grunewald C, et al. Association of cerebral perfusion pressure with headache in women with preeclampsia. Br J Obstet Gynecol. 1999;106:814-21.

65. Zeeman GG, Hatab MR, Twickler DM. Increased cerebral blood flow in preeclampsia using magnetic resonance imaging. Am J Obstet Gynecol. 2004;191:1425-9.

66. Belfort MA, Varner MW, Dizon-Townson DS, et al. Cerebral perfusion pressure and not cerebral blood flow, may be the critical determinant of intracranial injury in preeclampsia: a new hypothesis. Am J Obstet Gynecol. 2002;187:626-34.

67. Engelhardt T, Moodley J, Mothlabani B. Does antenatal care in developing countries prevent eclampsia? Hypertens Preg. 1996;15:87-94.

68. Lazard EM. A preliminary report on the intravenous use of magnesium sulphate in puerperal eclampsia. Am J Obstet Gynecol. 1925;9:178-88.

69. Kullberg G, Lindeberg S, Hanson U. Eclampsia in Sweden. Hypertens Preg. 2002;21:13-21.

70. The Magpie Trial Collaboration Group. Do women with preeclampsia and their babies, benefit from magnesium sulphate? The Magpie Trial: a randomized placebo-controlled trial. Lancet. 2002;359:1877-90.

71. Duley L, Gulmezoglu AM, Henderson-Smart DJ, et al. Magnesium sulphate and other anticonvulsants for women with pre-eclampsia. Cochrane Database Syst Rev. 2010;(11):CD000025.

72. Witlin AG, Friedman SA, Sibai BM. The effect of magnesium sulfate therapy on the duration of labor in women with mild preeclampsia at term: a randomized, double-blind, placebo-controlled trial. Am J Obstet Gynecol. 1997;176:623-7.

73. Livingston JC, Livingston LW, Ramsey R, et al. Magnesium sulfate in women with mild preeclampsia: a randomized controlled trial. Obstet Gynecol. 2003;101:217-20.

74. Sibai BM. Magnesium sulfate prophylaxis in preeclampsia: Lessons learned from recent trials. Am J Obstet Gynecol. 2004;190:1520-6.

75. Belfort MA, Anthony J, Saade GR, et al. Nimodipine Study Group. A comparison of magnesium sulfate and nimodipine for the prevention of eclampsia. N Engl J Med. 2003;348:304-11.

76. Duley L, Henderson-Smart DJ, Chou D. Magnesium sulphate versus phenytoin for eclampsia. Cochrane Database Syst Rev. 2010;(10):CD000128.

77. Duley L, Henderson-Smart DJ, Walker GJA, et al. Magnesium sulphate versus diazepam for eclampsia. Cochrane Database Syst Rev. 2010; (12) CD000127.

78. Duley L, Gulmezoglu AM, Chou D. Magnesium sulphate versus lytic cocktail for eclampsia. Cochrane Database Syst Rev. 2010;(9):CD002960.

79. Lean TH, Ratnam SS, Sivasamboo R. Use of benzodiazepines in the management of eclampsia. J Obstet Gynecol Br Comm. 1968;75:856-62.

80. Lubarsky S, Barton JR, Friedman SA, et al. Late postpartum eclampsia revisited. Obstet Gynecol. 1994;83:502-5.

81. Dineen R, Banks A, Lenthall R. Imaging of acute neurological conditions in pregnancy and puerperium. Clin Radiol. 2005;60:1156-70.

82. Hinchey I, Chaves C, Appignani B, et al. A reversible posterior leukoencephalopathy syndrome. N Engl J Med. 1996;334:494-500.

83. Witlin AG, Friedman SA, Egerman RS, et al. Cerebrovascular disorders complicating pregnancy-beyond eclampsia. Am J Obstet Gynecol. 1997; 176:1139-48.

84. Sibai BM. Imitators of severe preeclampsia. Obstet Gynecol. 2007;109:956-66.

85. George JN. The association of pregnancy with thrombotic thrombocytopenic purpura-hemolytic uremic syndrome. Curr Opin Hematol. 2003;10: 339-44.

86. George JN. Corticosteroids and rituximab as adjunctive treatments for thrombotic thrombocytopenic purpura. Am J Hematol. 2012; 87:S88-S91.

12 Timing and Mode of Delivery in Hypertensive Disorders of Pregnancy

Lavanya Rai

INTRODUCTION

Hypertensive disorders of pregnancy are common and an important cause of maternal mortality in both developed and developing world. It is also one of the most common causes of iatrogenic preterm birth. The National Institute of Health (NIH) system has classified these disorders into four categories.[1] Among them, gestational hypertension (GH) and preeclampsia (PE) are common while chronic hypertension preceding pregnancy and PE superimposed on chronic hypertension are less common. Preeclampsia is further subclassified into mild and severe types based on the American College of Obstetricians and Gynecologists (ACOG) criteria for prognostication and management.[2] Majority of the cases of GH and mild PE occur after 36–37 weeks' gestation. Progression of GH to PE depends on the gestational age at onset. Fifty percent of GH prior to 30 weeks will eventually progress to PE. However, the progression from mild to severe PE is variable, the risk being 10–25%.[3,4]

Preeclampsia is a pregnancy-specific, multi-system, progressive disorder of multifactorial etiology. Problems arise when severe disease occurs prior to 34 weeks. There is no therapy to alter the pathophysiology or treat the disease. Delivery is the only known cure for PE but "when" and "how", needs to be decided by the obstetrician caring for the mother. Delivery prior to 34 weeks' gestation poses a problem for the baby though it is appropriate for the mother. Conservative approach is an option today for preterm fetuses because of the available fetal surveillance techniques, steroid prophylaxis and remarkable advances in neonatal care. Timing and mode of delivery, however, needs to be individualized based on a combination of fetal and maternal factors.

The objectives of delivery in hypertensive disorders at the appropriate time are to prevent complications, restore mother's health with a birth of an infant who subsequently thrives. In severe PE, it also means prevention of eclampsia, hemolysis, elevated liver enzymes and low platelet count (HELLP) syndrome, intracranial hemorrhage and other related complications.

TIMING OF DELIVERY

Traditional approach to PE was to hasten delivery. After the advent of steroid prophylaxis for lung maturation in preterm labor, delivery was deferred for 48 hours. In some of these women the disease stabilized. When these pregnancies were continued, the neonatal morbidity lessened with increasing gestational age. This paved the way for adopting conservative line of management in some selected cases. Timing of delivery depends on severity of PE, period of gestation, presence of complications and fetal well-being. However, maternal status always takes a priority over fetus.

When a patient is admitted with PE or any hypertensive disorder in pregnancy, 24 hours of initial window period will be required for evaluation and observation. This evaluation window enables the doctors to categorize the patient and plan the management strategy.

A detailed work-up of the case with investigations is necessary to decide the time and route of delivery. As PE is a multisystem disorder, investigations are required to find out multiorgan involvement or fetal compromise as indicated by fetal well-being tests.

Evaluation/Stabilization Window

- *Assess severity of hypertension*: 4 hourly blood pressure (BP) recording or more frequently if situation demands
- Send PE profile consisting of blood counts, serum creatinine, uric acid, liver enzymes and 24 hour urine protein is also estimated. A coagulation screen [prothrombin time (PT), activated partial thromboplastin time (APTT)] is required if platelets are less than 100,000/μL or whenever liver enzymes are elevated.
- Antihypertensive therapy is started with labetalol or nifedipine to prevent maternal complications like stroke or intracranial hemorrhage. The aim is never to bring down the BP to normal as this would reduce uteroplacental perfusion that is harmful to the fetus.
- In severe PE, seizure prophylaxis with magnesium sulfate should be started. Cochrane database systematic review has proved beyond doubt that magnesium sulfate is beneficial in prevention of eclampsia.[5]
- *Fetal growth and surveillance tests*: Ultrasound to assess fetal growth is essential to rule out fetal growth restriction (FGR). Nonstress test (NST), biophysical profile (BPP) and amniotic fluid index (AFI) are done to assess the fetal well-being. Umbilical artery Doppler is done to assess the uteroplacental blood flow. The frequency of fetal testing is dictated by the clinical severity and fetal status.
- Monitor urinary output, symptoms and signs of imminent eclampsia such as epigastric pain, headache, vomiting and visual disturbances.
- Anesthesia consultation is useful for planning labor analgesia as well as anesthesia in the event of Cesarean delivery (CD). It will enable them to assess the airway, medications used and plan their management.
- *Arrange for corticosteroids*: Injection betamethasone 12 mg—two doses at 24 hour interval for pregnancies less than 34 weeks' gestation. A single course of antenatal corticosteroids is the standard of care for patients at risk of preterm labor.[6]

It is now clear that fetuses of preeclamptic women do not have accelerated lung maturity as was once believed. Delivery can be planned 24 hours after the second dose of steroids.

Corticosteroids for lung maturity in hypertensive disorders are safe.

A prospective randomized double blind trial has reported a significant reduction in respiratory distress syndrome (RDS) with the use of steroids in women with severe PE between 26 weeks and 34 weeks of gestation [23% vs. 43%; relative risk (RR), 0.53; 95% confidence interval (CI), 0.35–0.82]. Other neonatal morbidities such as intraventricular hemorrhage and perinatal infections were also less in the corticosteroid group.[7]

Factors to Decide Timing of Delivery

- Gestational age
- Severity of FGR
- Fetal well-being tests
- Maternal complications
- Severity of hypertension
- Response to therapy

After the initial thorough evaluation, patient and her family are counseled regarding the management strategy. Birth plan and indications for delivery should be documented in the file.

Delivery is considered in all women beyond 37 completed weeks of gestation in mild PE and GH. All cases of severe PE are delivered when they reach 34 weeks or earlier, if necessary, after a course of steroid prophylaxis.[6] Severe GH should be managed as severe PE.

▨ SEVERE PREECLAMPSIA/ GESTATIONAL HYPERTENSION PRIOR TO 34 WEEKS

The time of delivery in preterm cases with severe PE between 28 weeks and 34 weeks poses a problem. Immediate delivery before 34 weeks is associated with neonatal morbidity sometimes severe enough to cause death or survival with disability.

Two methods of management are now adopted for those with gestational ages less than 34 weeks, either expectant or aggressive management.

Aggressive management is one where delivery is planned either immediately or after a course of steroid prophylaxis. It is also known as interventionist care. Expeditious delivery may sometimes be warranted in the event of complications like abruptio placenta or eclampsia where there may not be sufficient time to give steroid prophylaxis.

Expectant management is one where pregnancy is continued under close surveillance so that the delivery is delayed to gain fetal maturity. It is beneficial to the fetus and has no benefits to the mother. It is recommended for severe PE less than 34 weeks provided mother and fetus are stable. In mild PE and GH, expectant monitoring continues up to 37 weeks. Monitoring during expectant approach in severe PE is to detect further deterioration and to plan delivery while in mild PE, it is to detect development of severe disease.

Aggressive Management

There is consensus that delivery is the only option in the presence of multiorgan dysfunction or fetal compromise in severe PE. Severe PE/severe GH beyond 34 weeks requires delivery.[8] Prior to 34 weeks, immediate delivery will depend on evidence of end organ damage for the mother.

Delivery may be planned after steroid prophylaxis or even before that in the event of a complication. Induction of labor may be done or CD may become essential if the fetus shows signs of compromise. Abnormal umbilical artery Doppler, flow absent or reversed, is an indication for delivery as fetal death risk is higher with expectant management.[8] Table 12.1 shows indications for immediate delivery with or without steroid prophylaxis.

Table 12.1: Indications for immediate delivery[1,8,9]	
Maternal	*Fetal*
Uncontrolled hypertension	Absent/reversed end diastole in Doppler
Imminent eclampsia/eclampsia	Variable decelerations or nonreassuring fetal trace
Labor/PROM	Decreased fetal movements/BPP < 4
Oliguria	Severe FGR (< 5th percentile)
Deteriorating liver or renal function	Severe oligoamnios (AFI < 5 cm)
Low platelet count	Gestation > 34 weeks in severe PE
Neurological complications	Gestational age > 37 weeks in mild PE/GH
HELLP syndrome	Abruption

Abbreviations: PROM, premature rupture of membranes; BPP, biophysical profile; FGR, fetal growth restriction; AFI, amniotic fluid index; HELLP, hemolysis, elevated liver enzymes and low platelet count; PE, preeclampsia; GH, gestational hypertension

Even in aggressive management, delivery is planned after stabilization with antihypertensives and magnesium sulfate for seizure prophylaxis for cases with severe PE. This has to be continued for 24 hours after delivery.

No attempt is made to stop preterm labor if it sets, in a patient with PE or hypertensive disorders. Proteinuria greater than 5 g per 24 hours is no longer a criterion for immediate delivery.

Presence of ascites by scan is regarded as a contraindication for expectant management. It indicates increased capillary leakage and these patients are more likely to develop cerebral edema and pulmonary edema.[10] Severe FGR (< 5th percentile) and HELLP are generally considered contraindications for expectant management but there have been some studies which have included these cases.[11,12] Admission to delivery interval is reduced in the presence of these problems compared to those without.

Expectant Management

Expectant management is one where the pregnancy is continued with close monitoring till the decision to deliver, which may be 34 weeks in severe PE and 37 weeks in mild PE. Delivery may be planned earlier if an immediate indication develops. The objective here is to prolong the pregnancy to improve gestational age and weight of the fetus without deterioration in the maternal status. For fetuses less than 32 weeks, every week gained will drastically reduce neonatal morbidity and duration of neonatal intensive care unit (NICU) admissions.[13]

Expectant management is also called as temporizing management by Ganzevoort et al. as they feel that this management requires close maternal and fetal surveillance in addition to antihypertensives and steroid prophylaxis.[14] Therefore, this is active management and not passive as the term "expectant" would suggest.

Where can Expectant Management be Done?

It should be carried out in a tertiary care center with an experienced dedicated team and facilities for monitoring mother and neonate. Hospitals with 24 hours anesthesia and operating room facility can carry out this management. As cases tend to suddenly deteriorate, there should be accessibility to a critical care unit. Expectant management can be started in a secondary level hospital and in utero transfer to a tertiary care center may then be considered.[15]

Who should Receive Expectant Management?

This management is reserved for selected cases of severe PE below 34 weeks where mother and fetus are stable. The indications for immediate delivery shown in Table 12.1 are contraindications and indications to stop the expectant management. Generally, two-thirds of patients who develop PE before 34 weeks are eligible for a conservative approach.[16,17] About 40% of women with severe PE less than 34 weeks are not eligible for expectant management. PE is an unpredictable disorder with endothelial injury affecting multiple organs with variable severity. If severe PE occurs in a patient with pre-existing medical disorders or when multiple organs are involved, they should not be included for expectant approach.

Guidelines for Expectant Management[13]

- Counseling the patient and her family regarding fetal prognosis and maternal risks is essential.

- Patient is kept on bed rest.
- Antihypertensive therapy is continued to maintain systolic BP between 130 mm Hg and 150 mm Hg and diastolic BP between 80 mm Hg and 100 mm Hg. Oral labetalol or nifedipine can be used.
- Fetal surveillance is done by keeping fetal movement count, NST and BPP, AFI and umbilical artery Doppler. These have to be done frequently based on the severity of patient's disease and fetal status.
- Monitor PE serum profile weekly or twice weekly depending on the severity of the disease.
- Maternal surveillance consists of BP monitoring, symptoms/signs of imminent eclampsia.
- Twenty-four hour urine output and daily maternal weight assessment may be done.
- Watch out for complications like abruptio placenta, renal failure and HELLP syndrome.
- Check whether steroid prophylaxis has been completed during the stabilization period.

Many prospective and retrospective trials have shown that expectant management is beneficial to some selected women as depicted in Table 12.2. There are only two randomized controlled trials (RCTs) that compared expectant with aggressive

Table 12.2: The results of various studies on expectant management

Author/Year	Type of Study	Number of Patients	Gesta-tional Age	Days Gained	Perinatal Outcome	Maternal Outcome
Sibai[19] (1994)	RCT Expectant vs aggressive	95	28–32	15.2	↓RDS 22% versus 50%; ↑baby weight; PNMR, 0	CD, 73% versus 85%; maternal morbidity, 8.1% vs 6.5%
Odendaal[18] (1990)	RCT Expectant vs aggressive	58	28–34	7.1	PNMR, 16.6%; neonatal morbidity, 33% vs 75%	CD, 76%; maternal morbidity, 17.8% vs 35%
Hall[20] (2000)	Prospective	340	24–34	11	PNMR, 2.4%	CD, 81.5%; maternal morbidity, 27%
Hall[10] (2006)	Prospective	169	20–34	12	> 1,000 g; PNMR, 0	
Haddad[21] (2004)	Prospective FGR	239	24–33	5	PNMR, 5,4%	CD, 95%; maternal morbidity, 25%
Oettle[15] (2005)	Prospective	131	24–34	11.6	PNMR, 13.7%	CD, 77%; maternal death, 1
Shear[22] (2005)	Retrospective 49% FGR	155	24–34	5.3	PNMR, 3.9%	CD, 75%; maternal morbidity, 36%
Visser[11] (1995)	With and without HELLP	128	24–34	5.3	PNMR, 14.1% vs 14.8%	CD, 79.6% vs. 85.9%; maternal morbidity, 14.1% vs. 11%

Abbreviations: RCT, randomized controlled trial; RDS, respiratory distress syndrome; PNMR, perinatal mortality rate; CD, Cesarean delivery; FGR, fetal growth restriction; HELLP, hemolysis, elevated liver enzymes and low platelet count treatment.[18,19] They showed improved perinatal outcome without major maternal morbidity for expectant treatment between 28 weeks and 34 weeks. In the randomized trial by Odendaal et al, 20 women in the aggressive management were compared to 18 women in expectant management. All were cases of severe PE; some were even with imminent eclampsia.[18] This study reported a significant increase of 7 days gained in utero which in turn reduced neonatal complications to 33% versus 75% with aggressive management. Maternal complication rate did not increase with expectant management. By reducing NICU stay, the cost of treatment reduces significantly with expectant management. Longer maternal hospitalization in the obstetric high-dependency unit costs much less than NICU stay.

Sibai et al. conducted another prospective randomized trial enrolling 46 for aggressive and 49 for expectant management.[19] They obtained a mean latency period of 15.4 days for their patients between 28 weeks and 34 weeks. Neonatal complications were significantly low in their study. There were no cases of eclampsia or perinatal death. The birth weight increased from 1,233 g to 1,622 g and gestational age from 30 weeks to 32 weeks. Expectant management reduced NICU admissions (76% vs. 100%; p = 0.002) and the total number of days there. Both the randomized trials excluded FGR fetuses and their lower limit of gestational age was 28 weeks.

Some trials later on decreased the lower limit to 24 weeks. These showed increased maternal morbidity, one maternal death with a perinatal mortality between 0% and 16.6%.[23] As the gestational age was lowered for expectant management, neonatal mortality and maternal complications increased. Two of the above studies included growth-restricted babies while one case controlled series included women with and without HELLP syndrome. In 43% of patients, reversal of HELLP was noted with median prolongation of pregnancy by 21 days. They concluded that temporizing treatment with HELLP that is not worsening may improve maternal, fetal and neonatal outcome. They used invasive hemodynamic monitoring plasma volume expansion and vasodilators.[11,21,22] One of the trials was conducted in secondary hospital and only the ones with complications were transferred to tertiary

care.[15] It is the gestational age at delivery rather than the severity of the disease which determines the perinatal outcome. Perinatal survival was 72% at 28 weeks and 92% at 32 weeks.[12,20,22] When perinatal outcome is studied in growth-restricted babies according to gestational age, neonatal morbidity was predicted better by gestational age rather than the degree of growth restriction. Presence of severe FGR resulted in higher fetal deaths during expectant management in fetuses prior to 30 weeks of gestation. Controlling for gestational age at delivery, fetal death was associated with severe intrauterine growth restriction (IUGR) [odds ratio (OR), 6.4; 95% CI, 1.05–39.35; p = 0.04].[12] Hence many suggest that severe FGR should be excluded from expectant management.[24] Longer expectant management and favorable outcome can be expected in fetuses without growth restriction or abnormal Doppler findings.[25,26]

■ SEVERE PREECLAMPSIA PRIOR TO 28 WEEKS

Many trials have been conducted for women between 24 weeks and 27 weeks of gestation with mixed results. A systematic review including observational data found in women less than 24 weeks went in favor of interventionist care by pregnancy termination due to high perinatal mortality and morbidity.[27] Serious maternal morbidity (62%) has also been reported.[28] In a group of survivors at 24 weeks gestation, 25% had moderate handicap.[29] Sibai reviewed all the studies on expectant management less than 25 weeks. The overall perinatal mortality rate was 83% and maternal complications were 57%. The lower limit for expectant management was thus set at 23 weeks below which termination should be offered to all women.[23] There was a report of gestation-specific perinatal and maternal outcome with expectant management which showed perinatal survival at 24 weeks ranging from 60% to 70%. At 25–26 weeks, it varied between 60% and 100%. Maternal complications ranged between 30% and 50%. Thus, with thorough counseling and good NICU facility, expectant management may be offered for gestational ages between 24 weeks and 26 weeks.[30]

Nevertheless, in developing countries where neonatal survival prior to 28 weeks is poor, termination of pregnancy would be a better option in the interests of the mother. Therefore, 24–27 weeks which is previable for most of the low-resource countries seems to be a grey zone.

Thus, factors influencing the duration and outcome of expectant management are presence of FGR, gestational age at onset, abnormal umbilical artery Doppler, NICU facility and presence of HELLP syndrome.[8]

Lower limit of gestational age for expectant management depends on the period of viability in a particular set up which in turn depends on the level of NICU care that is available. In most of the low-resource countries, this is at 28 weeks while in resource-rich countries, this may be earlier around 24–25 weeks and conservative management is therefore adopted. Most of the trials have shown prolongation of gestation by 1–2 weeks with expectant management.[15,19,20] This is beneficial for fetuses which are 1–2 weeks below the period of viability threshold. Even in those countries where period of viability is at 28 weeks, conservative management may be adopted if facilities exist because if a pregnancy continues by 2 weeks fetus has higher chance of survival.

It is essential to balance the risks and benefits while planning expectant management. Selection of patients for this management is done in the first 48 hours after admission. In severe PE beyond 34 weeks, there is no role for expectant management. In mild PE or GH with stable disease, expectant management is beneficial by prevention of late preterm morbidity for the neonate.

Demerits of expectant management include maternal complications like eclampsia, development of HELLP syndrome, renal failure and abruptio placenta (20%). There may be also a possibility of sudden fetal death. Incidence of small for gestational age (SGA) babies ranged from 24% to 61%.[20,22]

The structured review of literature by Magee et al. on expectant versus interventionist care noted that pregnancy prolongation of 2 weeks with good outcome for baby with minimal maternal morbidity is possible with expectant management for severe PE less than 34 weeks.[27] After having adopted this approach, 20% needed delivery within 48 hours due to maternal or fetal problems and only 20% reached 34 weeks or beyond. Expectant care for those with HELLP syndrome is associated with only prolongation of 5 days and therefore is of questionable benefit beyond 48 hours for steroid prophylaxis.

However, Cochrane review opinion is that there is not enough evidence from these trials to recommend either early delivery or expectant care for women with severe PE before 34 weeks of pregnancy.[31]

■ MILD PREECLAMPSIA/ GESTATIONAL HYPERTENSION

Though literature is clear in delivering severe PE after 34 weeks, many believe that 34–37 weeks of gestation in mild PE, GH or deteriorating chronic hypertension seems to be a grey zone where benefits of expectant management or induction of labor is not clear.[6]

Most of the guidelines suggest induction of labor around 37–38 weeks to avoid consequences of progression of disease and a small increased risk of complications like abruptio placenta and HELLP.[1,2,9] Forty-six percent of mild GH progresses to PE and 9.6% develop severe disease.[32]

There is no consensus regarding delivery of women with mild PE between 34 weeks and 36[+6] weeks of gestation. Barton et al. observed that in a group of mild and stable hypertension, 25% delivered electively at 34–37 weeks. They also had increased CDs. These late preterm infants have increased neonatal complications and prolonged length of stay as compared to those who delivered beyond 37 weeks.[33,34] Hence, it is advisable that patients with stable mild GH should be allowed to reach 37 weeks and beyond in the absence of any sudden indication for delivery. Pregnancy can be terminated if any of the indications mentioned in Table 12.1 occur during this expectant monitoring phase.[35] Expectant monitoring runs the risk of progression to severe disease and its associated complications. Thus, if this practice is adopted, close monitoring for severity, complications and fetal well-being is required. If they are stable, pregnancy can continue until 37 weeks.[35]

There is an ongoing hypertension and PE intervention trial in the almost term patient (HYPITAT-II), a multicenter, open-label RCT to investigate whether induction of labor at gestational ages 34–37 weeks in women with GH, mild PE or deteriorating chronic hypertension will reduce maternal morbidity and/or increase neonatal morbidity.[36]

Flow chart 12.1: Management protocol for preeclampsia/gestational hypertension

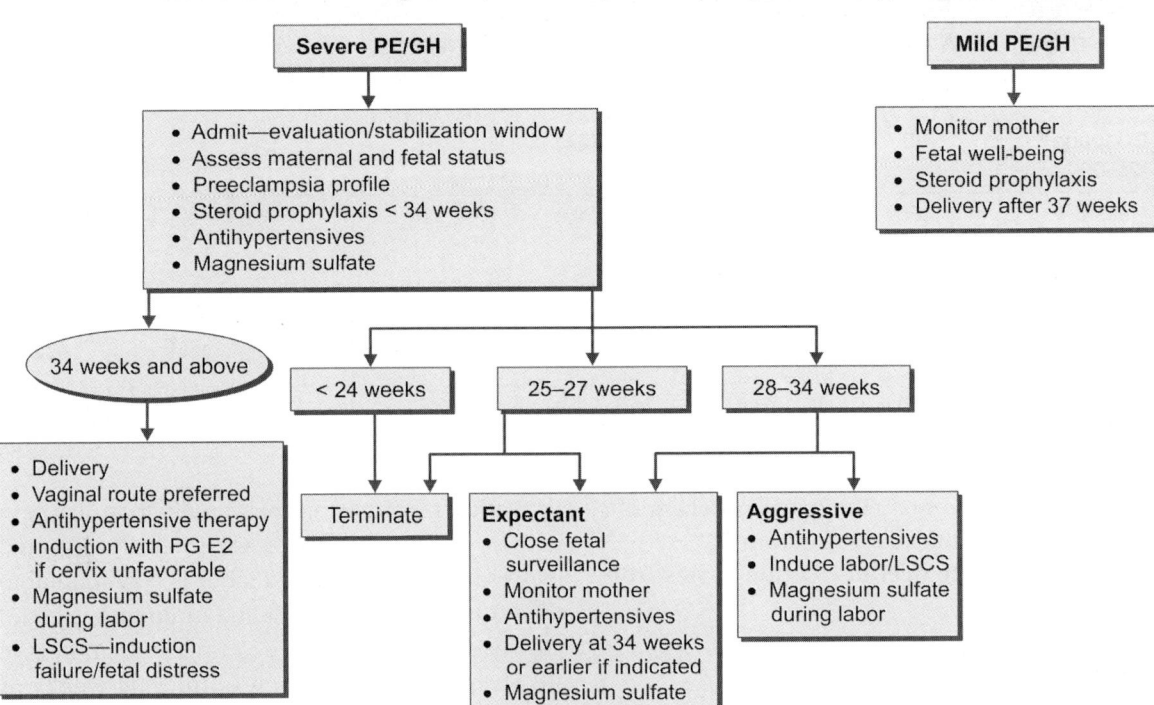

Abbreviations: PE, preeclampsia; GH, gestational hypertension; PG E2, prostaglandin E2; LSCS, lower segment Cesarean section

Summary of management protocol for hypertensive disorders is depicted in Flow chart 12.1.

ROUTE OF DELIVERY

The general dictum is to plan the delivery in the best place, by the best route, on the best day and with the best available team.[37] Team approach with obstetrician, neonatologist, anesthesiologist, midwife and a physician is ideal.

Factors to Decide Route of Delivery

- Fetal presentation
- Bishop score
- Fetal well-being
- Gestational age of the fetus
- Weight of fetus
- Presence of labor

Vaginal delivery is the option while CD is indicated for obstetric reasons.[38] There are no randomized trials to suggest the optimal route of delivery in hypertensive disorders of pregnancy. Some observational studies showed that immediate CD in severe PE did not confer any benefit to patients when compared with vaginal delivery.[39] The decision regarding route of delivery is generally made on a case-to-case basis.

Unfavorable cervix remote from term in cases of severe PE poses a dilemma. Cervical ripening is used to make it favorable.[38] Regardless of the Bishop score, induction of labor can be done and successful vaginal deliveries report range from 48% to 64% even with a Bishop score less than 2–4.[39-41]

Vaginal delivery has less morbidity compared to Cesarean and is safe provided the fetus is able to withstand labor. These patients may end up with CD for failed induction. Prolonged induction will be harmful for both mother and baby.

Response to induction is gestational age dependent with vaginal delivery being 7% (24–28 weeks), 26% (28–32 weeks) and 50% (32–34 weeks).[41] In another study, vaginal delivery was accomplished in 34% in the induced group of babies weighing less than 1,500 g. Their conclusion was that it is not harmful to induce women with low birth weight babies and that route of delivery had no effect on

Table 12.3: Route of delivery in severe preeclampsia

Author/Year	Number	Induced n	Vaginal Delivery n (%)	Emergency Cesarean n	Elective Cesarean n	Total Cesareans n (%)
Coppage[39] (2002)	93	59	37 (64)	22	34	56 (60)
Nassar[40] (1998)	306	145	70 (48)	75	161	236 (77)
Alanis[41] (2008)	491	282	151 (53.5)	131	209	340 (69)
Alexander[42] (1999)	278	145	50 (34.5)	95	133	228 (82)

the neonatal outcome.[42] The overall success rate of induction of labor may vary from 35% to 65% (Table 12.3), while overall CD rate varies from 60% to 80%.[39-41]

Cesarean Delivery

Though CD is for obstetric reasons, most of the trials have high incidence of CD (Table 12.3). Most of them are for fetal indications and it is significantly higher for fetuses with severe growth restriction (93% for ≤ 3rd percentile).[22] It is required if there is an urgency to deliver as in cases of abruptio placenta with a live baby. Regional anesthesia is preferred provided platelet counts are above 75,000/μL. Preloading prior to regional anesthesia predisposes to pulmonary edema.[5] General anesthesia causes increased BP during intubation and extubation. Most often, it may be associated with difficult or failed intubation. Parenteral labetalol is useful to attenuate the hypertensive response during intubation.

Indications for Cesarean Delivery in Hypertensive Disorders

- Fetuses less than 30 weeks with unfavorable cervix
- Severe FGR
- Absent or reversal of umbilical artery Doppler
- Failed induction
- Nonreassuring fetal status
- Associated complications with a live baby
- Pheochromocytoma
- Coarctation of aorta

Patients with gestational age less than 30 weeks with an unfavorable cervix are generally delivered by Cesarean as prolonged labor is detrimental to the fetus and the risk of failed induction is high.[3] However, many guidelines favor CD in severe PE with gestational age less than 34 weeks or 32 weeks because induction of labor is unlikely to be successful and it is done in the mother's interest to avoid prolonged induction.[37,43] Cesarean delivery is preferred in secondary hypertension due to coarctation of aorta. In pheochromocytoma, elective CD with tumor resection may be combined. Vaginal delivery is associated with catecholamine surge and related problems.

Prior to the Cesarean, platelet transfusion may be required if it is less than 50,000/μL.[16] Cesarean delivery is higher for fetuses with growth restriction.[22] Elective CD for an unfavorable cervix in severe PE less than 34 weeks accounts for nearly 33% of Cesareans. Very often CD is done for failed induction when there is failure to progress in the latent phase of labor itself. Women are not given enough time to enter active phase of labor.[40]

Induction of Labor

The earlier belief that women with PE respond better to induction is not true. A prospective study comparing induction of labor in women with and without PE showed that there is a higher risk of failure of induction and CD in PE pregnancies. Nevertheless, a significant number of women deliver vaginally.[44] The use of magnesium sulfate for seizure prophylaxis, gestational age, unfavorable cervix, higher maternal weight and parity are some of the risk factors for failed induction in PE.[45] Even when factors such as maternal age, Bishop score, gestational age and parity are matched, women with PE had longer induction delivery interval compared to non-preeclamptic group.[46] Induction of labor is successful and is safe in severe PE pregnancy greater than 28 weeks' gestation.[41] In women with PE at term, induction of labor is recommended by World Health Organization (WHO) as expectant management is associated with a substantial risk of maternal and fetal complications without much of a benefit.[47]

Evidence from randomized controlled HYPITAT trial reported that induction of labor is associated with improved maternal outcome in both GH and mild PE beyond 37 weeks of gestation (RR, 0.71; 95% CI, 0.59–0.86; $p < 0.0001$).[48] In this trial, induction of labor did not increase the rate of CD. Cesarean deliveries were less in the induced group compared to the expectant monitoring group because of decreased occurrence of maternal morbidity like severe hypertension or HELLP syndrome (19% vs. 14%; RR, 0.75; 95% CI, 0.55–1.04). This was true even for women with Bishop score less than 2. This multicenter trial included 756 women with mild GH and PE between 36 weeks and 41 weeks. Thirty percent of the expectant group progressed to severe disease. Vaginal prostaglandins (PGs) are used for cervical ripening in the presence of unfavorable cervix. A post hoc analysis of HYPITAT trial reported that mild PE and GH at term who have an unfavorable cervix benefited from labor induction as it shortens the time to delivery and risk of progression.[49] Even mild PE can deteriorate during labor. So close monitoring is required. Prolonged induction beyond 48 hours is not advisable.[3] Thus, induction beyond 37 weeks is generally not associated with increase in maternal morbidity or Cesarean rate.

Prostaglandin E2 induction of labor was successful in 75% of patients with hypertensive disorders and unfavorable cervix in a retrospective case controlled study from Israel.[50] Nevertheless, most often, preterm delivery prior to 34 weeks is achieved by Cesarean for failed induction. Fetal distress is another common indication for CD after induction of labor. Cesarean rate is high at 81% in a study when induction was tried for gestational age less than 30 weeks.[20]

Once decided, labor induction should be carried out with close monitoring of maternal and fetal status. Delivery is generally achieved within 24 hours. Serial induction must be avoided. Labor induction seems to be more successful with advancing gestational age.

ECLAMPSIA

Termination of pregnancy is the only option for eclampsia after initial stabilization, control of hypertension with antihypertensives and magnesium sulfate for control of seizures. Nevertheless, the route of delivery has been a controversy. There has been a steady rise of CD in eclampsia from 10.5% in 1995 to 49.5% in 2005.[51] Seizures may occur during labor in a severe PE or a patient may report to the labor room after onset of convulsions. If a patient is in labor, she may be allowed to progress with close monitoring of the fetus and progression of labor. Fetal heart tracing is likely to be abnormal during convulsions due to maternal hypoxemia and hypercarbia.[2] The trace may show fetal bradycardia, poor baseline variability and a compensatory tachycardia. These changes are due to decreased uteroplacental blood flow, maternal apnea and uterine contractions. The trace generally improves when the convulsions cease. Hence, it is not advisable to rush for a CD. It is better for the fetus to get resuscitated while in utero. It is inappropriate to deliver an unstable mother even in the presence of fetal distress.[37,52] If the cardiotocography (CTG) changes persist, abruption is a possibility.

Eclampsia itself is not an indication for CD. Recently an open-label RCT has compared maternal and neonatal outcomes of early Cesarean and planned vaginal delivery in eclampsia. Maternal event rate was similar in the Cesarean (10.89%) versus vaginal delivery (7.07%) (RR, 1.54; 95% CI, 0.62–3.81). Even for the neonatal events the difference was not statistically significant; although neonatal complications were marginally more in the vaginal delivery group (9.90% vs. 19.19%; RR, 0.52; 95% CI, 0.25–1.05). They concluded that early CD in eclampsia for greater than 34 weeks is not associated with better outcome.[53] Patients in labor should be monitored for progress and should be allowed to deliver by vaginal route. During labor, intensive monitoring, antihypertensive therapy and magnesium sulfate for control of seizures should continue. Pulse oximetry monitoring of oxygen saturation is useful.

However, it is believed that CD is a better option if the patient is not in labor or when remote from term with an unfavorable cervix.[37]

CHRONIC HYPERTENSION AND SUPERIMPOSED PREECLAMPSIA

In United States, a nationwide data showed a significant rise in the prevalence of chronic hypertension (from 0.01% to 1.78%) and secondary hypertension (from 0.07% to 0.24%).[54] This may be attributed to increasing age at conception, obesity and other related medical disorders. Mild essential hypertension without any organ damage is considered low risk, and may be treated like GH or mild PE with close maternal and fetal monitoring. Superimposed PE may occur here but the risk is lesser than high-risk chronic hypertension.

Essential hypertension with organ damage or secondary hypertension due to underlying disease is considered as high risk chronic hypertension and the risk of superimposed PE is 50%.[55]

Chronic hypertension with superimposed PE has worse prognosis than either of them occurring singly. Maternal mortality and morbidity is higher in superimposed PE than GH or severe PE. Perinatal mortality, preterm delivery, abruptio placenta and FGR were also believed to be higher.[56] However, recent literature reports that perinatal outcomes of superimposed PE were not different from severe PE when expectant management was adopted. Rates of abruption, stillbirth and eclampsia were not significantly different with superimposed PE and PE.[57,58]

There are no RCTs to guide time and route of delivery in superimposed PE. So the same principle as in severe PE is adopted. Expectant management in superimposed PE with close fetal and maternal surveillance was not associated with poor outcome.[57] Delivery is encouraged only when BP is not under control despite adequate antihypertensive therapy or when fetal compromise is noted during surveillance tests. If the chronic hypertension is well controlled and there is no imminent danger to the fetus, delivery

is planned only after 37 weeks. In uncomplicated chronic hypertension or GH with good control, delivery can be offered after 39 weeks.[59] As in PE, vaginal delivery is ideal but when circumstances require immediate delivery Cesarean is adopted. Higher incidence of postpartum hemorrhage and pulmonary edema has been reported in superimposed PE.[60] A population-based analysis quantified fetal and neonatal risks following induction of labor between 36 weeks and 41 weeks in women with chronic hypertension and pregnancy. Serious neonatal morbidity or mortality following induction of labor decreased five-fold from 36 weeks to 38 weeks with only minimal increase in risk of stillbirth. The optimal timing of delivery appeared to be at 38–39 weeks.[61]

MANAGEMENT OF LABOR

First Stage

- *Pain management*: Epidural analgesia is preferred because it lowers BP. It also prevents pain-induced increase in cardiac output. It decreases catecholamine release, promotes peripheral vasodilatation and improves renal perfusion. However, platelet counts should be checked before epidural analgesia.
- Close monitoring of BP, urine output and imminent symptoms/signs is essential. Even mild hypertension can progress to severe disease during labor due to increase in cardiac output and stress hormones. Blood pressure should be maintained less than 160 mm Hg systolic and less than 110 mm Hg diastolic through labor using antihypertensives.
- *Antihypertensives*: Parenteral labetalol or hydralazine has an important role in the intrapartum management of acute severe hypertension.[2]
- *Magnesium sulfate*: It is required for seizure prophylaxis during labor and 24 hours after delivery as risk of eclampsia is high.[2,37] This does not alter the length of labor.
- Partogram to monitor for progress of labor
- Continuous fetal monitoring for evidence of fetal distress
- Watch for signs of abruptio placenta
- Fluid management is important because pulmonary edema is a common complication. Fluid intake of 1 mL/kg/hour will be ideal.

Second Stage

Traditional concept of cutting the duration of second stage with assisted instrumental delivery in all hypertensive disorders is no longer true. There is no need to limit the duration of second stage routinely in women with stable mild (140/90–149/99 mm Hg) or moderate (BP 150/100–159/109 mm Hg) hypertension. This is applicable even to severe PE or hypertension if the BP is within the target range. Operative birth in second stage is reserved for women with severe hypertension whose BP has not responded to the initial treatment.[6]

Third Stage

- Oxytocin is used for active management either as 5 units intravenously or 10 units intramuscularly.[38] Ergometrine is contraindicated as it can cause severe hypertensive crisis.
- Postpartum collapse is likely even with minimum amount of blood loss. Any fall in BP after delivery does not mean resolution of the disease. Magnesium sulfate infusion should continue for 24 hours post partum. Thromboprophylaxis is essential.

■ POSTPARTUM MANAGEMENT

Though the cure for PE is delivery, 25% of women deteriorate in the early postpartum period.[38] Some of the anticipated complications in the postpartum period are:
- Eclampsia
- Pulmonary edema
- HELLP syndrome
- Thromboembolism
- Puerperal psychosis

■ INDICATIONS FOR CRITICAL CARE UNIT AND INVASIVE MONITORING

As severe preeclampsia/eclampsia patients are prone to multiorgan failure, they require intensive surveillance in critical care unit. Complications like renal failure, pulmonary edema and massive hemorrhage with coagulation failure, recurrent seizures, sepsis or pre-existing cardiac disease are indications for admission to critical care unit. Central venous pressure monitoring is not helpful.

Intra-arterial BP monitoring is useful during operative delivery.[8]

Management of delivery in hypertensive disorders requires facilities for maternal and fetal surveillance along with an experienced team and sound clinical judgment. PE at any gestation carries potential for severe risk for both baby and mother and even late-onset disease can have complications.[62] Delivery being the only curative treatment poses a dilemma for early onset disease. Expectant management is advocated to gain fetal maturity in preterm cases with severe hypertension, provided the mother is stable. It has shown to be a safe option in carefully selected cases provided intensive maternal and fetal surveillance is available. Fetal benefits and maternal risks of conservative management have to be weighed against risks and benefits of immediate delivery. Optimal timing and mode of delivery for hypertensive disorders in pregnancy has to be individualized to get the best for both mother and her neonate.

■ KEY POINTS

- In mild PE and GH, induction of labor after 37 weeks improves obstetrical outcomes.
- Expectant monitoring is preferred for mild PE between 34 weeks and 37 weeks as delivery at this gestational age will result in late preterm infants which have higher morbidity than term infants.
- In severe PE, there is an initial stabilization window period where intensive monitoring, investigations, antihypertensive therapy, seizure prophylaxis with magnesium sulfate and steroid prophylaxis is adopted prior to decision regarding delivery.
- Expectant management is possible for a selected group of patients with severe PE between 28 weeks and 34 weeks.
- In one-third of patients, aggressive management which is delivery with or without steroid prophylaxis is required.
- Expectant approach requires close monitoring of mother and fetus, an experienced team and a good NICU facility.
- Vaginal delivery is the favored route and CD is done for obstetrical reasons. Nevertheless, CD rates are high for nonreassuring fetal status and failed induction.

REFERENCES

1. Report of the National High Blood Pressure Education Program Working Group on High Blood Pressure in Pregnancy. Am J Obstet Gynecol. 2000; 183(1):S1-S22.

2. ACOG Committee on Practice Bulletins--Obstetrics. ACOG practice bulletin. Diagnosis and management of preeclampsia and eclampsia Obstet Gynecol. 2002;99(1):159-67.

3. Sibai BM. Diagnosis and management of gestational hypertension and preeclampsia. Obstet Gynecol. 2003;102(1):181-92.

4. Sibai BM. Induction of labour improves maternal outcomes compared with expectant monitoring in women with gestational hypertension or mild pre-eclampsia. Evid Based Med. 2010;15(1):11-2.

5. Duley L, Gülmezoglu AM, Hendenog-Smart DJ, et al. Magnesium sulphate and other anticonvulsants for women with pre-eclampsia. Cochrane Database Syst Rev. 2010;(11):CD000025.

6. National Institute for Health and Clinical Excellence. (2010). Hypertension in pregnancy: The management of hypertensive disorders during pregnancy. NICE clinical guideline 107. [online] Available from www.nice.org.uk/nicemedia/live/13098/50418/50418.pdf. [Accessed May, 2013].

7. Amorim MM, Santos LC, Faúndes A. Corticosteroid therapy for prevention of respiratory distress syndrome in severe preeclampsia. Am J Obstet Gynecol. 1999;180(5):1283-8.

8. Haddad B, Sibai BM. Expectant management in pregnancies with severe pre-eclampsia. Semin Perinatol. 2009;33(3):143-51.

9. Lowe SA, Brown MA, Dekker GA, et al. Guidelines for the management of hypertensive disorders of pregnancy 2008. Aust N Z J Obstet Gynaecol. 2009;49(3):242-6.

10. Hall DR, Grové D, Carstens E. Early pre-eclampsia: what proportion of women qualify for expectant management and if not, why not? Eur J Obstet Gynecol Reprod Biol. 2006;128(1-2):169-74.

11. Visser W, Wallenburg HC. Temporising management of severe pre-eclampsia with and without the HELLP syndrome. Br J Obstet Gynaecol. 1995;102(2):111-7.

12. Haddad B, Kayem G, Deis S, et al. Are perinatal and maternal outcomes different during expectant management of severe preeclampsia in the presence of intrauterine growth restriction? Am J Obstet Gynecol. 2007;196(3):237.e1-5.

13. Haddad B, Sibai BM. Expectant management of severe preeclampsia: proper candidates and pregnancy outcome. Clin Obstet Gynecol. 2005; 48(2):430-40.

14. Ganzevoort W, Sibai BM. Temporising versus interventionist management (preterm and at term). Best Pract Res Clin Obstet Gynaecol. 2011;25(4):463-76.

15. Oettle C, Hall D, Roux A, et al. Early onset severe pre-eclampsia: expectant management at a secondary hospital in close association with a tertiary institution. BJOG. 2005;112(1):84-8.

16. Abramovici D, Mattar F, Sibai BM. Conservative management of severe preeclampsia contemporary. Obstet Gynecol. 1998;43:80-105.

17. Schiff E, Friedman SA, Sibai BM. Conservative management of severe preeclampsia remote from term. Obstet Gynecol. 1994;84(4):626-30.

18. Odendaal HJ, Pattinson RC, Bam R, et al. Aggressive or expectant management for patients with severe preeclampsia between 28-34 weeks' of gestation: a randomized controlled trial. Obstet Gynecol. 1990;76(6):1070-5.

19. Sibai BM, Mercer BM, Schiff E, et al. Aggressive versus expectant management of severe preeclampsia at 28 to 32 weeks' gestation: a randomized controlled trial. Am J Obstet Gynecol. 1994;171(3):818-22.

20. Hall DR, Odendaal HJ, Kirsten GF, et al. Expectant management of early onset, severe pre-eclampsia: perinatal outcome. BJOG. 2000;107(10):1258-64.

21. Haddad B, Deis S, Goffinet F, et al. Maternal and perinatal outcomes during expectant management of 239 severe preeclamptic women between 24 and 33 weeks' gestation. Am J Obstet Gynecol. 2004; 190(6):1590-5.

22. Shear RM, Rinfret D, Leduc L. Should we offer expectant management in cases of severe preterm preeclampsia with fetal growth restriction? Am J Obstet Gynecol. 2005;192(4):1119-25.

23. Sibai BM, Barton JR. Expectant management of severe preeclampsia remote from term: patient selection, treatment, and delivery indications. Am J Obstet Gynecol. 2007;196(6):514.e1-9.

24. Witlin AG, Saade GR, Mattar F, et al. Predictors of neonatal outcome in women with severe pre-eclampsia or eclampsia between 24 and 33 weeks' gestation. Am J Obstet Gynecol. 2000;182(3):607-11.

25. Geerts L, Odendaal HJ. Severe early onset pre-eclampsia: prognostic value of ultrasound and Doppler assessment. J Perinatol. 2007;27(6):335-42.

26. Chammas MF, Nguyen TM, Li MA, et al. Expectant management of severe preterm preeclampsia: is intrauterine growth restriction an indication for immediate delivery? Am J Obstet Gynecol. 2000;183(4):853-8.

27. Magee LA, Yong PJ, Espinosa V, et al. Expectant management of severe preeclampsia remote from term: a structured systematic review. Hypertens Pregnancy. 2009;28(3):312-47.

28. Gaugler-Senden IP, Huijssoon AG, Visser W, et al. Maternal and perinatal outcome of preeclampsia with an onset before 24 weeks' gestation. Audit in a

tertiary referral center. Eur J Obstet Gynecol Reprod Biol. 2006;128(1-2):216-21.

29. Budden A, Wilkinson L, Buksh MJ, et al. Pregnancy outcome in women presenting with pre-eclampsia at less than 25 weeks gestation. Aust N Z J Obstet Gynecol. 2006;46(5):407-12.

30. Bombrys AE, Barton JR, Nowacki EA, et al. Expectant management of severe preeclampsia at less than 27 weeks' gestation: maternal and perinatal outcomes according to gestational age by weeks at onset of expectant management. Am J Obstet Gynecol. 2008;199(3):247.e1-6.

31. Churchill D, Duley L. Interventionist versus expectant care for severe pre-eclampsia before term. Cochrane Database Syst Rev. 2002;(3):CD003106.

32. Barton JR, O'brien JM, Bergauer NK, et al. Mild gestational hypertension remote from term: progression and outcome. Am J Obstet Gynecol. 2001; 184(5):979-83.

33. Barton JR, Barton LA, Istwan NB, et al. Elective delivery at $34^0(/)^7$ to $36^6(/)^7$ weeks' gestation and its impact on neonatal outcomes in women with stable mild gestational hypertension. Am J Obstet Gynecol. 2011;204(1):44.e1-5.

34. Spong CY, Mercer BM, D'alton M, et al. Timing of indicated late-preterm and early-term birth. Obstet Gynecol. 2011;118(2 Pt 1):323-33.

35. Sibai BM. Management of late preterm and early-term pregnancies complicated by mild gestational hypertension/pre-eclampsia. Semin Perinatol. 2011;35(5):292-6.

36. Langenveld J, Broekhuijsen K, van Barren GV, et al. (2011). Induction of labor versus expectant monitoring for gestational hypertension or mild pre-eclampsia between 34 and 37 weeks' gestation (HYPITAT-II): a multicentre, open-label randomized controlled trial. [online] Available from www.biomedcentral.com/1471-2393/11/50. [Accessed May, 2013].

37. Tuffnell DJ, Shennan AH, Waugh JJ, et al. (2006). The management of severe preeclampsia/eclampsia. Royal College of Obstetricians and Gynaecologists Guideline No 10 (A). [online] Available from www.neonatalformulary.com/pdfs/uk_guidelines/MAGNESIUM-SULPHATE-RCOG_preeclampsia_guideline.pdf. [Accessed May, 2013].

38. Magee LA, Helewa M, Moutquin JM, et al. Diagnosis, evaluation, and management of the hypertensive disorders of pregnancy. J Obstet Gynaecol Can. 2008;30(3 Suppl):S1-48.

39. Coppage KH, Polzin WJ. Severe preeclampsia and delivery outcomes: is immediate cesarean delivery beneficial? Am J Obstet Gynecol. 2002;186(5):921-3.

40. Nassar AH, Adra AM, Chakhtoura N, et al. Severe preeclampsia remote from term: labor induction or elective cesarean delivery? Am J Obstet Gynecol. 1998;179(5):1210-3.

41. Alanis MC, Robinson CJ, Hulsey TC, et al. Early-onset severe preeclampsia: induction of labor vs elective cesarean delivery and neonatal outcomes. Am J Obstet Gynecol. 2008;199(3):262.e1-6.

42. Alexander JM, Bloom SL, McIntire DD, et al. Severe preeclampsia and the very low birth weight infant: is induction of labor harmful? Obstet Gynecol. 1999;93(4):485-8.

43. Institute of Obstetricians and Gynecologists, Royal College of Physicians of Ireland, Clinical Strategy and Programmes Directorate, Health Service Executive. (2011). The Diagnosis and Management of Pre-eclampsia and Eclampsia. Clinical Practice Guideline No 3. Version 1.0. [online] Available from www.rcpi.ie/content/docs/000001/649_5_media.pdf. [Accessed May, 2013].

44. Xenakis EM, Piper JM, Field N, et al. Preeclampsia: is induction of labor more successful? Obstet Gynecol. 1997;89(4):600-3.

45. Park KH, Cho YK, Lee CM, et al. Effect of pre-eclampsia, magnesium sulfate prophylaxis, and maternal weight on labor induction: a retrospective analysis. Gynecol Obstet Invest. 2006;61(1):40-4.

46. Griffiths AN, Hikary N, Sizer AR. Induction to delivery time interval in patients with and without preeclampsia: a retrospective analysis. Acta Obstet Gynecol Scand. 2002;81(9):867-9.

47. World Health Organization. (2012). WHO recommendations for prevention and treatment of pre-eclampsia and eclampsia. [online] Available from www.who.int/reproductivehealth/publications/maternal_perinatal_health/9789241548335/en/. [Accessed May, 2013].

48. Koopmans CM, Bijlenga D, Groen H, et al. Induction of labour versus expectant monitoring for gestational hypertension or mild pre-eclampsia after 36 weeks' gestation (HYPITAT): a multicentre, open-label randomised controlled trial. Lancet. 2009;374(9694):979-88.

49. Tajik P, van der Tuuk K, Koopmans CM, et al. Should cervical favourability play a role in the decision for labor induction in gestational hypertension or mild pre-eclampsia at term? An exploratory analysis of the HYPITAT trial. BJOG. 2012;119(9):1123-30.

50. Ben-Haroush A, Yogev Y, Glickman H, et al. Mode of delivery in pregnant women with hypertensive disorders and unfavorable cervix following induction of labor with vaginal application of prostaglandin E. Acta Obstet Gynecol Scand. 2005; 84(7):665-71.

51. Kamilya G, Bharracharyya SK, Mukherji J. Changing trends in the management of eclampsia from a teaching hospital. J Indian Med Assoc. 2005;103(3):132, 134-5.

52. Sibai BM. Diagnosis, prevention, and management of eclampsia. Obstet Gynecol. 2005;105(2):402-10.

53. Seal SL, Ghosh D, Kamilya G, et al. Does route of delivery affect maternal and perinatal outcome in women with eclampsia? A randomized controlled pilot study. Am J Obstet Gynecol. 2012;206(6):484.e1-7.

54. Bateman BT, Bansil P, Hernandez-Diaz S, et al. Prevalence, trends, and outcomes of chronic hypertension: a nationwide sample of delivery admissions. Am J Obstet Gynecol. 2012;206(2):134.e1-8.

55. Sibai BM. Chronic hypertension in pregnancy. Obstet Gynecol. 2002;100(2):369-77.

56. Chronic hypertension in pregnancy. ACOG Practice Bulletin No 29. Obstet Gynecol. 2001;98:177-85.

57. Vigil-De Gracia P, Montufar-Rueda C, Ruiz J. Expectant management of severe preeclampsia and preeclampsia superimposed on chronic hypertension between 24 and 34 weeks' gestation. Eur J Obstet Gynecol Reprod Biol. 2003;107(1):24-7.

58. Tuuli MG, Rampersad R, Stamilio D, et al. Perinatal outcomes in women with preeclampsia and superimposed preeclampsia: do they differ? Am J Obstet Gynecol. 2011;204(6):508.e1-7.

59. Chandiramani M, Joash K, Shennan AH. Options and decision-making: hypertensive disorders of pregnancy. Future Cardiol. 2010;6(4):535-46.

60. Samuel A, Lin C, Parviainen K, et al. Expectant management of preeclampsia superimposed on chronic hypertension. J Matern Fetal Neonatal Med. 2011;24(7):907-11.

61. Hutcheon J, Lisonkova S, Magee L, et al. Optimal timing of delivery in pregnancies with pre-existing hypertension. BJOG. 2011;118(1):49-54.

62. Pettit F, Brown MA. The management of pre-eclampsia: what we think we know. Eur J Obstet Gynecol Reprod Biol. 2012;160(1):6-12.

13 Anesthetic Considerations for Hypertensive Disease in Pregnancy

Anthony Addei

INTRODUCTION

Hypertensive disease in pregnancy is a leading cause of maternal morbidity and mortality worldwide and it remains one of the leading causes of maternal mortality in the UK. In the 2006–2008 Center for Maternal and Child Enquiries (CMACE) report there were 19 deaths directly attributed to eclampsia or preeclampsia, an increase from the previous report. Substandard care could be demonstrated in the majority of cases.[1]

Women with severe disease need effective team care based on clear communication and common understanding. A team-based approach with early consultant obstetric, neonatal and anesthetic involvement and the engagement of intensive care specialists where appropriate should optimize maternal and fetal outcomes.

DEFINITIONS AND CLASSIFICATION

The use of multiple and conflicting systems to classify the hypertensive disorders of pregnancy not only leads to confusion but also makes comparison of clinical studies difficult. The most important consideration is to distinguish hypertension that predates pregnancy from preeclampsia (Tables 13.1 and 13.2).[2-4]

Preeclampsia

A multisystem disorder unique to human pregnancy characterized by hypertension and involvement of one or more other organ systems and/or the fetus.

Table 13.1: Classification of hypertension in pregnancy

	Hypertension	Proteinuria	Onset
Chronic hypertension	Y	N	Before 20 weeks
Gestational hypertension	Y	N	After 20 weeks
Preeclampsia	Y	Y	After 20 weeks
Preeclampsia superimposed on chronic hypertension	Y	N to Y	Typically third trimester proteinuria

Table 13.2: Severity of hypertension

	Mild (mm Hg)	Moderate (mm Hg)	Severe (mm Hg)
Systolic blood pressure	140–149	150–159	> 160
Diastolic blood pressure	90–99	100–109	> 110

Severe Preeclampsia

Severe preeclampsia is defined as preeclampsia with severe hypertension and/or with symptom and/or biochemical and/or hematological impairments.

Eclampsia

A convulsive condition associated with preeclampsia.

Hemolysis, Elevated Liver Enzymes and Low Platelet Count (HELLP) Syndrome

A variant of severe preeclampsia where hypertension is less marked but there is severe involvement of both the liver and the coagulation system.[5]

▓ EFFECT OF PREECLAMPSIA ON ORGAN SYSTEMS AND ANESTHETIC IMPLICATIONS

Central Nervous System

Central nervous system manifestations include cerebral vasospasm, thrombosis, cerebral edema, severe headache, visual disturbances, hyperexcitability, hyperreflexia and eclampsia. Eclampsia is a marker for severe disease and the seizures also carry intrinsic risks associated with loss of the airway, aspiration, hypoxia and brain damage.[1] The administration of magnesium sulfate for seizure prophylaxis may also contribute to depressed levels of consciousness.

Respiratory System

Airway

Marked pharyngolaryngeal edema because of mucosal capillary engorgement may make intubation of the airway difficult or impossible. Airway obstruction may follow extubation because of subglottic edema.

Lungs

Pulmonary edema results in respiratory distress and hypoxemia. The most common reasons for the development of pulmonary edema are decreased colloid osmotic pressure, elevated left ventricular filling pressures (as reflected by the pulmonary artery wedge pressure) and increased capillary permeability.[6]

Generally, it is noted that older patients, multigravidas and those patients with underlying chronic hypertension are more likely to develop pulmonary edema associated with preeclampsia. The reported incidence is around 2.9% with 70% of these developing in the postpartum period.[7]

The reduction of colloid osmotic pressure, alteration of capillary membrane permeability and elevated pulmonary vascular hydrostatic pressure may lead to extravasation of fluid into the pulmonary interstitium and alveolar spaces. It is thought that although the causes of pulmonary edema in preeclampsia are multifactorial, the nonhydrostatic elements play a more important role in preeclampsia.

Some patients with pulmonary edema require mechanical ventilation.

Cardiovascular System

Hypertension is the defining clinical feature but the hemodynamic explanation for hypertension in preeclampsia is still controversial. Hypertension is determined by cardiac output (CO) and systemic vascular resistance. Hypertension in untreated preeclampsia is due to increased CO and mild vasoconstriction, with increased inotropy and reduced diastolic function.[8] The 2006–2008 CMACE report noted that inadequate treatment of systolic hypertension in several women resulted in a fatal intracranial hemorrhage. Systolic hypertension was also a key factor in most of the deaths from aortic dissection.

Hepatic System

Hemolysis, elevated liver enzymes, low platelets syndrome may present before the other symptoms of preeclampsia. It has a poor prognosis and often requires immediate delivery of the baby to prevent rapid deterioration of maternal liver function. In addition to the usual complications of severe preeclampsia there is a risk of liver failure and bleeding. This may have implications for regional analgesia/anesthesia.

Epigastric pain in the second half of pregnancy should be considered to be the result of preeclampsia until proven otherwise.[1]

Renal System

Oliguria is the main manifestation of renal dysfunction in preeclampsia. Acute renal failure is relatively uncommon in preeclampsia. Acute tubular necrosis is the most common cause of reversible renal failure, while cortical necrosis, fortunately quite rare, causes permanent renal failure. Precipitating factors include abruption, coagulopathy, hemorrhage and severe hypotension.[9]

Hematologic System

Thrombocytopenia is common in preeclampsia and downward trends in platelet counts indicate increasing disease severity. HELLP syndrome results in low platelets and deranged clotting from impaired liver function. This may have implications for regional analgesia/anesthesia.

Uteroplacental System

Uteroplacental perfusion is decreased in preeclampsia. In contrast to normal pregnancy, downstream resistance in the uteroplacental bed increases. This leads to increases in the systolic/diastolic ratio. These changes are commonly seen in association with intrauterine growth restriction (IUGR) and the fetus of a preeclamptic woman must be assumed to be at risk for compromise. For the baby, risks include fetal distress due to vasoconstriction reducing the blood supply across the placenta and placental abruption (separation of the placenta from the wall of the womb before birth).

◼ ANTENATAL MANAGEMENT

Whenever possible, an anesthetist should be informed about a woman with severe preeclampsia well in advance of labor or operative delivery, because appropriate anesthetic management is associated with a reduction in both fetal and maternal morbidity.[10] Relevant issues include high dependency care, monitoring, blood pressure (BP) control, fluid management, eclampsia prophylaxis and planning of analgesia or anesthesia.[11-14]

High Dependency Care

A subgroup of women with preeclampsia develops severe disease and may require critical care to manage complications including severe hypertension, acute kidney injury, liver dysfunction, pulmonary edema and intracranial hemorrhage. Critical care is a crucial part of the care of these women, both in the management after life-threatening events and in optimizing management of women at the highest risk of developing complications. It is important to have an understanding of what critical care can offer, and how best to utilize these services in a timely fashion when such a patient becomes unwell. The goal of critical care management is to correct abnormal physiology whilst the underlying disease process is treated. Early warning scores modified for obstetrics are useful to detect clinical deterioration.[15]

Monitoring

Routine monitoring should include noninvasive systemic arterial BP and heart rate, oxygen saturation, urinary output and tococardiography. Some automated BP monitoring systems systematically underestimate systolic pressure in preeclampsia.[16-18] Direct intra-arterial BP monitoring is often useful, including during anesthesia and operative delivery. However, establishing an arterial line should not delay treatment for acute severe hypertension. Central venous pressure correlates poorly with pulmonary capillary wedge pressure and although it may provide trend monitoring, it is infrequently used to complement clinical indicators of intravascular volume. Some recommend pulmonary artery catheters for assessment of left ventricular preload but they can cause serious complications and are not of proven outcome benefit in preeclampsia.[19] Cardiac output monitoring provides valuable information about the patient's hemodynamic status and may be useful in patients with complicated severe preeclampsia. Arterial waveform analysis is a minimally invasive technique for measuring CO whilst transthoracic echocardiography and suprasternal aortic Doppler are noninvasive methods for measuring CO.

Blood Pressure Control

Effective and safe control of severe hypertension is the most important aspect of critical care management because the main cause of maternal death is the consequence of poorly controlled hypertension. The BP must be adequately controlled before inducing anesthesia for cesarean section. The choice of antihypertensive treatment in severe hypertension in the critical care setting has evolved historically rather than scientifically. There is no clear evidence that one antihypertensive is preferable to the others for improving outcome for women with very high BP during pregnancy and their babies.[20] The commonly used antihypertensives are labetalol (oral or intravenous), hydralazine (intravenous) and nifedipine (oral). A precipitous drop in BP may occur with any antihypertensive agent used to treat the severe hypertension of preeclampsia. Response to treatment should therefore be monitored to assess the fall in BP, identify adverse effects for both the woman and the fetus and treatment should be modified according to response.

Labetalol is a combined alpha (α) and beta (β)-adrenergic blocking agent. It may cause neonatal bradycardia and should be avoided in women with asthma or heart failure.

Nifedipine is a calcium channel blocker that blocks the entry of calcium ions through the L-type channels. This relaxes arterial smooth muscle. Caution is required with concomitant use of magnesium sulfate as this combination can lead to hypotension and potentiation of neuromuscular blockade.

Hydralazine is a hydrazinophtalazine. It acts through the activation of guanylate cyclase and increase in intracellular cyclic GMP leading to a decrease in intracellular calcium. It is a direct acting smooth muscle relaxant of arteries and arterioles, causing peripheral vasodilation and decreasing peripheral vascular resistance. These actions decrease BP and increase heart rate, stroke volume and CO. Hydralazine has side effects of headache, flushing, light head, nausea and palpitations; these are similar to symptoms of worsening preeclampsia and so may make the clinical management more difficult. Consider giving 250–500 mL crystalloid fluid bolus before or at the same time as the first dose of intravenous hydralazine in the antenatal period.

In the rare event when intravenous labetalol or hydralazine or both fail to relieve acute onset severe hypertension, the anesthetists and critical care doctors should be involved. Other drug options to consider would be glyceryl trinitrate and sodium nitroprusside. These should be reserved for extreme emergencies and used for the shortest amount of time possible. Sodium nitroprusside may cause cyanide and thiocynate toxicity in the mother and fetus or newborn and increase intracranial pressure with the potential worsening of vertebral edema in the mother.

Fluid Management

Fluid management is a challenging area in pre-eclampsia and there is no clear evidence regarding optimal type or volume of fluid. The aim of fluid therapy is to maintain organ perfusion without causing acute pulmonary edema in the setting of vasoconstriction, endothelial dysfunction and in some parturients severe left ventricular diastolic dysfunction.[21-26] There are generally three groups of oliguria in preeclamptic patients. The first group is found to have low pulmonary capillary wedge pressure (PCWP), hyperdynamic left ventricular function and mild to moderately increased systemic vascular resistance (SVR). These patients respond to further volume replacement and the oliguria is felt to be due to intravascular volume depletion. The second group of oliguric patients has normal or increased PCWP, normal CO and normal SVR accompanied by intense urine concentration. It is thought that the pathological basis in this case is intrinsic renal artery spasm out of proportion to the degree of generalized systemic vasospasm. Low-dose vasodilators such as dopamine have been described to raise the urine output in the group of preeclamptic women. The final group of oliguric patients has markedly elevated PCWP and SVR with depressed ventricular function. In many cases, this is accompanied by incipient pulmonary edema with fluid accumulation in the pulmonary interstitium. This is generally thought to be due to intense systemic vasospasm and the management would be fluid restriction and aggressive after-load reduction.[9,19]

Intravenous fluid should be administered incrementally in small volumes (e.g. crystalloid 250 mL) with monitoring of maternal hemodynamics, urine output and fetal heart rate, because fluid overload contributes to maternal mortality from pulmonary edema and adult respiratory distress syndrome. Particular caution is necessary in women with oliguria, renal impairment or pulmonary edema, in whom the left ventricle may adapt less well to volume load. Fluid loading is not necessary before regional analgesia during labor when low-dose local anesthetic and opioid methods are used.

Eclampsia Prophylaxis

If a woman in a critical care setting has severe hypertension or severe preeclampsia or previously had an eclamptic fit, she should be given intravenous magnesium sulfate. Consider giving intravenous magnesium sulfate to women with severe preeclampsia who are in a critical care setting if birth is planned within 24 hours.

Use the Collaborative Eclampsia Trial regimen for administration of magnesium sulfate:

- Loading dose of 4 g should be given intravenously over 5 minutes, followed by an infusion of 1 g/hour maintained for 24 hours.
- Recurrent seizures should be treated with a further dose of 2–4 g given over 5 minutes.

It is recommended that diazepam, phenytoin or lytic cocktail should not be used as an alternative to magnesium sulfate in women with eclampsia.[27-32]

Analgesia and Anesthesia

Labor is an intense and painful experience for most women. Painful labor produces several adverse changes in maternal physiology and biochemistry including surges in BP during labor.[33]

Labor Analgesia

Regional analgesia using low-dose epidural analgesia or combined spinal epidural analgesia is a useful adjunct to antihypertensive therapy for BP control. It provides superior pain relief when compared to systemic or inhalational analgesia and prevents further surges in BP associated with autonomic activity. Epidural analgesia promotes uteroplacental blood flow and results in improved umbilical blood gases. It can be readily extended to provide regional anesthesia for instrumental delivery or cesarean section.[34-36]

Contraindications to regional blocks include severe thrombocytopenia and coagulopathy which may be present in a subgroup of women. A recent platelet count should be available and for those with severe disease, repeated every 6 hours. If the platelet count falls below $100 \times 10^9/L$,

clotting studies should be performed. If the platelet count is more than $75 \times 10^9/L$ evidence from thromboelastograph studies suggests that spinal anesthesia is safe. The absolute number and rate of decline guides the anesthetist to the risk of spinal hematoma. If the total platelet count is below $75 \times 10^9/L$ or the number has dropped by more than $50 \times 10^9/L$ in the previous 12 hours, many anesthetists would avoid performing a regional block. The risks and benefits should be assessed on an individual basis and senior clinicians should be involved.[37-39]

Remifentanil has superseded meperidine and fentanyl as the opioid of choice for intravenous analgesia if epidural analgesia is unavailable or contraindicated. Remifentanil is a synthetic opioid with direct agonist action specifically on mu-opioid receptors. Its rapid hydrolysis by nonspecific blood and tissue esterases to an inactive metabolite results in a very short duration of action. The metabolism of remifentanil is independent of renal and hepatic function and there is no accumulation during repeat bolus injection. Placental transfer of remifentanil does occur but in the neonate it appears to be rapidly metabolized, redistributed, or both.[40] Remifentanil is set up via a pump as patient controlled analgesia by an anesthetist.

Anesthesia for Operative Interventions

Early anticipation and preoperative preparation reduces the risk of anesthesia in women with preeclampsia. BP control, fluid management, eclampsia prophylaxis and in utero resuscitation are important in stabilizing the patient and should be instituted as soon as possible as part of the preparation for anesthesia and surgery to avoid causing unnecessary delay.

Epidural, spinal, combined spinal epidural and general anesthesia (GA) techniques have all been used successfully to manage patients with severe preeclampsia. The decision whether to use regional or GA is based both on the severity of preeclampsia and the urgency of delivery. Regional anesthesia is preferred to GA for cesarean section, especially as airway problems including laryngeal edema may be increased. However, well-conducted GA is also suitable and may be indicated in the presence of severe fetal compromise; pulmonary edema; hemodynamic instability; epidural, subdural and spinal hematoma risk (e.g. coagulopathy and severe thrombocytopenia); or after eclampsia where altered consciousness or neurological deficit persists. Emergency cesarean section is associated with increased maternal morbidity, so early anesthetic notification by the obstetrician and in utero resuscitation provide additional time for assessment, planning and establishment of regional anesthesia.[41-47] In the presence of severe preeclampsia, when a well-functioning epidural catheter is in situ, GA is achieved only marginally more rapidly than conversion to epidural anesthesia.[48]

Drugs that are best avoided in severe preeclampsia include ergometrine, ketamine (hypertension), and the nonsteroidal anti-inflammatory drugs (NSAIDs) and cyclooxygenase-2 (COX-2) specific inhibitors (impaired renal function and hypertension). Oxytocin should be given slowly in small doses to minimize its significant hemodynamic effects.

General anesthesia: Preoperative assessment should be as thorough as time permits. Prophylaxis against pulmonary aspiration is recommended using clear antacid and ranitidine, with or without metoclopramide. Ensure left uterine displacement with a pelvic displacement wedge or table tilt to minimize aortocaval compression. Marked pharyngolaryngeal edema may make laryngoscopy and intubation of the airway difficult. Optimizing the initial intubating conditions is preferable in attempting to reposition the patient when intubation and ventilation attempts are hampered by poor positioning. Skilled anesthetic assistance and equipment to manage difficult intubation is mandatory. Laryngoscopy and tracheal intubation present a particularly dangerous time for the preeclamptic woman, especially if the intracranial pressure is elevated or the BP is inadequately controlled. The transient but severe hypertension that usually accompanies intubation can cause myocardial ischemia, cerebral hemorrhage or pulmonary edema and may result in maternal death.[43,44,49]

Attenuation of pressor responses at general anesthesia for cesarean section: Attenuation of this pressor response is best achieved with additional induction drugs. Supplementary doses of induction agents, short-acting opiates (e.g. remifentanil, alfentanil and fentanyl), local anesthetics (e.g. lidocaine), magnesium sulfate, β-blockers (e.g. esmolol) and vasodilators (e.g. hydralazine, glyceryl trinitrate, sodium nitroprusside and diazoxide) have all been used successfully but no method guarantees the complete absence of pressor responses at doses free of side effects. Alfentanil and more recently remifentanil are the more widely used drugs in the UK. Neuromuscular block must always be monitored closely after intravenous magnesium administration. The hypertensive response may also occur at extubation and should be controlled.[50-57]

Regional anesthesia: All the regional anesthetic techniques (spinal, epidural or combined spinal-epidural) appear safe provided meticulous attention is paid to fluid management, preventing aortocaval compression and dealing with hypotension.

Compared with healthy pregnant women, matched for gestational age, women with untreated preeclampsia have increased cardiac output as well as increased entropy and mild vasoconstriction, with reduced diastolic function. Cardiac output is well maintained and regional anesthesia is associated with less hypotension and lower vasopressor requirements than among healthy parturients. Combined spinal-epidural anesthesia appears to offer further advantages in specific cases. The preferred vasoconstrictor in preeclampsia has yet to be determined. Treatment or prevention of hypotension with drugs, such as phenylephrine or metaraminol, is effective and appears safe if used with caution in preeclamptic women. Women with relatively low platelet counts or impaired clotting should be assessed on an individual basis (considering patient risks, coagulation tests and thromboelastography or platelet function if available) and risk reduction strategies (experienced anesthetist, single-shot spinal anesthesia or flexible tip epidural catheter) should be used.[58-63]

■ POSTPARTUM MANAGEMENT

Women with severe preeclampsia remain unwell after delivery and require close monitoring. They should be cared for in an appropriate environment; usually in a level 2 or sometimes level 3 care setting. Antenatal hypertension may persist in the postpartum period and should be treated. The risk of pulmonary edema is high in the early postpartum period when fluid is mobilized. This may be further complicated by overzealous fluid administration to address the oliguria that may be associated with preeclampsia, or by prolonged infusion of oxytocin to augment labor. Such patients may require ventilatory support (either noninvasive or invasive) if significant respiratory compromise persists despite pharmacological therapy. Intravenous glyceryl trinitrate may be of benefit if hypertension also requires treatment. The appropriate fluid management in the setting of major hemorrhage and pulmonary edema is challenging and requires very careful fluid balance.

There is usually a further reduction in the platelet count in women with HELLP syndrome. These women can also develop hematoma of the liver and capsular rupture, acidosis and disseminated intravascular coagulation. The risk of eclampsia is highest in the postpartum period. Magnesium sulfate seizure prophylaxis is usually continued for 24 hours after delivery. Up to 10% of women develop repeated seizures despite magnesium sulfate administration, and if repeated boluses of magnesium fail to control seizures, intravenous phenytoin or diazepam may be used. Seizures refractory to treatment require sedation and intubation. Typical anesthetic agents used in this setting include thiopentone, propofol and midazolam, which have anticonvulsant properties.

The highest risk period for venous thromboembolism in obstetric patients is in the first 6 weeks postpartum, so the appropriate dose of low molecular weight heparin should be used unless clearly contraindicated. Consideration should be given to the timing of anticoagulants in relation to neuraxial anesthesia.

▓ REFERENCES

1. Lewis G. Saving mothers' lives: reviewing maternal deaths to make motherhood safer-2006–2008. The Eighth Report of the Confidential Enquiries into Maternal Deaths in the United Kingdom. Br J Obstet Gynecol. 2011;118 (Suppl. 1):1-203.
2. National High Blood Pressure Education Program Working Group on High Blood Pressure in Pregnancy. Report of the national high blood pressure education program working group on high blood pressure in pregnancy. Am J Obstet Gynecol. 2000; 183:S1-S22.
3. ACOG practice bulletin. Diagnosis and management of preeclampsia and eclampsia. Obstet Gynecol. 2002;99:159-67.
4. Sibai BM. Diagnosis and management of gestational hypertension and preeclampsia. Obstet Gynecol. 2003;102:181-92.
5. Brown MA, Lindheimer MD, de Swiet M, et al. The classification and diagnosis of the hypertensive disorders of pregnancy: statement from the International Society for the Study of Hypertension in Pregnancy (ISSHP). Hypertension in Pregnancy. 2001;20(1):IX-XIV.
6. Benedetti TJ, Kates R, Williams V. Hemodynamic observations in severe preeclampsia complicated by pulmonary edema. Am J Obstet Gynecol. 1985; 152:330-4.
7. Sibai BM, Mabie BC, Harvey CJ, et al. Pulmonary edema in severe preeclampsia-eclampsia: analysis of thirty-seven consecutive cases. Am J Obstet Gynecol. 1987;156:1174-9.
8. Dennis AT, Castro J, Carr C, et al. Hemodynamics in women with untreated pre-eclampsia. Anesthesia. 2012;67:646-59.
9. Deering SH, Seiken GL. Acute renal failure. In: Belfort MA, Saade G, Foley MR, Phelan JP, Dildy GA (Eds). Critical Care Obstetrics, 5th edition. Oxford: Wiley-Blackwell; 2010. pp. 376-84.
10. Gatt S. Clinical management of established pre-eclampsia/gestational hypertension perspectives of the midwife, neonatologist and anesthetist. In: Brown M (Ed). Bailliere's Clinical Obstetrics and Gynecology, Pregnancy and Hypertension. London: Tindall; 1999. pp. 95-105.
11. Mortl MG, Schneider MC. Key issues in assessing, managing and treating patients presenting with severe preeclampsia. Int J Obstet Anesth. 2000;9: 39-44.
12. Royal College of Obstetricians and Gynecologists Guidelines. (2003). Preeclampsia study group statement. [online] Available from www.rcog.org. uk/index.asp. [Accessed Sept 2003].
13. Dyer RA, Piercy JL, Reed AR. The role of the anesthetist in the management of the pre-eclamptic patient. Curr Opin Anesthesiol. 2007;20:168-74.
14. Engelhardt T, MacLennan FM. Fluid management in pre-eclampsia. Int J Obstet Anesth. 1999;8:253-9.
15. Price LC, Slack A, Nelson-Piercy C. Aims of obstetric critical care management. Best Pract Res Clin Obstet Gynaecol 2008; 22:775-99.
16. Brown MA, Robinson A, Buddle ML. Accuracy of automated blood pressure recorders in pregnancy. Aust N Z J Obstet Gynaecol. 1998;38:262-5.
17. Gupta M, Shennan AH, Halligan A, et al. Accuracy of oscillometric blood pressure monitoring in pregnancy and pre-eclampsia. Br J Obstet Gynecol. 1997;104:350-55.

18. Pickering TG, Hall JE, Appel LJ, et al. Recommendations for blood pressure measurement in humans and experimental animals: part 1: blood pressure measurement in humans: a statement for professionals from the Subcommittee of Professional and Public Education of the American Heart Association Council on High Blood Pressure Research. Hypertension. 2005;45:142-61.

19. Li YH, Novikova N. Pulmonary artery flow catheters for directing management in pre-eclampsia. Cochrane Database Syst Rev. 2012;6:CD008882. doi: 10.1002/14651858.CD008882.pub2.

20. Duley L, Henderson-Smart DJ, Meher S. Drugs for treatment of very high blood pressure during pregnancy. Cochrane Database Syst Rev. 2006; (3):CD001449.

21. Duley L, Williams J, Henderson-Smart DJ. Plasma volume expansion for treatment of pre-eclampsia. Cochrane Database Syst Rev. 1999;4:CD001805.

22. Ganzevoort W, Rep A, Bonsel GJ, et al. A randomized controlled trial comparing two temporizing management strategies, one with and one without plasma volume expansion, for severe and early onset pre-eclampsia. Br J Obstet and Gynecol. 2005;112:1358-68.

23. Sriram S, Robertson MS. Critically ill obstetric patients in Australia: a retrospective audit of 8 years' experience in a tertiary intensive care unit. Crit Care Resusc. 2008;10:124.

24. Dunne C, Meriano A. Acute postpartum pulmonary edema in a 23-year-old woman 5 days after caesarean delivery. CJEM. 2009;11:178-81.

25. Sibai BM, Mabie BC, Harvey CJ, et al. Pulmonary edema in severe preeclampsia-eclampsia: analysis of thirty-seven consecutive cases. Am J Obstet Gynecol. 1987;156:1174-9.

26. Dennis AT, Solnordal CB. Acute pulmonary edema in pregnant women. Anesthesia. 2012;67:646-59.

27. Knight M. Eclampsia in the United Kingdom 2005. BJOG. 2007;114:1072-8.

28. Duley L, Gülmezoglu AM, Chou D. Magnesium sulphate versus lytic cocktail for eclampsia. Cochrane Database Syst Rev. 2010;9:CD002960.

29. Duley L, Gülmezoglu AM, Henderson-Smart DJ, et al. Magnesium sulphate and other anticonvulsants for women with preeclampsia. Cochrane Database Syst Rev. 2010;11:CD000025.

30. The Collaborative Eclampsia Trial Group. Which anticonvulsant for women with eclampsia? Evidence from the Collaborative Eclampsia Trial. Lancet. 1995;345:1455-63.

31. Duley L, Henderson-Smart DJ, Chou D. Magnesium sulphate versus phenytoin for eclampsia. Cochrane Database Syst Rev. 2010;10:CD000128.

32. Duley L, Henderson-Smart DJ, Walker GJA, et al. Magnesium sulphate versus diazepam for eclampsia. Cochrane Database Syst Rev. 2010;12: CD000127.

33. Loo CC, Irestedt L. The benefits of labor analgesia. In: Reynolds F. (Ed). Regional Analgesia in Obstetrics: a Millennium Update. London: Springer; 2000. pp. 205-17.

34. Halpern SH, Leighton BL, Ohlsson A, et al. Effect of epidural vs parenteral opioids analgesia on the progress of labor. JAMA. 1998;280:2105-10.

35. Jouppila P, Jouppila R, Hollmen A, et al. Lumbar epidural analgesia to improve intervillous blood flow during labor in severe pre-eclampsia. Obstet Gynecol. 1982;59:158-61.

36. Reynolds F, Sharma SK, Seed PT. Analgesia in labor and fetal acid-base balance: a meta-analysis comparing epidural with systemic opioid analgesia. BJOG. 2002;109:1344-53.

37. Regional Anesthesia in Patients with Abnormalities in Coagulation. A guidance document produced by a joint working party of the Association of Anesthetists of Great Britain & Ireland (AAGBI), Obstetric Anesthetists' Association (OAA) and Regional Anesthesia UK (RAUK). 2011.

38. Douglas MJ. The use of neuraxial anesthesia in parturients with thrombocytopenia: what is an adequate platelet count? In: Halpern SH, Douglas MJ, (Eds). Evidence Based Obstetric Anesthesia. Massachusetts: Blackwell; 2005. pp. 165-77.

39. Sharma SK, Philip J, Whitten CW, et al. Assessment in changes in coagulation in parturients with preeclampsia using thromboelastography. Anesthesia. 1999;90;385-90.

40. Douma MR, Verwey RA, Kam-Endtz CE, et al. Obstetric analgesia: a comparison of patient-controlled meperidine, remifentanil, and fentanyl in labor. Br J Anesth. 2010;104(2):209-15.

41. Visalyaputra S, Rodanant O, Somboonviboon W, et al. Spinal versus epidural anesthesia for cesarean delivery in severe preeclampsia: a prospective, randomized, multicenter study. Anesth Analg. 2005;101:862e8.

42. Aya AG, Vialles N, Tanoubi I, et al. Spinal anesthesia-induced hypotension: a risk comparison between patients with severe preeclampsia and healthy women undergoing preterm cesarean delivery. Anesth Analg. 2005;101:869-75.

43. Cormack RS. Failed intubation in obstetric anesthesia. Int J Obstet Anesth. 2006;61:505-6.

44. Russell R. Failed intubation in obstetrics: a self-fulfilling prophecy? Int J Obstet Anesth. 2007;16:1-3.

45. Wallace DH, Leveno KJ, Cunningham FG, et al. Randomized comparison of general and regional anesthesia for cesarean delivery in pregnancies complicated by severe preeclampsia. Obstet Gynecol. 1995;86:193-9.

46. Dyer RA, Els I, Farbas J, et al. Prospective, randomized trial comparing general with spinal anesthesia

for cesarean delivery in preeclamptic patients with a non-reassuring fetal heart trace. Anesthesiology. 2003;99:561-9.

47. Popham P, Buettner A, Mendola M. Anesthesia for emergency caesarean section, 2000-2004, at the Royal Women's Hospital, Melbourne. Anesth Intensive Care. 2007;35:74-9.

48. Allam J, Malhotra S, Hemingway C, et al. Epidural lidocaine-bicarbonate-adrenaline vs levobupivacaine for emergency Caesarean section: a randomized controlled trial. Anesthesia. 2008; 63:243-9.

49. Munnur U, de Boisblanc, Surech MS. Airway problems in pregnancy. Crit Care Med. 2005;33: S259-68.

50. O'Hare R, McAtamney D, Mirakhur RK, et al. Bolus dose remifentanil for control of haemodynamic response to tracheal intubation during rapid sequence induction of anesthesia. Br J Anesth. 1999;82:283-5.

51. Ngan Kee WD, Khaw KS, Ma KC, et al. Maternal and neonatal effects of remifentanil at induction of general anesthesia for cesarean delivery: a randomized, double-blind, controlled trial. Anesthesiology. 2006;104:14-20.

52. Yoo KY, Jeong CW, Park BY, et al. Effects of remifentanil on cardiovascular and bispectral indexresponses to endotracheal intubation in severe pre-eclamptic patients undergoing caesarean delivery under general anesthesia. Br J Anesth. 2009;102:812-9.

53. Alanoglu Z, Ates Y, Abbas Yilmaz A, et al. Is there an ideal approach for rapid-sequence induction in hypertensive patients? J Clin Anesth. 2006;18:34-40.

54. Ashton WB, James MJ, Janicki P, et al. Attenuation of the pressor response to tracheal intubation by magnesium sulphate with and without alfentanil in hypertensive proteinuric patients undergoing cesarean section. Br J Anesth. 1991;67:741-7.

55. Ramanathan J, Sibai BM, Pillai R, et al. Neuromuscular transmission studies in preeclamptic women receiving magnesium sulfate. Am J Obstet Gynecol. 1988;158:40-6.

56. Rout CC, Rocke DA. Effects of alfentanil and fentanyl on induction of anesthesia in patients with severe pregnancy-induced hypertension. Br J Anesth. 1990;65:468-74.

57. Liu PL, Gatt S, Gugino LD, et al. Esmolol for control of increases in heart rate and blood pressure during tracheal intubation after thiopental and succinylcholine. Can Anesth Soc J. 1986;33:556-62.

58. Mortl MG, Schneider MC. Key issues in assessing, managing and treating patients presenting with severe preeclampsia. Int J Obstet Anesth. 2000;9: 39-44.

59. Engelhardt T, MacLennan FM. Fluid management in pre-eclampsia. Int J Obstet Anesth. 1999;8:253-9.

60. Aya AG, Mangin R, Vialles N, et al. Patients with severe preeclampsia experience less hypotension than healthy parturients. Anesth Analg. 2003;97: 867-72.

61. Clark VA, Sharwood-Smith GH, Stewart AV. Ephedrine requirement are reduced during spinal anesthesia for cesarean section in preeclampsia. Int J Obstet Anesth. 2004;14:9-13.

62. Aya AG, Vialles N, Tanoubi I, et al. Spinal anesthesia-induced hypotension: a risk comparison between patients with severe preeclampsia and healthy women undergoing preterm cesarean delivery. Anesth Analg. 2005;101:869-75.

63. Dyer RA, Piercy JL, Reed AR, et al. Hemodynamic changes associated with spinal anesthesia for cesarean delivery in severe preeclampsia. Anesthesiology. 2008;108:802-11.

14 Management of Second and Third Stages of Labor in Hypertensive Disorders

Hema Divakar, Girija Wagh, Jarita Deb

◼ INTRODUCTION

Despite enormous amount of literature available in the recent past and relatively uniform management practices, we were unable to present the best practices for the management of second and third stages of labor in women with hypertensive disorders. Answering this question is difficult because of the many potential confounding variables that affect morbidity in the mother and the very immature infants. In this chapter, we will outline the preferred contemporary practice.

During the second stage of labor, worsening or new manifestations of maternal hypertension leading to eclampsia may occur. The forceful maternal efforts may jeopardize the cardiovascular system and the hemodynamics leading to complications. In addition, the use of epidural analgesia, necessity of instrumental delivery and possibilities of hematomas due to altered coagulation make the management of the second stage a specialized period needing close vigilance. Many a times there is sufficient reserve to maintain oxygenation of the fetus during the second stage of labor even though the uteroplacental circulation is reduced, but in pregnancies complicated with preeclampsia, both the fetal and maternal condition can deteriorate rapidly.[1] An already compromised fetus along with the pressure effects due to strong expulsive uterine contractions is at risk of asphyxia and death.

Likewise the third stage of labor needs prophylactic management to prevent complications, such as postpartum hemorrhage (PPH), cerebrovascular accidents, etc. with specific caution to be exercised related to use of drugs.

This chapter addresses the management of second and third stages of labor in hypertensive disorders with the constraint of relative dearth of standard recommendations and available evidence in literature under the following headings:
- Dynamics of the second and third stage of labor—difference in hypertensive disorder
  - Maternal considerations—second stage delays
  - Fetal considerations—fetal hypoxia
- Maternofetal considerations during an eclamptic convulsion
- Risk assessment in second stage of labor in pregnancy hypertension
  - The monitoring of mother and fetus
  - Obstetric assessment
- Management in second stage of labor in pregnancy hypertension
  - Prevention of seizures and control of hypertension
  - Reducing the duration of the second stage
  - Management in second stage of labor in HELLP syndrome
  - Interventions that may be needed and caution to be exercised
  - Pregnant women with chronic hypertension
- Third stage management in pregnancy hypertension
- Summary points and conclusions

◼ DYNAMICS OF THE SECOND AND THIRD STAGE OF LABOR— DIFFERENCE IN HYPERTENSIVE DISORDER

Vaginal delivery is associated with important changes in maternal circulation parameters.

In particular, pain at birth causes a raise of about 50% in heart rate and in cardiac output (CO), along with an increase of more than 20% in blood pressure (BP). When the baby is expelled at the end of the second stage of labor, systolic blood pressure (SBP) may reach the level of 200 mm Hg through Valsalva mechanism.[2] Uterine contractions cause increased left ventricular stroke volume by 16% (75 ± 15 mL per beat–89 ± 17 mL per beat, p < 0.001) and increased cardiac output by 11% (6.31 ± 1.79 L/min–7.12 ± 1.93 L/min, p < 0.001). The contraction-induced increase in the CO is phase dependent and is more after full cervical dilatation approximately 1–2 L/min more than prelabor values. Oxygen consumption also increases approximately by 23% during labor.[3]

The second stage of labor is divided in two phases: (1) passive or pelvic phase when the presenting part descends within the pelvis and (2) the active or perineal phase when the presenting part descends through the pelvic floor and is then finally expelled out of the vagina and the perineum. The cervical distension at the end of the first stage and the vaginal distension when the presenting part negotiates the pelvic floor causes the release of oxytocin in large quantums (Fergusson reflex) leading to enhanced uterine contractions. Approximation of the presenting part to the pelvic floor initiates a cascade of muscular reflexes which result in the voluntary expulsive efforts by the mother. Physiologically this phase is more demanding for the mother and the fetus. The uterine contractions during this phase are intense and long lasting. The uteroplacental circulation has less time to replenish its oxygenation before the onset of the next contraction. The maternal skeletal activity due to bearing down efforts generates metabolic products, such as lactic acid, which can be transferred to the fetus. Fetal head and eyeball compression can cause heart decelerations due to raised intracranial pressure and vagal stimulation which are early or variable decelerations (Fig. 14.1). If the decelerations remain for a longer time compared with the duration at the baseline heart rate (Fig. 14.2) the gas exchange at the placental intervillous perfusion is compromised.[4]

The rate of fall of the pH in the fetus is much faster in the active phase of the second stage of labor compared to the first stage.[5]

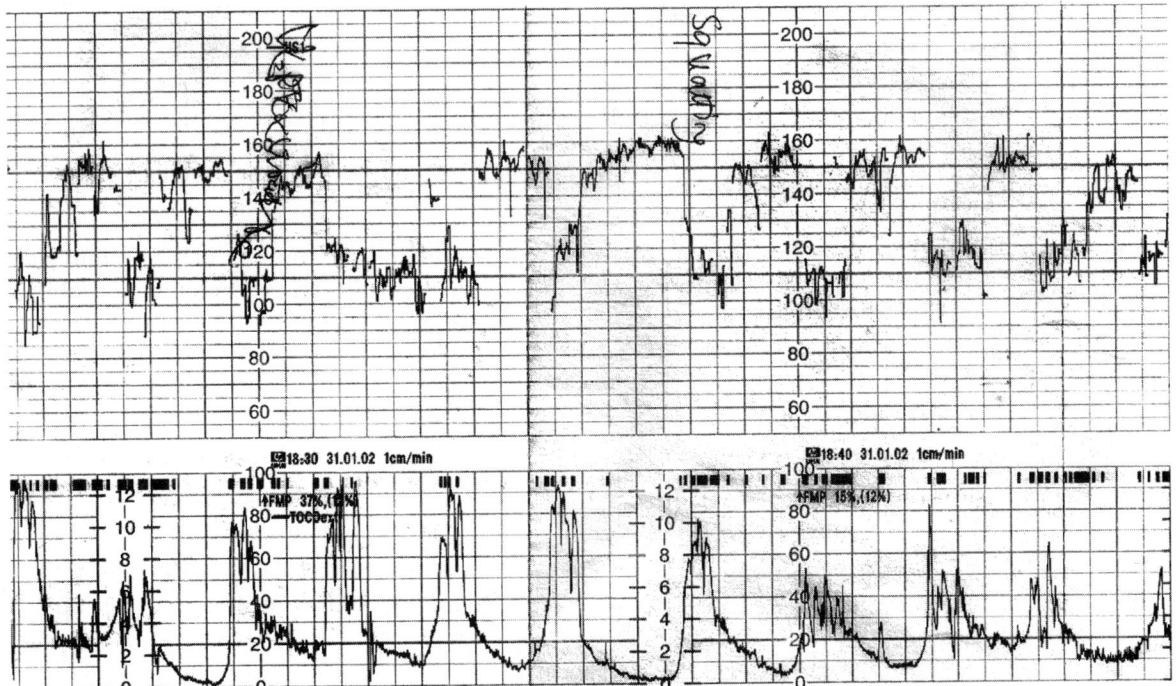

Fig. 14.1: The head compression variable decelerations—the duration of decelerations does not exceed the duration of contractions; the interval between the decelerations is greater than during the decelerations; there is no rise or fall in the baseline rate and the baseline variability is normal second stage trace that is unlikely to cause compromise

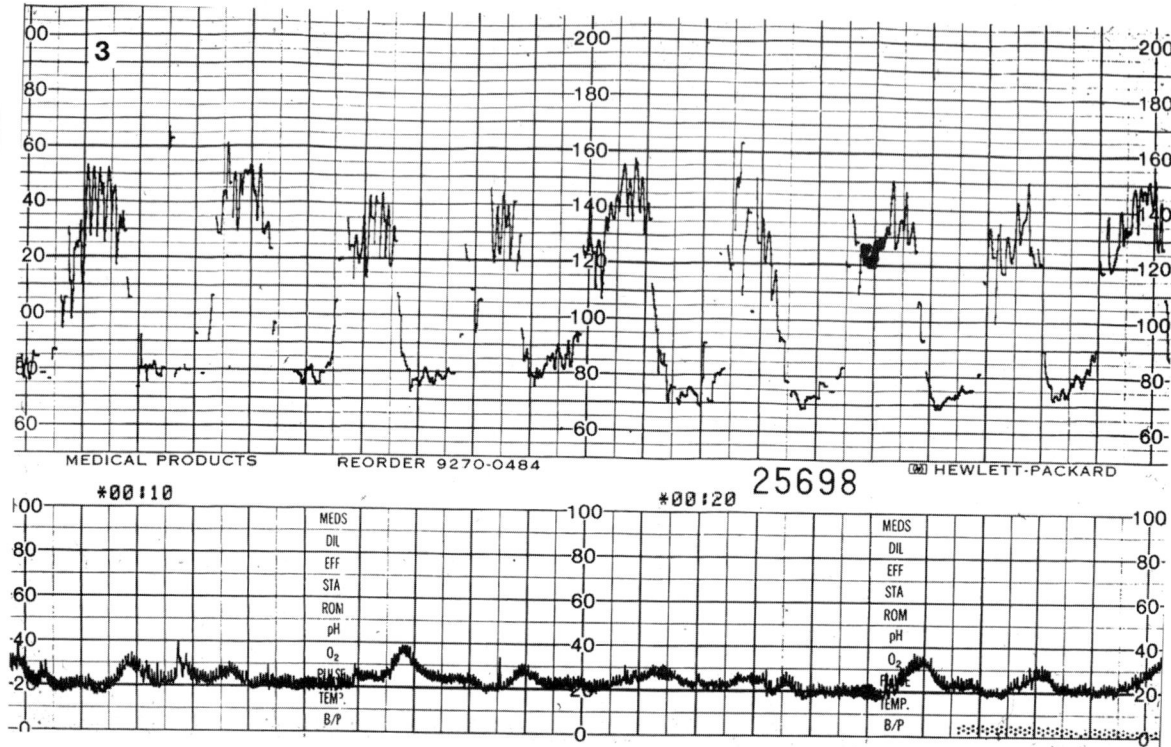

Fig. 14.2: The deceleration lasts for a longer duration than the time spent at the baseline rate; there is exaggerated baseline variability (salutatory) and the depth of duration descends less than 80 beats per minute (bpm)—a case of suboptimal perfusion that can lead to rapid development of acidosis

All these factors together bring about fetal hypoxia. In an already compromised fetus these can be more profound leading to poor neonatal outcomes. Antenatally compromised fetus such as the one with hypertensive disorders in the mother may not be able to compensate adequately to these effects.

Maternal Considerations— Second Stage Delays

In mothers with hypertension, second stage delays can be due to uterine dysfunction. Feinstein et al. (2002) in a multivariate study observed that hypertensive disorders can be one of the risk factors for the delay in second stage of labor. The other risk factors observed were gestational diabetes, nulliparity, epidural analgesia, macrosomia and maternal obesity. These patients needed cesarean sections (20.4%) or instrumental delivery (74.4% vacuum and 5.4% forceps) with significantly low Apgar scores in the neonates compared to the controls.[6]

Fetal Considerations—Fetal Hypoxia

Uterine contractions intermittently reduce the flow of oxygenated maternal blood into the intervillous space. During the second stage of labor, delivery of the oxygenated blood to the intervillous space is further reduced due to the increased frequency, amplitude and the durations of the uterine contractions. Eventually the oxygen available to the fetus through the intervillous space is reduced. The fetus responds to this hypoxia through myriad of adrenergic responses which cause a shift of aerobic metabolism to anaerobic metabolism to maintain cellular function which results in lactic acidosis. The ability of the fetus to protect itself from this metabolic acidosis is very low as the fetal kidney and the placenta cannot efficiently eliminate lactic acid compared with the better elimination of carbon dioxide. These indices of fetal acidosis, flow pH, high base deficit and lactate concentrations were correlated to the duration of the second stage of labor by Wood et al. in 1987.[7]

MATERNOFETAL CONSIDERATIONS DURING AN ECLAMPTIC CONVULSION

Increased uterine activity is seen to be associated with eclamptic seizure in the form of increased tone and frequency and may last from 2 minutes to 14 minutes. Persistent bradycardia with heightened uterine tone after a seizure should make one suspect placental abruption.

Fetal circulation may get compromised during a convulsion. The electronic fetal monitoring often reveals prolonged bradycardia followed by transient tachycardia. In addition, the recovery phase is observed to have a loss of baseline variability and late decelerations. These changes are a reflection of fetal hypoxia due to uterine contraction and lack of maternal respiration during convulsion. Also a sick baby, like a growth restricted or preterm baby, with reduced reserves may have exaggerated response to these changes.

RISK ASSESSMENT IN SECOND STAGE OF LABOR IN PREGNANCY HYPERTENSION

At the onset of second stage it is a good practice to carefully evaluate the condition of the women and vigilance for any complications should continue.

Monitoring of Mother and Fetus in Second Stage of Labor

The goals are early detection of progression from mild to severe disease and prevention of maternal complications and early detection of fetal heart rate abnormalities;[8] progression to severe disease may lead to eclampsia, cerebrovascular complications or cardiovascular complications. Monitoring will help to identify severe hypertension, pulmonary edema and possibility of an eclamptic fit. There could also be a risk of abruptio placentae. Hemolysis, elevated liver enzyme, low platelet count (HELLP) syndrome is associated with its own risks and complications.

Fetal distress in a fetus with already reduced reserve may lead to adverse outcome in the neonate.

Maternal Monitoring during Second Stage

Measurement of Blood Pressure
- Hourly in women with mild or moderate hypertension
- Continually in women with severe hypertension
- Continue use of antenatal antihypertensive treatment during labor.[9]

Onset of New Symptoms Suggesting Severe Disease

Be vigilant about the onset of new symptoms suggesting severe disease. Those who develop severe hypertension and/or symptoms and signs of severe preeclampsia should be managed promptly.[8]

Additional Maternal Monitoring during Second Stage of Labor in Patients with Severe Preeclampsia/Eclampsia

- Strict charting of fluid balance
- An indwelling urinary catheter with urometer to observe for oliguria would be useful. Urinary output of less than 20 mL/hour for 3 or more hours suggests impending renal failure
- Observe for pulmonary edema
- Pulse rate and oxygen saturation

Although there are no randomized control trials to support routine use of invasive hemodynamic monitoring in patients with severe preeclampsia, it may prove beneficial in preeclamptic women with severe cardiac disease, severe renal disease, refractory hypertension, oliguria or pulmonary edema.[10]

Additional Maternal Monitoring for Patients on Magnesium Sulfate

- Half hourly BP, pulse and respiratory rate in the acute phase
- Hourly patellar reflexes
- Hourly urine output measurement + 4 hourly testing of urinary protein
- Two hourly temperature
- Continuous oxygen saturation monitoring.

Fetal Monitoring during Second Stage of Labor

Continuous fetal heart rate monitoring with electronic monitor is preferred. The American

College of Obstetricians and Gynecologists (ACOG) recommends continuous electronic fetal monitoring (EFM) for women with high-risk conditions.[11] The Royal College of Obstetricians and Gynaecologists (RCOG) and the Royal Australian and New Zealand College of Obstetricians and Gynaecologists (RANZCOG) recommend continuous EFM for high-risk women.[12,13] In the absence of facilities for continuous fetal monitoring auscultation of the fetal heart with stethoscope or with a hand-held Doppler every 5 minutes after each contraction and during the interval is preferred.

Obstetric Assessment

Monitoring of progress of labor is similar to an uncomplicated pregnancy except in those with preeclampsia there should be continuous monitoring of uterine activity. Watch for hyper-stimulation and/or development of vaginal bleeding. Uterine irritability and/or recurrent variable or late decelerations may be the first sign of abruptio placentae in these women.[8]

Monitoring fetal condition facilities available for neonatal resuscitation need to be checked. It is preferable to have a neonatal pediatrician in attendance if assistance for a compromised baby becomes a necessity.

▪ MANAGEMENT IN SECOND STAGE OF LABOR IN PREGNANCY HYPERTENSION

Prevention of Seizure and Control of Hypertension

There is enough evidence to suggest that intravenous magnesium sulfate is beneficial in preventing seizures in women with severe preeclampsia and also recurrent seizures. However, its benefit in mild preeclampsia remains unclear.[8,14] Intravenous magnesium sulfate should be given to women with severe hypertension or severe preeclampsia who have or previously had an eclamptic fit. If magnesium sulfate is given, it should be continued for 24 hours following delivery or 24 hours after the last seizure, whichever is later.[15]

If the patient is already on antihypertensive it should be continued during labor.[9] The objective of treating acute severe hypertension is to prevent potential cerebrovascular and cardiovascular

complications such as encephalopathy, hemorrhage and congestive heart failure.[8,16] Immediate antihypertensive therapy should be started if the BP is 160/105–110 mm Hg. Aim of treatment should be to keep SBP below 150 mm Hg and diastolic blood pressure (DBP) between 80 mm Hg and 100 mm Hg. Labetalol (oral or intravenous), hydralazine (intravenous) or nifedipine (oral) may be used. Labetalol should not be used in case of asthma.[9]

Women with chronic hypertension who develop severe hypertension with or without other evidence for preeclampsia should be given magnesium sulfate prophylaxis for prevention of eclampsia.[17]

Reduction of the Duration of the Second Stage of Labor

The lactic acidosis is time dependent and is directly proportional to the length of the second stage of labor. Katz et al. in 1987 observed that the delay of over 30 minutes in the second stage of labor was associated with increased occurrence of lactic acidosis in the fetus.[5] Based on this it is recommended that expulsive forces of second stage of labor should not last for more than 20–30 minutes, especially in hypertensive patients.

Evidence does not support the need that the second stage of labor should routinely be shortened in women with stable mild or moderate hypertension. Consideration should be given to limiting the duration of the second stage of labor in women with severe hypertension that is unresponsive to initial treatment in view of the hemodynamic alterations that ensue in the second stage of labor.[9]

In cases of chronic hypertension, vaginal delivery is usually preferable. Cesarean delivery is performed for usual obstetrical indications. It is recommended that the duration of the second stage is reduced in uncontrolled severe hypertension, impending eclampsia or for fetomaternal indications.

Management in Second Stage of Labor in HELLP Syndrome

- Prophylactic transfusion of platelets is not recommended, even prior to cesarean section, when platelet count is more than $50 \times 10^9/L$, there is no excessive bleeding or platelet dysfunction. (II-2D)

- Consideration should be given to ordering blood products, including platelets, when platelet count is less than 50×10^9/L, platelet count is falling rapidly and/or there is coagulopathy. (III-I)
- Platelet transfusion should be strongly considered prior to vaginal delivery when platelet count is less than 20×10^9/L. (III-B)
- Platelet transfusion is recommended prior to cesarean section when platelet count is less than 20×10^9/L. (III-B)
- Corticosteriods may be considered for women with platelet count of less than 50×10^9/L. (III-I)
- There is insufficient evidence to make a recommendation regarding the usefulness of plasma exchange or plasmapheresis.[18] (III-I)

Interventions that may be needed and Caution to be exercised

Oxytocins and Fluids

Active management of labor with oxytocin augmentation may be required to overcome uterine inertia set in due to hypertension[19] or usage of magnesium sulfate. It is a good practice to deliver the oxytocin through a microdrip as it is observed that the drop rates counted on a regular intravenous line may not be correct. This helps to limit undue fluid overload that is best avoided in hypertension as it may add further to "flooding" of the lungs. It is important that the fluids are administered judiciously. The rate preferred is 80/mL/hour and titrated against the urinary output.[9] These patients are susceptible to pulmonary edema due to endothelial dysfunction, increased permeability and increased capillary wedge pressure. Ringer's lactate is the preferred crystalloid. Use of colloids has not been demonstrated to be of better benefit.

Pain Relief

Epidural analgesia offers superior pain relief over parenteral narcotics in labor. It also causes beneficial hemodynamic effects such as 20% reduction in BP with a small reduction in systemic vascular resistance and maintenance of cardiac input.[20] Doppler velocimetry has been performed in such cases and epidural analgesia is shown to reduce the systolic/diastolic flow ratio in the uterine artery by 25% to levels seen in nonpreeclamptics.[21]

It also has advantages such as reduction in the vascular resistance and relief of vasospasm. Also there is increase in the intervillous blood flow by 77% in severe preeclamptics without maternal BP or fetal heart rate abnormalities.[22]

There are limited data to address the issue of analgesia or anesthesia in pregnant women with chronic hypertension. General anesthesia is associated with risks such as difficult intubation due to laryngeal edema and drug interactions. Regional anesthesia administered by clinicians with specialized training in obstetric anesthesia is preferred. Labetalol should be given to minimize acute and significant elevations in BP during intubation and extubation in case general anesthesia needs to be administered.[23] Coagulopathy needs to be ruled out before administering epidural anesthesia.

Positioning during Labor

Women can adopt any position they like while preferably avoiding long periods lying supine. They should be encouraged to experiment with what feels most comfortable and should be supported in their choice. Birth attendants need training in coaching and performing births in other positions than the supine in order to not be an inhibiting factor in the choice of position.[24]

Instrumental delivery may be essential to reduce the duration of the second stage in a very sick parturient or in cases of fetal distress or prolonged labor. Risk of hematomas should be born in cases of compromised coagulation profile.

Pregnant Women with Chronic Hypertension

The majority of pregnant women with chronic hypertension have uncomplicated mild hypertension and can be managed in the same way as normal, nonhypertensive women during the intrapartum period. In contrast, women with severe hypertension/or hypertension that is complicated by cardiovascular or renal disease may present special problems during the intrapartum period.[23] These women are at increased risk for placental abruption and cerebral hemorrhage.[25,26] Pulmonary edema from peripartum heart failure is common at this time. They require special attention regarding fluid load and urine output. When the patient presents late in pregnancy it is usually difficult to distinguish worsening chronic hypertension from severe preeclampsia.

Severe hypertension with or without super-imposed preeclampsia should be treated with antihypertensives. It is generally recommended that immediate antihypertensive medications should be given to women with preeclampsia for SBP more than 160 mm Hg or DBP 105–110 mm Hg or greater.[27]

Intravenous labetalol is the drug of first choice but it should be avoided in asthma and/or congestive heart failure. Intravenous hydralazine may also be used.[28]

THIRD STAGE MANAGEMENT IN HYPERTENSION

Hypertensive disorder, failure to progress during the second stage of labor, oxytocin augmentation and vacuum extraction were found to be major risk factors for severe PPH.[29]

Active management of third stage of labor is strongly recommended in hypertensive patients, because even a small blood loss may alter the hemodynamics in the patient resulting in shock. Secondly, the uterine inertia may prevent effective uterine retraction. Thirdly, the underlying coagulation defects or thrombocytopenia will prevent effective hemostasis.

The preferred method is intramuscular administration of oxytocin 10 IU at the delivery of the anterior shoulder or within a minute of the birth of the baby. Intravenous methylergometrine is best avoided for the possibility of sudden rise in BP and convulsions. Prostaglandins should be used with caution. 15 methyl F 2 alpha is best deferred in situations where respiratory system compromise or affliction is suspected. Misoprostol (prostaglandin E1 compound) can be used for maintenance of sustained uterine contraction.[9,30]

Cord clamping can be undertaken based on the condition of the fetus. It is preferred to delay the clamping of cord by 1–2 minutes for better neonatal outcome.[31] When faced with a sick neonate, early clamping and early initiation of resuscitative measures appears to be the norm. Recent trend appears to encourage resuscitation with the intact umbilical cord to enable more blood to enter the fetal circulation that may help the neonate to respond better. This concept needs further study.

Careful confirmation of uterine retraction, hemostasis and ruling out of soft tissue injuries and hematomas should be taken. The maternal condition should be carefully evaluated. Close monitoring for PPH, hypertension, eclampsia, cardiovascular accidents and pulmonary edema should be continued for the first 24 hours post delivery.

SUMMARY POINTS AND CONCLUSION

- Second stage of labor uterine contractions can cause significant alterations in the hemo-dynamics leading to hypertension, eclampsia and precipitation of other complications of hypertension.
- The compromised fetus due to deficient placental perfusion needs close monitoring.
- Epidural analgesia is a preferred intervention with many benefits in hypertensive deliveries.
- Active management of third stage of labor is essential.
- Delivery is preferred in a well-equipped facility.

Knowledge about the pathological changes associated with the baseline disease and the changing dynamics due to labor have to be born in mind. The mother needs close monitoring and so does the fetus and the essential interventions should be undertaken with this understanding. There has to be vigilant surveillance for occurrence of complications and efforts taken to prevent them.

REFERENCES

1. Janni W, Schiessl B, Peschers U, et al. The prognostic impact of a prolonged second stage of labor on maternal and fetal outcome. Acta Obstet Gynecol Scand. 2002;81(3):214-21.
2. Ueland K. Maternal cardiovascular dynamics. VII. Intrapartum blood volume changes. Am J Obstet Gynecol. 1976;126(6):671-7.
3. Ueland K, Hansen JM. Maternal cardiovascular dynamics. 3. Labor and delivery under local and caudal analgesia. Am J Obstet Gynecol. 1969; 103(1):8-18.
4. Bhatt R, Sabaratnam A, Sarala G, et al. Management of spontaneous labor. Obstetrics and Gynecology for Postgraduates. Hyderabad: Universities Press (India) Pvt. Ltd. 2009. pp. 346-63.
5. Katz M, Lunenfield E, Meizner I, et al. The effect of the duration of the second stage of labour on the

acid-base state of the fetus. Br J Obstet Gynecol. 1987;94(5):425-30.

6. Feinstein U, Sheiner E, Levy A, et al. Risk factors for arrest of descent during the second stage of labor. Int J Gynecol Obstet. 2002;77(1):7-14.

7. Wood C, Ng KH, Hounslow D, et al. Time—an important variable in normal delivery. J Obstet Gynaecol Br Commnw. 1973;80(4):295-300.

8. Sibai BM. Diagnosis and management of gestational hypertension and preeclampsia. Obstet Gynecol. 2003;102(1):181-92.

9. National Collaborating Centre for Women's and Children's Health (UK). (2010). Hypertension in Pregnancy: The Management of Hypertensive Disorders During Pregnancy. [online] Available from http://www.ncbi.nlm.nih.gov/books/NBK62652/. [Accessed Aug, 2010].

10. ACOG Committee on Practice Bulletins-Obstetrics. ACOG practice bulletin. Diagnosis and management of eclampsia and preeclampsia. Number 33, January 2002. Obstet Gynecol. 2002;99:159-67.

11. American College of Obstetricians and Gynecologists. ACOG Practice Bulletin no. 106: Intrapartum fetal heart rate monitoring: nomenclature, interpretation, and general management principles. Obstet Gynecol. 2009;114(1):192-202.

12. National Institute for Health and Clinical Excellence (NICE). Intrapartum Care–Management and Delivery of Care to Women in Labor. London: NICE; 2007. (Nice clinical guideline 55).

13. The Royal Australian and New Zealand College of Obstetricians and Gynecologists. Clinical Guidelines. Intrapartum Fetal Surveillance Guidelines. May 2006.

14. Sibai BM. Diagnosis, prevention and management of eclampsia. Obstet Gynecol. 2005;105(2):402-10.

15. Royal College of Obstetricians and Gynecologists (RCOG). (2006). The Management of Severe pre-eclampsia/Eclampsia, Guideline No. 10(A). [online] March 2006. http://www.rcog.org.uk/womens-health/clinical-guidance/management-severe-pre-eclampsiaeclampsia-green-top-10a. [Accessed March, 2006].

16. Report of the National High Blood Pressure Education Program. Working group report on high blood pressure in pregnancy. Am J Obstet Gynecol. 2000;183:S1-22.

17. Alexander JM, McIntire DD, Leveno KJ, et al. Selective magnesium sulfate prophylaxis for the prevention of eclampsia in women with gestational hypertension. Obstet Gynecol. 2006;108(4):826-32.

18. Society of Obstetricians and Gynecologists. (2008). Diagnosis, evaluation and management of the hypertensive disorders of pregnancy. [online]

Available from http://www.sogc.org/guidelines/documents/gui206CPG0803_001.pdf

19. Leushuis E, Tromp M, Ravelli AC, et al. Indicators for intervention during the expulsive second-stage arrest of labour. BJOG. 2009;116(13):1773-81.

20. Newsome LR, Bramwell RS, Curling PE. Severe preeclampsia: hemodynamic effects of lumbar epidural anesthesia. Ancsth Analg. 1986;65(1):31-6.

21. Ramos-Santos E, Devoe LD, Wakefield ML, et al. The effects of epidural anesthesia on the Doppler velocimetry of umbilical and uterine arteries in normal and hypertensive patients during active term labor. Obstet Gynecol. 1991;77(1):20-6.

22. Jouppila P, Jouppila R, Hollmen A, et al. Lumbar epidural analgesia to improve intervillous blood flow during labor in severe preeclampsia. Obstet Gynecol. 1982;59(2):158-61.

23. ACOG Practice Bulletin No. 29. Chronic Hypertension in Pregnancy. Obstet Gynecol. 2001;98 (1):177-85.

24. World Health Organization. (1996). Maternal and Newborn Health/Safe Motherhood Unit. Care in normal birth: a practical guide. [online] Available from:http://www.who.int/maternal_child_adolescent/documents/who_frh_msm_9624/en/ [Accessed May, 2013].

25. Cunningham FG. Severe preeclampsia and eclampsia: systolic hypertension is also important. Obstet Gynecol. 2005;105(2):237-8.

26. Martin JN, Thigpen BD, Moore RC, et al. Stroke and severe preeclampsia and eclampsia: a paradigm shift focusing on systolic blood pressure. Obstet Gynecol. 2005;105(2):246-54.

27. National high blood pressure education program working group report on high blood pressure in pregnancy. Am J Obstet Gynecol. 1990;163(5 Pt 1): 1691-712.

28. Podymow T, August P. Update on the use of anti-hypertensive drugs in pregnancy. Hypertension. 2008;51(29):960-6.

29. Sheiner E, Sarid L, Levy A, et al. Obstetric risk factors and outcome of pregnancies complicated with early postpartum hemorrhage: a population-based study. J Matern Fetal Neonatal Med. 2005;18(3):149-54.

30. Leduc D, Senikas V, Lalonde AB. Active management of the third stage of labor: prevention and treatment of postpartum hemorrhage. J Obstet Gynaecol Can. 2009;31(10):980-93.

31. Abalos E. Effect of timing of umbilical cord clamping of term infants on maternal and neonatal outcomes: RHL commentary (last revised: 2 March 2009). The WHO Reproductive Health Library; Geneva: World Health Organization.

15

Care of the Critically ill Mother

Nishkantha Arulkumaran

■ INTRODUCTION

Most women of childbearing age are healthy with no chronic comorbidity. However, in a small proportion of women, severe and sometimes life-threatening complications do occur. This cohort of patients is unique as their management requires consideration of the physiological changes associated with pregnancy and the well-being of the fetus.

Hypertension during pregnancy is a relatively common disorder. Majority of cases are managed successfully in the community or in the obstetric ward. Occasionally, high blood pressure and its associated complications may be life threatening. Along with hemorrhage and thromboembolism, preeclampsia accounts for majority of maternal mortality,[1] and hypertensive disorders account for the greatest proportion of intensive care unit (ICU) admissions among pregnant patients globally.[2] The maternal mortality rate is significantly higher in those admitted to the ICU, and is 14% in the under-resourced countries compared to 3.3% in developed countries despite similar rates of ICU admission and profile of obstetric patients admitted to ICUs.[2] One of the key factors associated with poor outcomes is a delay in accessing ICU within 24 hours of illness.[3] Patients admitted to ICUs from under-resourced countries tend to have higher illness severity scores, suggesting delayed admission to ICU.[2] It is likely that the majority of maternal deaths in under-resourced countries do not reach ICU services at all.[4]

ICU services and multidisciplinary team involvement should be considered early to ensure that mothers with preeclampsia are stabilized prior to delivery. Despite wide heterogeneity in resources available globally and the number of ICU beds per capita,[5] one of the defining features is the higher nurse to patient ratio. The increased nursing care available allows regular monitoring of clinical vital signs and early identification of perturbations. Up to 50% of maternal deaths have preventable factors, including failure to recognize severity of illness and delay in receiving appropriate treatment.[6] Early warning scores, critical care outreach services and close monitoring on ICU may facilitate timely recognition and management of acute illness.

In this chapter, we review the diagnosis and management of severe preeclampsia and its associated life-threatening complications. Maternal complications associated with severe preeclampsia are not uncommon, and include hemolysis, elevated liver enzymes and low platelet count (HELLP) syndrome (10–25%), acute kidney injury (AKI) (1–5%), pulmonary edema (2–5%) and placental abruption (1–4%).[1,7,8]

■ SEVERE PREECLAMPSIA

Hypertension in pregnancy is defined as high blood pressure occurring before 20 weeks of gestation. Pregnancy-induced hypertension [a systolic blood pressure (SBP) ≥ 140 mm Hg and/or diastolic blood pressure (DBP) ≥ 90 mm Hg] occurs after this period, and when associated with proteinuria (> 300 mg in a 24 hour urine collection), preeclampsia is diagnosed.[9] In addition, the condition must resolve within 6 weeks of the postpartum period. Rarely, preeclampsia may occur in the immediate postpartum period. Further details on the definitions and diagnosis of hypertensive disorders in pregnancy can be found in Chapter 1. Other causes of hypertension including recreational drugs, pheochromocytoma and thyrotoxicosis are much less common, but should always be considered.

Approximately 3–8% women in developed countries develop preeclampsia[9,10] and approximately 0.56 per 1,000 births are complicated by eclampsia.[11] The clinical features for the diagnosis of preeclampsia and severe preeclampsia are summarized in Table 15.1. Critical care services should consider admitting any mother with severe preeclampsia.

The general management of severe preeclampsia should include the following:

- Appropriate monitoring and management of maternal blood pressure (detailed further)
- Monitoring of other vital signs including heart rate, urine output, oxygen saturation, respiratory rate, deep tendon reflexes and Glasgow Coma Scale
- Twenty-four hour urine collection for protein estimation
- Thromboembolism-deterrent (TED) stockings
- Ultrasound assessment of the fetus to assess fetal size, umbilical artery Doppler and liquor volume
- Prevention and management of complications, including infusion of magnesium sulfate
- Continuous fetal monitoring
- Consideration for steroids for those less than 34 weeks of gestation and of delivery of the baby.

Since automated blood pressure monitors lack accuracy in women with preeclampsia,[12] standard manual aneroid sphygmomanometers should be used. When rapidly-acting intravenous infusions of antihypertensive agents are used, invasive blood pressure measurements should be considered.

Cerebral autoregulation is impaired and the risk of cerebral hemorrhage is increased when the mean arterial pressure exceeds 145 mm Hg. Targeting a SBP lower than 140–150 mm Hg and DBP less than 80–90 mm Hg is prudent to minimize the risk of hemorrhagic stroke.[6]

If oral agents have failed to adequately reduce blood pressure, intravenous antihypertensives should be considered. Rapid reduction in SBP should be avoided as it may result in acute hypoperfusion and ischemia of vital organs and a reduction in SBP of 10 mm Hg every 20 min is adequate. Commonly used intravenous antihypertensives include hydralazine, labetalol and glyceryl trinitrate. In addition to this, oral nifedipine is also administered.

Hydralazine

Intravenous hydralazine, a potent vasodilator, is often used in hypertensive crises and can be administered as a bolus (5 mg) repeated after 20 min up to a total cumulative dose of 20 mg or as a continuous infusion (0.5–10.0 mg/hour). Repeated boluses of hydralazine may be required once target blood pressure has been achieved. Hydralazine may cause reflex tachycardia and should therefore be avoided if the maternal heart rate exceeds 120 beats per minute (bpm).

Table 15.1: Features of preeclampsia and severe preeclampsia	
Preeclampsia	*Severe Preeclampsia*
• Systolic blood pressure (SBP) ≥ 140 mm Hg or diastolic blood pressure (DBP) ≥ 90 mm Hg after 20 weeks of gestation in a previously normotensive woman	• SBP ≥ 160 mm Hg or DBP ≥ 110 mm Hg on two separate occasions at least 6 hours apart
• Proteinuria ≥ 300 mg in 24 hour urine collection	• Proteinuria ≥ 1 g in a 24 hour urine collection
	• End organ involvement: – Oliguria (< 400 mL/day) – Thrombocytopenia – Impared liver function tests – Epigastric/right upper quadrant pain (liver capsule distension) – Cerebral or visual disturbances – Pulmonary edema

Labetalol

Labetalol acts on both alpha and beta adrenoceptors to result in a reduction in heart rate and vasodilation. In emergencies, it may be used as an alternative to hydralazine with an initial bolus dose of 20 mg. If required, this dose is doubled every 10 min to a maximum cumulative dose of 220 mg. Alternatively, labetalol may be administered as a continuous infusion started at 2 mg/min followed by 5–10 mg/hour up to cumulative dose of 200 mg. Bradycardia (fetal and maternal) is a potential side effect and heart rate should therefore be monitored.

Nitrates

Intravenous glyceryl trinitrate is a particularly useful intravenous antihypertensive agent in the context of acute pulmonary edema. An infusion of 1–10 mg/hour is often effective, though prolonged use may result in tachyphylaxis. Sodium nitroprusside has a very short half-life, facilitating rapid titration. Accumulation of cyanide or thiocyanate may occur, usually with more than 24 hours of sodium nitroprusside infusion and in patients with renal insufficiency.[13] Sodium nitroprusside is therefore rarely used in preeclampsia.

Nifedipine

Nifedipine is a calcium channel blocker that results in vascular smooth muscle relaxation and vasodilation. It is administered orally as a slow release preparation starting at 10 mg BD and may be increased to 40 mg BD. Although there is less experience and evidence behind the use of nifedipine compared to methyldopa, there is no evidence to suggest long-term fetal harm.

The renal response to intense vasoconstriction is increased salt and water elimination (pressure natriuresis), with a reduction in circulating volume. Therefore, when a vasodilator is administered, "preloading" with up to 500 mL of intravenous crystalloids may be required to prevent precipitous fall in blood pressure and to maintain organ perfusion. The volume and rate of fluid administration needs to be closely monitored to avoid iatrogenic pulmonary edema.

In severe preeclampsia, delivery of the baby should always be considered in the interest of maternal health. Antihypertensive therapy should not be considered as definitive therapy. In almost all cases, preeclampsia resolves on delivery of the baby.

ECLAMPSIA

Eclampsia is the occurrence of generalized tonic-clonic seizures in the absence of other neurologic disorders. It is a relatively rare complication of preeclampsia and up to 40% of cases occur after delivery. Convulsions occur as a result of intracranial vasospasm, raised intracranial pressure and endothelial dysfunction associated with vasogenic edema.

Magnesium sulfate is superior to phenytoin, diazepam and lytic cocktails in preventing initial and recurrent seizures in severe preeclampsia.[14-16] The use of magnesium sulfate may be beneficial even in cases of less severe preeclampsia, and compared to placebo, halves the rate of eclampsia.[17] A dose of 4 g should be administered intravenously over 15 min (or 5 min if actively seizing) followed by an infusion of 1 g/hour for 24 hours, and should be maintained for 24 hours following delivery of the baby or from the last seizure. Serum levels should be maintained between 2 mmol/L and 3.5 mmol/L.[3]

Magnesium toxicity is uncommon, particularly in the absence of any renal dysfunction. It may manifest as myopathy, hyporeflexia and respiratory depression, and tends to occur with serum levels greater than or equal to 3.5 mmol/L. As such, urine output, respiratory rate, oxygen saturation and deep tendon reflexes should be monitored regularly. In cases of toxicity, the infusion should be stopped and 1 g of 10% intravenous calcium gluconate should be administered over 10 min.

All patients suffering from an eclamptic fit should be referred to critical care, as between 5% and 20% of eclamptic seizures recur. If a recurrent seizure occurs despite initial magnesium sulfate, a further 2 g should be given. If seizures persist despite this, intravenous diazepam (10 mg as a bolus) or thiopentone (50 mg) should be administered.

In addition to blood pressure control, airway management should take priority if seizures occur. Where the patient has a reduced level of consciousness, supplemental oxygen should be administered with the patient in the left lateral decubitus position. Any oral secretions should be suctioned and an oropharyngeal airway adjunct may be required. If consciousness does not improve or if recurrent seizures occur, endotracheal intubation, ventilation and sedation should be considered. The patients with recurrent seizures will lose their ability to protect their airway during the seizure or the postictal phase, leading to possible airway obstruction or aspiration of gastric contents. Furthermore, anticonvulsants including benzodiazepines and thiopentone cause a reduction in consciousness. A Glasgow Coma Scale score of less than 8 is usually an indication to intubate the patient, though endotracheal intubation may also be appropriate with higher levels of Glasgow Coma Scale scores.

Intubation of the pregnant patient is particularly challenging, with failed intubation up to eight times more commonly in this population.[18] Due to mechanical effects of the gravid uterus on the vena cava, the pregnant patient should be positioned on a left lateral tilt. Airway hyperemia may impair visualization. Adequate preoxygenation is vital, as reduced functional residual capacity due to diaphragmatic splinting and increased oxygen demand predisposes to rapid desaturation. The risk of aspiration of gastric contents is increased due to delayed gastric emptying and raised intra-abdominal pressure. Although cricoid pressure may impair visualization during laryngoscopy, it is still considered an important precaution in a patient with a high risk of aspiration. Preintubation blood pressure should always be adequately controlled, as the profound hypertensive response to laryngoscopy has been reported to result in intracranial hemorrhage.[6]

■ COMPLICATIONS RELATED TO SEVERE PREECLAMPSIA

Acute Respiratory Failure

Acute pulmonary edema may complicate severe preeclampsia, and is a frequent reason for critical care unit admission associated with high maternal and perinatal mortality and morbidity.[6,19] It is often the consequence of left ventricular failure, "noncardiogenic pulmonary edema" and iatrogenic fluid overload. Although it may be difficult to ascertain the relative contribution of each etiology, the fundamental management is similar.

Severe hypertension may result in left ventricular failure due to an increased afterload, resulting in acute pulmonary edema (cardiogenic pulmonary edema). A transthoracic echocardiogram should be performed to exclude any pre-existing undiagnosed structural cardiac lesions that may have led to acute pulmonary edema. Gradual reduction in SBP will improve cardiac function and aid resolution of pulmonary edema. As mentioned previously, glyceryl trinitrate is a useful therapeutic agent in such circumstances.

Traditionally, acute respiratory distress syndrome (ARDS) has been considered "noncardiogenic" pulmonary edema. However, it is recognized that cardiogenic and "noncardiogenic" pulmonary edema coexist and the definition of ARDS has recently been updated.[20] Acute respiratory distress syndrome may complicate severe preeclampsia. The incidence of ARDS associated with preeclampsia is unclear, due in part to the varying definitions of ARDS in pregnancy.[21] Due to an increase in capillary permeability associated with endothelial dysfunction, an increase in hydrostatic pressure associated with hypertension and a reduction in plasma oncotic pressure in the postpartum period, patients with severe preeclampsia are at risk of ARDS.[19,22]

Supplemental oxygen should be used to maintain oxygen saturations well above 92% and serial arterial blood gas analyses should be performed. In addition, fluid balance and respiratory rate should be monitored on an hourly basis, thus continuous monitoring in a high dependency unit may be required. The patient should be managed in the head up position to facilitate ventilation. Loop diuretics (furosemide) should be administered either as a slow bolus (40–80 mg) over 2 min, repeated after 30 min if required or as a continuous infusion (5–120 mg/hour) to achieve a negative fluid balance.

The patient may require ventilatory support in addition to supplemental oxygen. In circumstances where relatively rapid reversal of the underlying pathology is likely, noninvasive ventilation (NIV) may help maintain oxygenation and aid carbon dioxide clearance. Gastric insufflation due to the positive pressure may increase the risk of aspiration of gastric contents, and NIV should therefore only be considered when the patient is fully conscious. Noninvasive ventilation avoids the potential complications of endotracheal intubation, ventilation and sedation. When there is no improvement in gas exchange (within an hour of starting NIV), if respiratory effort is causing exhaustion, the underlying pathology is unlikely to resolve rapidly or when consciousness is impaired, endotracheal intubation and mechanical ventilation should be considered.

The mainstay in the management of ARDS is the management of the underlying disease. Due to rarity of the condition, clinical evidence specific to the management of pregnant patients with ARDS is lacking. Management strategies in ARDS, including protective ventilation with limited tidal volumes and plateau pressures, prone positioning and restrictive fluid strategies have not been assessed in pregnancy.

The central venous pressure (CVP) has traditionally been used as a surrogate of cardiac preload. However, absolute CVP readings are unreliable in predicting fluid responsiveness among critically ill patients[23] and there is little correlation between right atrial and left atrial pressures (measured by the pulmonary artery catheter) among critically ill pregnant patients.[24] Trends in CVP measurements, however, may offer information on response to intravenous fluid therapy. A CVP rise of greater than 2 cm H_2O in response to a fluid challenge (3 mL/kg intravenous fluid) may suggest that the patient has adequate intravascular volume and further fluid challenges should be stopped. Although the use of the pulmonary artery catheter has the benefit of being able to measure left atrial pressure, the use of the pulmonary artery catheter has significantly declined due to concerns that the invasive procedure does not reduce mortality.[25] No cardiac output monitor has been shown to improve clinical outcome in this cohort of patients.

Altered Neurology

Although the overall occurrence of intracranial hemorrhage is low, cerebral complications account for approximately half the deaths in pregnancies complicated by hypertensive disorders.[26] The possibility of intracranial hemorrhage, infarcts or cerebral edema should be considered as a cause of seizures, particularly if associated with focal neurologic signs, prolonged coma, atypical or recurrent convulsions or who continue to have seizures for a prolonged time following delivery

of the baby. In such circumstances, neuroimaging should be performed. Although headache is a typical feature of severer preeclampsia, it may be the only manifestation of intracerebral hemorrhage; therefore, a low index of suspicion should be held.

In hospitals with limited resources, a non-contrast computerized tomography (CT) head scan should be performed, as fresh intracranial blood will be identified. Magnetic resonance imaging (MRI) is superior to CT in soft tissue contrast and resolution, and for imaging the subcortical areas. Magnetic resonance imaging can rule out small infarcts, cerebral edema and venous thrombosis in addition to acute intracranial hemorrhage.[27]

As mentioned above, patients with reduced level of consciousness may need to be intubated in order to protect the airway. Continuous sedation is required for tolerance of the endotracheal tube. The ideal long-term intravenous sedative is not known as data on long-term sedation in pregnancy is lacking. Propofol has been used for induction of anesthesia but the effects with prolonged used are unclear. Benzodiazepines are able to cross the placenta and diazepam has been associated with cleft lip and palate when used in early pregnancy. The clinical effects of lorazepam and midazolam are unclear. Opiates including morphine and fentanyl have also been associated with the occurrence of congenital malformations but severe preeclampsia and eclampsia occurs only in late gestation after the period of organogenesis and the use of these drugs should not pose a problem. Neuromuscular blocking agents are able to cross the placenta. In utero, this is unlikely to have any significant consequence. However, if intravenous sedatives or neuromuscular blocking agents are given just prior to delivery, the newborn may require a period of ventilatory support and the neonatologist should be alerted.

Acute Kidney Injury

Occasionally, AKI may occur in the context of severe preeclampsia. Consistent with underlying endothelial dysfunction in preeclampsia, the predominant abnormalities seen on renal histology are to the endothelium and glomeruli.[28] In practice, due to the risks of bleeding, a renal biopsy is rarely performed.

There are varying diagnostic criteria of AKI in pregnancy. Formulas for estimating glomerular filtration rate (GFR) lack accuracy in pregnant patients.[29,30] Creatinine clearance by measurement of 24 hour urine creatinine remains the gold standard of GFR estimation in pregnancy. Similarly, renal protein excretion is best estimated by a 24 hour urine collection, as urine protein to creatinine ratios in this population are less reliable.[31] Any sustained fall in urine output (< 0.5 mL/kg/hour) or a rising serum creatinine should alert the clinician to the likelihood of AKI.

The management of AKI is largely supportive, and includes management of the underlying condition, ensuring adequate circulating volume and avoidance of nephrotoxic drugs. Attempting to increase urine output with frusemide or dopamine in the absence of fluid overload should be avoided, as increasing the urine output with diuretics does not improve renal function or outcome.[32-34] Magnesium levels should be monitored closely as toxicity, though uncommon, tends to occur in patients with renal impairment.

If supportive measures do not prevent further deterioration of renal function, renal replacement therapy (hemodialysis, or more commonly, continuous venovenous haemofiltration) may be required. Indications for renal replacement therapy are similar to the general population:

- Hyperkalemia resistant to medical therapy
- Metabolic acidosis resistant to medical therapy
- Uremic pericarditis
- Uremic encephalopathy

HELLP Syndrome

The combination of hemolysis, elevated liver enzymes and low platelets is known as HELLP syndrome and occurs in up to 20% of patients with severe preeclampsia. It occurs in the postpartum period in approximately 30% of cases. This condition is thought to arise as a consequence of endothelial and microvascular injury, increased vascular tone and platelet aggregation. The criteria for the diagnosis of HELLP include the following:

- Microangiopathic hemolysis as evidenced by schistocytes and red cell fragments on blood film
- Lactate dehydrogenase greater than 600 U/L
- Total bilirubin greater than 20 μmol/L
- Aspartate transaminase greater than 70 U/L
- Platelet count less than 50,000/mm³

Renal dysfunction often coexists with HELLP syndrome. It is important to exclude other causes of a thrombotic microangiopathy [thrombotic thrombocytopenic purpura (TTP) and hemolytic uremic syndrome (HUS)] and acute fatty liver of pregnancy. Compared to acute fatty liver of pregnancy, liver dysfunction associated with HELLP tends to be more severe and hepatic infarctions and subcapsular hematomas are features. As such, a liver ultrasound scan should always be performed.

Life-threatening complications of HELLP include hepatic hemorrhage, parenchymal necrosis and subcapsular hematoma leading to hepatic rupture; the latter condition associated with significant maternal and fetal mortality. A surgical consult should be sought early, as drainage of hematoma, packing and oversewing of lacerations is required for imminent or actual hepatic rupture. Radiological embolization may also be considered as an alternative.

A consultant hematologist must be involved at an early stage. Platelet transfusion should be considered if the platelet count falls below 20,000/mm³ or 50,000/mm³ if an interventional procedure is being carried out. The risk of bleeding into the epidural space is significantly reduced with a platelet count of greater than 75,000/mm³.[35] Administration of steroids does not improve outcome in HELLP syndrome.[36]

Definitive treatment is delivery of the baby, though the condition may deteriorate in the following 48 hours. Maternal mortality associated with HELP is approximately 1%, whereas quoted perinatal mortality rates vary from 7% to 60%. Further details on HELLP syndrome are detailed in Chapter 10.

■ SUMMARY

Hypertensive disorders during pregnancy are relatively prevalent and majority of cases are managed well in the community or obstetric ward. However, preeclampsia may be life threatening, and is one of the leading causes of maternal mortality worldwide. Severe preeclampsia is a multisystem disorder. Early involvement of other specialties and allied healthcare professionals to provide a multidisciplinary approach to patient care is therefore important. Continuous monitoring of maternal vital signs and provision of supportive care for multiple organ dysfunctions is best done in ICU. The key to management is early recognition of severe preeclampsia and early admission to ICUs, as this may facilitate appropriate care and improve mortality rates.

REFERENCES

1. Sibai B, Dekker G, Kupferminc M. Pre-eclampsia. Lancet. 2005;365(9461):785-99.
2. Pollock W, Rose L, Dennis CL. Pregnant and postpartum admissions to the intensive care unit: a systematic review. Intensive Care Med. 2010;36(9):1465-74.
3. Zeeman GG. Obstetric critical care: a blueprint for improved outcomes. Crit Care Med. 2006;34(9 Suppl):S208-14.
4. Ronsmans C, Graham WJ. Lancet Maternal Survival Series steering group. Maternal mortality: who, when, where, and why. Lancet. 2006;368(9542):1189-200.
5. Adhikari NK, Fowler RA, Bhagwanjee S, et al. Critical care and the global burden of critical illness in adults. Lancet. 2010;376(9749):1339-46.
6. Lewis G. (2007). Confidential Enquiry into Maternal and Child Health (CEMACH). Saving Mothers' Lives. Reviewing maternal deaths to make motherhood safer: 2003-2005. The Seventh Report of the Confidential Enquiries into Maternal Deaths in the United Kingdom. [online] Available from www.publichealth.hscni.net/sites/default/files/Saving%20Mothers%27%20Lives%202003-05%20.pdf. [Accessed May 2013].
7. Hauth JC, Ewell MG, Levine RJ, et al. Pregnancy outcomes in healthy nulliparas who developed hypertension. Calcium for Preeclampsia Prevention Study Group. Obstet Gynecol. 2000;95(1):24-8.
8. Bombrys AE, Barton JR, Nowacki EA, et al. Expectant management of severe preeclampsia at less than 27 weeks' gestation: maternal and perinatal outcomes according to gestational age by weeks at onset of expectant management. Am J Obstet Gynecol. 2008;199(3):247.e1-6.
9. Carty DM, Delles C, Dominiczak AF. Preeclampsia and future maternal health. J Hypertens. 2010;28(7):1349-55.
10. Khalil AA, Cooper DJ, Harrington KF. Pulse wave analysis: a preliminary study of a novel technique for the prediction of pre-eclampsia. BJOG. 2009;116(2):268-76.
11. Saftlas AF, Olson DR, Franks AL, et al. Epidemiology of preeclampsia and eclampsia in the United States, 1979-1986. Am J Obstet Gynecol. 1990;163(2):460-5.
12. Shennan AH, Halligan AW. Measuring blood pressure in normal and hypertensive pregnancy. Baillieres Best Pract Res Clin Obstet Gynaecol. 1999;13(1):1-26.
13. Hollenberg SM. Vasodilators in acute heart failure. Heart Fail Rev. 2007;12(2):143-7.
14. Duley L, Gülmezoglu AM, Chou D. Magnesium sulphate versus lytic cocktail for eclampsia. Cochrane Database Syst Rev. 2010;(9):CD002960.
15. Duley L, Henderson-Smart DJ, Walker GJ, et al. Magnesium sulphate versus diazepam for eclampsia. Cochrane Database Syst Rev. 2010;(12):CD000127.
16. Duley L, Henderson-Smart DJ, Chou D. Magnesium sulphate versus phenytoin for eclampsia. Cochrane Database Syst Rev. 2010;(10):CD000128.
17. Altman D, Carroli G, Duley L, et al. Do women with pre-eclampsia, and their babies, benefit from magnesium sulphate? The Magpie Trial: a randomised placebo-controlled trial. Lancet. 2002;359(9321):1877-90.
18. King TA, Adams AP. Failed tracheal intubation. Br J Anaesth. 1990;65(3):400-14.
19. Sibai BM, Mabie BC, Harvey CJ, et al. Pulmonary edema in severe preeclampsia-eclampsia: analysis of thirty-seven consecutive cases. Am J Obstet Gynecol. 1987;156(5):1174-9.
20. ARDS Definition Task Force, Ranieri VM, Rubenfeld GD, et al. Acute respiratory distress syndrome: the Berlin Definition. JAMA. 2012;307(23):2526-33.
21. Cole DE, Taylor TL, McCullough DM, et al. Acute respiratory distress syndrome in pregnancy. Crit Care Med. 2005;33(10 Suppl):S269-78.
22. Yeast JD, Halberstadt C, Meyer BA, et al. The risk of pulmonary edema and colloid osmotic pressure changes during magnesium sulfate infusion. Am J Obstet Gynecol. 1993;169(6):1566-71.
23. Osman D, Ridel C, Ray P, et al. Cardiac filling pressures are not appropriate to predict hemodynamic response to volume challenge. Crit Care Med. 2007;35(1):64-8.
24. Young P, Johanson R. Haemodynamic, invasive and echocardiographic monitoring in the hypertensive parturient. Best Pract Res Clin Obstet Gynaecol. 2001;15(4):605-22.
25. Wiener RS, Welch HG. Trends in the use of the pulmonary artery catheter in the United States, 1993-2004. JAMA. 2007;298(4):423-9.
26. Moodley J. Maternal deaths associated with hypertensive disorders of pregnancy: a population-based study. Hypertens Pregnancy. 2004;23(3):247-56.
27. Zeeman GG, Fleckenstein JL, Twickler DM, et al. Cerebral infarction in eclampsia. Am J Obstet Gynecol. 2004;190(3):714-20.
28. Tribe CR, Smart GE, Davies DR, et al. A renal biopsy study in toxaemia of pregnancy. J Clin Pathol. 1979;32(7):681-92.

29. Smith MC, Moran P, Ward MK, et al. Assessment of glomerular filtration rate during pregnancy using the MDRD formula. BJOG. 2008;115(1):109-12.

30. Alper AB, Yi Y, Webber LS, et al. Estimation of glomerular filtration rate in preeclamptic patients. Am J Perinatol. 2007;24(10):569-74.

31. Rodriguez-Thompson D, Lieberman ES. Use of a random urinary protein-to-creatinine ratio for the diagnosis of significant proteinuria during pregnancy. Am J Obstet Gynecol. 2001;185(4):808-11.

32. Steyn DW, Steyn P. Low-dose dopamine for women with severe pre-eclampsia. Cochrane Database Syst Rev. 2007;(1):CD003515.

33. Keiseb J, Moodley J, Connolly CA. Comparison of the efficacy of continuous furosemide and low-dose dopamine infusion in preeclampsia/eclampsia-related oliguria in the immediate postpartum period. Hypertens Pregnancy. 2002;21(3):225-34.

34. Nasu K, Yoshimatsu J, Anai T, et al. Low-dose dopamine in treating acute renal failure caused by preeclampsia. Gynecol Obstet Invest. 1996; 42(2):140-1.

35. Vigil-De Gracia P, Silva S, Montufar C, et al. Anesthesia in pregnant women with HELLP syndrome. Int J Gynaecol Obstet. 2001;74(1):23-7.

36. Fonseca JE, Méndez F, Cataño C, et al. Dexamethasone treatment does not improve the outcome of women with HELLP syndrome: a double-blind, placebo-controlled, randomized clinical trial. Am J Obstet Gynecol. 2005;193(5):1591-8.

16 Immediate Postpartum and Long-Term Care following Hypertension Disease in Pregnancy

Nirmala Chandrasekaran, Basky Thilaganathan

◼ INTRODUCTION

Hypertensive disorders of pregnancy are the most common causes of maternal mortality and morbidity in the developing countries. They are responsible for 12% of maternal mortality during pregnancy and the puerperium. Even though preeclampsia is presumed to be a vascular placental pathology, it continues to pose a threat in the postpartum period and also in the long term. This chapter focuses on the immediate and the long-term care after delivery following hypertensive disorders of pregnancy.

◼ CARDIOVASCULAR PHYSIOLOGY IN THE POSTPARTUM PERIOD

Following a normal pregnancy, the arterial blood pressure (BP) rises progressively during the first 3–5 days of the postpartum period. It has been reported that 12–20% of the normotensive women exceed BP readings of 150/100 mm Hg during this period. This is mainly because this period is characterized by profound fluid shifts from the extravascular space into the intravascular compartments causing a rise in the arterial pressure. In pregnancies complicated with hypertensive diseases, there is a compromised vascular system with diffuse vasospasm secondary to endothelial cell damage and contraction of the intravascular volume. Hence, this fluid shift in these women can lead to pulmonary and cerebral edema and eclampsia. In the postpartum period, Doppler studies have shown that preeclamptic women show persistently elevated central retinal artery systolic velocity, which suggests distal vasoconstriction. These changes take around 6 weeks to resolve. Hence, all of these should be considered whilst discharging women with hypertensive disorders early. Also the time period taken for the BP to normalize varies among the different groups of women. Women who have had gestational hypertension normalize their BP sooner than those with preeclampsia (6 days on an average versus 16 days). The duration of hypertension could reflect well the recovery time of endothelial injury in cases of preeclampsia. Women who have had chronic hypertension also tend to deteriorate during the immediate postpartum period, the severity of which is directly proportional to the severity of the hypertension, the presence of other comorbidities like obesity and renal disease, etc.

Hypertension during puerperium can be due to the persistence of the gestational hypertension or preeclampsia or it can be due to pre-existent hypertension or a hypertension that arise de novo during this period. The latter is due to either late onset preeclampsia or an unmasking of pre-existing hypertension. During normal pregnancy there is an increase in plasma volume and also an associated sodium and water retention in the interstitial tissue. This can be aggravated by the fact that many women tend to receive large volumes of fluids during the intrapartum period and tend to receive drugs that can cause vasoconstriction, e.g. ergot or that compromise renal function, e.g. nonsteroidal anti-inflammatory drugs (NSAIDs). All these can aggravate or cause hypertension but these are rather transient.

IMMEDIATE CARE DURING THE PUERPERIUM

It is well recognized that the immediate postpartum period still continues to pose a risk of developing eclampsia. The British eclamptic survey showed that majority of the fits occurred during the first 48 hours after delivery and only 12% of fits occurred after that period and only 2% occurred 7 days after delivery. Ninty percent of these fits were heralded by prodromal symptoms like headaches and visual disturbances. Hence in the immediate postpartum period women who had preeclampsia should be continued to be monitored for symptomatology, BP and urine output as clinical indicators of disease resolution. The presence of persistent hypertension (> 150/100 mm Hg), prodromal symptoms and hyper-reflexia justifies continuing admission after the 4th postpartum day.

ANALGESIA AND THROMBOPROPHYLAXIS

There are a few studies that examined the different analgesic options for women with gestational hypertension and preeclampsia after a Cesarean section. NSAIDs may contribute to postpartum hypertension as per few case reports and thus their use should be avoided in patients who are already hypertensive. They are absolutely contraindicated if preeclampsia has been complicated by hemorrhage, or there is concern about adequacy of hemostasis (e.g. uterine atony). In women with mild renal disease (good urine output and no serum indices of renal failure), there seems little reason to deny women the benefit of the morphine-sparing effect of NSAID. However, successive doses should not be given without repeated confirmation of sustained satisfactory urine output.

Pregnancy being a hypercoagulable state increases the risk of both arterial and venous thrombosis to 3–4 fold than nonpregnant population. In women with hypertensive disorders, there is widespread endothelial damage thereby destroying the integrity of the vascular compartments. Also there is a state of generalized volume contraction. These factors along with the hypercoagulability due to proteinuria, make the preeclamptic women more prone to both arterial and venous thrombosis. Thromboprophylaxis should be considered for all women with hypertensive disorders of pregnancy, the duration of which will depend on the associated additional risk factors.

MONITORING

As the puerperium continues to pose a risk, it is important that these women are monitored more frequently. There is no evidence identified in relation to the frequency of monitoring that these patients need and it should be based on the clinical picture and the severity of the disease. The National Institute of Clinical Excellence (NICE) recommends that women who had preeclampsia during pregnancy should continue to be monitored with 4 hourly BP and urine output whilst they stay as inpatient if the serum creatinine is normal, fluid balance need not be measured. The BP should be checked at least once a day between day 3 and 5 and if the BP was abnormal at that point the checks should be carried out every alternate day until it normalizes. If the BP warranted treatment antenatally with antihypertensive, in addition to the 4 hourly monitoring whilst staying as inpatient, the BP should be monitored every 1–2 days for up to 2 weeks after transfer to community care until the woman is off treatment and has no hypertension. In women with preeclampsia, the platelet count and serum transaminases should be repeated 48–72 hours after birth unless clinical conditions warrant an early blood test. If they are normal there is no benefit in repeating them after. Women who had hypertension without proteinuria should be monitored for the signs and symptoms of preeclampsia including the trends in renal and liver functions, although there could be physiological elevation in the liver enzymes due to uterine involution. If biochemical and hematological indices are not improving relative to pregnancy ranges in women with preeclampsia who have given birth, repeat platelet count, transaminases and serum creatinine measurements as clinically indicated and if they are improving but still abnormal, they need to be repeated at 6–8 weeks check. Proteinuria should be estimated with a protein reagent strip at 6 weeks review and if it is persistent at this stage, renal functions should be assessed further at 3 months postnatal in order to eliminate primary renal disease.

Women who have had hypertensive disease should only be discharged to the community if the BP is well under control (i.e. < 140/99 mm Hg), the blood tests are stable and there are no symptoms of preeclampsia. Whilst discharge, a clear written plan is essential informing who provides the care in the community, the symptoms and signs of preeclampsia that the patient needs to watch for, the threshold for treatment and to stop the medication and indications for referral to the hospital during the postnatal period. Women who were treated with antihypertensive need a postnatal medical review in 2 weeks after delivery and all women who have had preeclampsia need a 6–8 week medical review.

Blood Pressure Control

The principles of management of hypertension in the postnatal period are the same as in the antenatal period, i.e. to prevent severe hypertension. Severe hypertension can cause direct arterial injury and lead to cerebral hemorrhage. The aim of emergency treatment is to maintain the BP less than 160 mm Hg systolic and 110 mm Hg diastolic, in order that the mean arterial pressure is less than 125 mm Hg, thereby preventing cerebral injury from occurring. Hence in women who are on antihypertensives antenatally, the medications need to be continued during the postnatal period as well and if the BP falls below 140/80 mm Hg, consideration should be given to reduce the dose. For women who were not treated during the antenatal period, treatment should be commenced if the BP is higher than 149/99 mm Hg.

A Cochrane review of the prevention and treatment of postpartum hypertension concludes that there were no reliable data to guide the management of women who are hypertensive postpartum or at an increased risk of becoming so. It concludes by saying that if a clinician feels that hypertension is severe enough to treat, the agent used should be based on his/her familiarity with the drug. Severe hypertension can be treated acutely with labetalol orally or intravenously, intravenous hydralazine or nifedipine orally.

Labetalol has the advantage of using orally and also intravenously. It is not clear as to whether labetalol or hydrazine is superior in treating acute hypertension as the evidence for the use of short-acting antihypertensives for the treatment of severe hypertension is not robust enough to guide clinical practice. Hence clinicians could choose the drug they are familiar and comfortable with. Once control of acute hypertension is achieved, the choice of antihypertensives is varied. Even though methyldopa is the drug of choice in the antenatal period, it should be avoided in the postpartum period as it causes depression and psychosis. If the patient was on methyldopa originally it must be switched to some other medication within the 2nd postnatal day which could include a beta blocker (atenolol, metoprolol, labetalol, calcium channel blocker (nifedipine) or an angiotensin converting enzyme (ACE) inhibitor (e.g. enalapril, captopril) which are all safe with breastfeeding. As a general rule diuretics should be avoided in women who breastfeed as it causes volume contraction and reduces milk production and there is insufficient evidence on the safety with amlodipine and ACE inhibitors other than captopril and enalapril. The clinical well-being and the adequacy of feeding of the babies should be assessed at least daily for the first 2 days after the birth. The antihypertensive for women who had gestational hypertension should be continued for at least 2–3 weeks postnatally after which they can either be reduced or withdrawn in the primary care setting. For women who need antihypertensive after 6 weeks postpartum, consideration should be given to investigate the woman appropriately for essential hypertension.

Other Therapeutic Strategies

Postpartum curettage was first attempted in the 1960s and revisited again later in an attempt to remove all the trophoblast associated toxins to accelerate the recovery from preeclampsia. Even though small randomized trials have concluded that the mean arterial pressures were significantly lower with curettage, follow-up studies comparing nifedipine and postnatal curettage failed to demonstrate the effectiveness of curettage in accelerated recovery. Also, curettage adds the risk of putting a preeclamptic woman to the risk of general anesthesia and also the associated complications of curettage. Hence, it is not widely practised in the developed world.

■ LONG-TERM RISKS ASSOCIATED WITH HYPERTENSIVE DISEASES OF PREGNANCY

Risk of Recurrence in Subsequent Pregnancies

Preeclampsia was originally thought to be predominantly a disease of first birth. But it has been understood now that women with a history of previous preeclampsia are at increased risk of preeclampsia and other adverse pregnancy outcomes in subsequent pregnancies. The magnitude of this risk is dependent on gestational age at time of disease onset, severity of disease, presence or absence of pre-existing medical disorders including a raised body mass index (BMI), pre-existing renal disease and advanced maternal age. In women who have had gestational hypertension in their first pregnancies, the risk of recurrence of gestational hypertension in the subsequent pregnancies is quoted to be between 16% and 47%. The risk of preeclampsia in the same group of women is between 2% and 7%. For women who have had pregnancies complicated with preeclampsia, the risk of recurrence is about 16%. If it had been an early onset preeclampsia (leading to a delivery before 34 weeks) or one that was complicated by HELLP syndrome, the risk of recurrence is about 25%. The interpregnancy interval does not increase this risk unless it is more than 10 years. It was also thought that a change in partner increases the risk of preeclampsia in the subsequent pregnancies. A large Danish cohort study suggested that the change in partner does not increase the risk of subsequent preeclampsia. It also concluded that women who had preeclampsia in their first pregnancy did not seem to increase their risk with increased interpregnancy intervals but those who had no preeclampsia in their first pregnancy had increasing risk with increased interpregnancy interval. The least risk in both groups was with an interpregnancy interval of less than 3 years. Also the maternal BMI seems to have a linear relationship with the risk of recurrence in

subsequent pregnancies. Hence, women should be advised to maintain a healthy weight prior to getting pregnant again.

Risk of Cardiovascular Diseases and Stroke

It is well known that pregnancy is a stress test of life. The risk factors for preeclampsia and coronary artery diseases are similar namely obesity, family history, dyslipidemia, abnormal angiogenesis, diabetes and hypertension. Hence, it is not surprising that preeclampsia being a vascular pathology increases the risk of all cardiovascular events like ischemic heart disease, chronic hypertension, stroke and venous thromboembolism. A systematic review which included 3,488,160 women concluded that the risk of chronic hypertension after preeclamptic pregnancy was four times more than the controls. This risk tends to vary depending on the severity and the gestation of onset. It also added that the risk of ischemic heart disease is twice that of the controls and the risk of both fatal and nonfatal stroke increased by 1.8 times that of controls. It is possible that much of the excess risk of future ischemic heart disease and stroke is explained by the link between preeclampsia and BP. Similarly the risk of developing a venous thromboembolism was 1.8 times more than the controls when followed-up for 7 years. A Danish registry-based cohort study also concluded strong association of preeclampsia and subsequent type 2 diabetes mellitus. The severity, parity and recurrence of these hypertensive pregnancy disorders increase the risk of subsequent cardiovascular events.

■ PREDICTING FUTURE DISEASE

As the history of preeclampsia exerts an independent risk for future cardiovascular disease, it may increase the risk of cardiovascular disease in midlife in affected women, which would render them eligible for preventive therapies at an earlier age than usual. There is an increasing understanding that cardiovascular diseases are generally progressive disorders which proceed through asymptomatic to symptomatic stages. One of the principal manifestations of this progression is the change in the geometry and function of the left ventricle. There has been a prospective longitudinal case control study which has shown that women with preterm preeclampsia, and to a lesser extent term preeclampsia, are at a significantly increased risk of asymptomatic left ventricle dysfunction/ hypertrophy and essential hypertension within 1–2 years after delivery. Hence, it is possible to identify these women early before the disease becomes clinically apparent and introduce measures in order to prevent progression of the disease.

▓ PREVENTATIVE STRATEGIES

Preeclampsia should be used as an independent risk factor for cardiovascular risk stratification. Women should be educated regarding the long-term health consequences and advised to maintain a healthy lifestyle at the postnatal visit including stopping smoking, lifestyle modification (physical activity, diet, alcohol consumption and weight), BP control (to below 140/85 mm Hg) and strict diabetic control (meticulous control of BP and glucose). Treating hyperlipidemia when identified would help although there is no strong evidence to suggest primary prevention with statins or aspirin is advantageous. The other most important aspect is good communication between primary and secondary care practitioners.

▓ CONCLUSION

Preeclampsia is an endothelial dysfunction which originates from complex interactions among maternal constitutional factors, including pre-existing metabolic abnormalities, placenta-derived products, and the exaggerated adaptive mechanisms that normally occur during pregnancy. It does not "resolve" once the baby and the placenta are delivered. Hence, the care of pregnant hypertensive women does not stop by delivering the baby but it is a long-term process.

▓ BIBLIOGRAPHY

1. Bellamy L, Casas JP, Hingorani AD, et al. Pre-eclampsia and risk of cardiovascular disease and cancer in later life: systematic review and meta-analysis. BMJ. 2007;335(7627):974.
2. Fejgin MD, Charles AG. Immediate postpartum curettage: accelerated recovery from severe preeclampsia. Obstet Gynecol. 1993;82(1):163-4.
3. Garovic VD, Bailey KR, Boerwinkle E, et al. Hypertension in pregnancy as a risk factor for cardiovascular disease later in life. J Hypertens. 2010;28(4):826-33.
4. Ghuman N, Rhiener J, Tendler BE, et al. Hypertension in the postpartum woman: clinical update for the hypertension specialist. J Clin Hypertens (Greenwich). 2009;11(12):726-33.
5. Giannina G, Belfort MA, Arcardia L, et al. Persistent cerebrovascular changes in postpartum pre-eclamptic women: a Doppler evaluation. Am J Obstet Gynecol. 1997;177(5):1213-18.
6. Green A, Loughna P, Pipkin FB. New-onset hypertension in pregnancy: a review of the long-term maternal effects. Obstet Gynecol. 2012;14:99-105.
7. Lykke JA, Langhoff-Roos J, Sibai BM, et al. Hypertensive pregnancy disorders and subsequent cardiovascular morbidity and type 2 diabetes mellitus in the mother. Hypertension. 2009;53(6):944-51.
8. Magee L, Sadeghi S. Prevention and treatment of postpartum hypertension. Cochrane Database Syst Rev. 2005;(1):CD004351.
9. Makris A, Thornton C, Hennessy A. Postpartum hypertension and nonsteroidal analgesia. Am J Obstet Gynecol. 2004;190(2):577-8.
10. Melchiorre K, Sutherland GR, Liberati M. Pre-eclampsia is associated with persistent postpartum cardiovascular impairment. Hypertension. 2011;58(4):709-15.
11. McDonald SD, Best C, Lam K. The recurrence risk of severe de novo pre-eclampsia in singleton pregnancies: a population-based cohort. BJOG. 2009;116(12):1578-84.
12. National Institute for Health and Clinical Excellence (2010). Hypertension in pregnancy: the management of hypertensive disorders during pregnancy. Clinical Guideline 107. [online] Available from http://www.nice.org.uk/cg107 [Accessed June, 2013].
13. Sibai BM. Thrombophilia and severe preeclampsia: time to screen and treat in future pregnancies? Hypertension. 2005;46(6):1252-3.
14. Tan LK, de Swiet M. The management of postpartum hypertension. BJOG. 2002;109(7):733-6.
15. Walters BN, Thompson ME, Lee A, et al. Blood pressure in the puerperium. Clin Sci (Lond). 1986; 71(5):589-94.

17

Lesson Learnt from Confidential Enquiries

Adele Zito, Boon H Lim

■ INTRODUCTION

Hypertensive disease in pregnancy still poses major challenges in the management and outcome for obstetric services around the world. Evidence from various confidential enquiries into maternal deaths show that deaths from complications of preeclampsia and eclampsia remain high on the list of direct causes of maternal mortality. Many important lessons have been learnt from the confidential enquiries and these have led to improvements of provision of care and outcome for pregnant women. However, there is still room for improvement in the understanding and management of hypertensive disease in pregnancy and the complications in order to reduce avoidable deaths from a potentially treatable condition.

Pregnancy is a time associated with great hope and prospect of new life and motherhood for most women. Despite advances in obstetric care, women still die of causes directly or indirectly related to pregnancy.[1,2] In the developed world, it is estimated that 1 in every 2,800 women will die of complications related to pregnancy, while in some of the developing countries, this figure is an astounding one in 16. It can be easy to become complacent, particularly in the developed world as maternal death has become a relatively uncommon event. However, with changing demographics and lifestyle, modern obstetrics is now facing new challenges of a greater proportion of older

and obese women, with associated complex medical problems, becoming pregnant.[3] It is an alarming fact that lifestyle choices have significant impacts on maternal health. Over 50% of women who died in the United Kingdom (UK) between 2003 and 2005 were classed as overweight or obese.[4]

It is important to realize that good maternal health is not a universal right, even in countries with high quality maternity services and low maternal morbidity and mortality rates.[1] Disappointingly, substandard care is often associated with maternal mortality, in spite of highly trained health professionals providing maternity care.[1,2] As maternal mortality has a significant social impact, it is understandably subject to rigorous review in developed countries as lessons learnt provide a stimulus for change in healthcare provision and clinical practice. This process in the UK is known as the Confidential Enquiries into Maternal Deaths.

Confidential enquiries into maternal deaths have been a regular and integral part of assessing maternal mortality in the UK since 1952.[1,2,5] The confidential enquiry process is the most longstanding example of a maternal mortality or morbidity surveillance cycle (Fig. 17.1). Over the 60 years of review, these enquiries have gained international recognition as the "gold standard" in evaluating maternal mortality, and have resulted in improvements in clinical practice in order to prevent and reduce maternal deaths.[1,2,5-7]

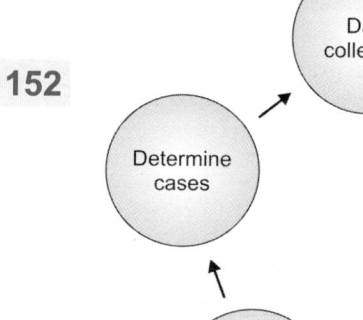

Fig. 17.1: Maternal morbidity or mortality surveillance cycle
Source: Modified from Lewis G. (2011). Centre for Maternal and Child Enquiries (CMACE). Saving Mothers' Lives. Reviewing maternal deaths to make motherhood safer: 2006-2008. The Eighth Report on Confidential Enquiries into Maternal Deaths in the United Kingdom. [online] Available from www.cdph.ca.gov/data/statistics/Documents/MO-CAPAMR-CMACE-2006-08-BJOG-2011.pdf. [Accessed May, 2013].

Many countries have now adopted this methodology to review and improve outcomes.[1,8] A fundamental aspect of the enquiry process is the significance of the confidentiality, anonymous and nonthreatening environment, allowing for complete analysis of each maternal death, with the principal objective to save lives rather than attribute blame.[3] A confidential enquiry into maternal death is defined as "a systematic multidisciplinary anonymous investigation of all or a representative sample of maternal deaths occurring at an area, regional or national level; it identifies the numbers, causes and avoidable or remediable factors associated with them".[3,9] The most recent enquiries in the UK were overseen by the Centre for Maternal and Child Enquiries (CMACE), which produced the triennial report, known as "Saving Mothers' Lives".[1,2] The title "Saving Mothers' Lives" (previously known as "Why Mothers Die") is a recent change since the seventh report of the confidential enquiries, and was made to reflect the significance of understanding each maternal death, the importance of going beyond the statistics and exploring the stories of each

maternal death so that lessons can be learnt from each of the tragic events.[1,2] This methodology and philosophy has also been adopted by the World Health Organization (WHO) in their maternal mortality review "Beyond the numbers".[3]

Recent UK reports not only contain detailed recommendations, but also "top 10 recommendations", which are considered top priority areas for improvement, implementation and audit in maternity services and the "back to basics" section, consisting of checklists to aid recognition and action for signs and symptoms of potentially life-threatening conditions. They are by no means aimed at covering every possibility, but serve as good practice points to help identify and exclude the more common disorders of pregnancy.[1,2]

These practice points can be considered in three categories:
1. Improving basic medical and midwifery practice such as taking a history, undertaking basic observations and understanding normality.
2. Attributing signs and symptoms of emerging serious illness to commonplace symptoms in pregnancy.
3. Improving communication and referrals.

As the numbers of maternal deaths continue to decrease in developed countries, it is increasingly recognized that the understanding of maternal morbidity and "near miss" events can provide integral information for the prevention and management of potentially life-threatening conditions.[1] The United Kingdom Obstetric Surveillance System (UKOSS) was established in 2005 to evaluate rare events of pregnancy.[1,4] Data obtained from the UKOSS can be used to quantify risk and prognostic factors, audit national management and prevention guidelines, and describe disease management as well as outcomes for both mothers and infants. Examples of information obtained from UKOSS studies include estimating disease incidence; describing the prevalence factors associated with "near miss" morbidity; quantifying risk factors for severe morbidity; auditing national guidelines; investigating different management techniques and describing the outcomes of severe morbidity. Eclampsia is one of the conditions under surveillance by UKOSS, which confirmed a 45% reduction in the incidence of eclampsia in the UK between 1992 and 2005. In 1992 the incidence of eclampsia was 4.9 per 100,000 maternities, while in 2005 this had decreased to 2.7 per 100,000 maternities. This dramatic reduction in the incidence of eclampsia was attributed to the introduction of magnesium sulfate ($MgSO_4$) into protocols for the management of preeclampsia and eclampsia in maternity units in the UK.[1] This highlighted the useful benefits of translating evidence from audit and research into practice thereby improving outcomes for women.[1] There are similar organizations around the world including the Australasian Maternal Outcome Surveillance System (AMOSS).

MATERNAL MORTALITY

Maternal mortality is defined by the ninth and tenth revisions of the International Classification of Diseases, Injuries and Causes of Death (ICD 9/10) as "the death of a woman while pregnant or within 42 days of termination of pregnancy, from any cause related to or aggravated by the pregnancy or its management but not from accidental or incidental causes". Maternal deaths are further classified as direct, indirect, late, coincidental (fortuitous) or nonpregnancy-related deaths.

Direct maternal death is defined as "deaths resulting from obstetric complications of the pregnant state (pregnancy, labor and puerperium), from interventions, omissions, incorrect treatment or a chain of events resulting from any of the above". Maternal deaths which arise as a result of

pre-existing disease, or disease that developed during pregnancy and which was not due to direct obstetric causes, but which was aggravated by the physiological effects of pregnancy are classified as indirect maternal deaths. Any maternal death occurring between 42 days and 1 year after abortion, miscarriage or delivery that was due to direct or indirect maternal causes is known as a late maternal death. Coincidental maternal deaths refer to any maternal death from unrelated causes which happen to occur in pregnancy or the puerperium, while a pregnancy-related death is defined as, "death occurring in women while pregnant or within 42 days of termination of pregnancy, irrespective of the cause of death".[4,10-13]

Definitions of maternal mortality ratios are also important to understand, as they are used frequently in reports such as the UK confidential enquiries into maternal deaths as well as internationally but their definitions vary slightly. The discrepancy in definitions is a result of difficulties experienced in many countries, particularly those in the developing world, when collecting reliable data relating to maternal death as well as basic denominator data.[1] In the UK, the maternal mortality rate (MMR) is defined as "the number of direct and indirect deaths per 100,000 maternities", while internationally, the MMR is "the number of direct and indirect deaths per 100,000 live births" (Table 17.1). Maternities are the

Table 17.1: Maternal mortality by direct and indirect deaths in the United Kingdom in the different triennia from 1985 (maternal mortality rates per 100,000 maternities)

Triennium	Direct Deaths		Indirect Deaths		Total Direct and Indirect Deaths	
	Number (N)	Rate	Number (N)	Rate	Number (N)	Rate
1985–1987	139	6.13	84	3.70	223	9.83
1988–1990	145	6.14	93	3.94	238	10.08
1991–1993	128	5.53	100	4.32	228	9.85
1994–1996	134	6.10	134	6.10	268	12.19
1997–1999	106	4.99	136	6.40	242	11.40
2000–2002	106	5.31	155	7.76	261	13.07
2003–2005	132	6.24	163	7.71	295	13.95
2006–2008	107	4.67	154	6.72	261	11.39

Source: Lewis G. (2011). Centre for Maternal and Child Enquiries (CMACE). Saving Mothers' Lives. Reviewing maternal deaths to make motherhood safer: 2006–2008. The Eighth Report on Confidential Enquiries into Maternal Deaths in the United Kingdom. [online] Available from www.cdph.ca.gov/data/statistics/Documents/MO-CAPAMR-CMACE-2006-08-BJOG-2011.pdf. [Accessed May, 2013].

"number of pregnancies that result in a live birth at any gestation or stillbirths occurring at or after 24 completed weeks of gestation, and are required to be notified by law".[4,10-13]

Measuring maternal mortality in many countries can be difficult, notably in the developing countries.[14] Some countries lack civil registration systems, and thus routine registration of death, and in particular maternal deaths does not occur.[14] In countries where deaths are recorded, the pregnancy status of a woman at the time of her death may not be recognized, and thus is not recorded as a maternal death.[14] Finally in many developing countries, death is not medically certified and thus again maternal deaths can go unrecorded.[14] Problems in accurately representing maternal mortality are not confined to the developing world, as misclassification of death using the ICD 9/10 can result in misrepresentation of the actual number of maternal deaths.[14]

For decades, preeclampsia and eclampsia have been the leading causes of maternal death. Over the years, with developments and changes in obstetric practice there has been a global decline in maternal deaths from hypertensive disorders of pregnancy. This chapter explores the trends in maternal mortality attributed to hypertensive disease with a focus on the confidential enquiries into maternal deaths, particularly those arising from the UK and more broadly what has been reflected in the international community. Key learning points and recommendations in relation to hypertensive disease in pregnancy and trends from each of the reports have been highlighted (Box 17.1).

> **Box 17.1:** Key learning points—
> maternal mortality
>
> • A confidential enquiry is an anonymous, systematic review of maternal deaths to determine cause and prevent future mortality rather than attribute blame
> • Internationally, the UK confidential enquiries into maternal deaths are considered as the gold standard and are the longest running reviews of its kind
> • Understanding maternal morbidity complements knowledge and lessons learnt from maternal mortality

THE UNITED KINGDOM PERSPECTIVE

The Early Years

Hypertensive disease in pregnancy was the leading cause of direct maternal deaths in England and Wales between 1952 and 1957. Over 50% of these deaths had avoidable origins, with the most common being suboptimal antenatal care. Other issues surrounding hypertensive maternal deaths in this time period included maternal refusal of medical advice, failing to attend follow-up reviews as well as hospital bed shortages. With improving antenatal care, the number of deaths attributed to hypertensive disease in pregnancy got more than halved by the next triennium (1958–1960). In 1928, the overall MMR was an alarming 400 per 100,000 births![15]

The Early 1990s (1994–1996)

The overall MMR was 12.2 per 100,000 maternities in this triennium which was the same as the preceding report. This report showed that hypertensive disease was the second highest cause of direct maternal deaths, with thromboembolic disease being the leading cause. Twenty maternal deaths were attributed to hypertensive disease of pregnancy during this time. Eight women died of eclamptic seizures, six of whom had their first seizure outside of hospital.[10]

From this triennium, deaths due to hypertension in pregnancy continued to decrease, mainly due to a reduction in deaths from pulmonary and cerebral edema. Maternal death arising from fluid balance disparity in the setting of hypertensive disease became less of an issue toward the end of the 1990s. Substandard care however was an ongoing concern in 80% of the maternal deaths.[15]

Specific recommendations arising in the triennium included an emphasis on clinical leadership in the management of these cases, particularly in relation to fluid balance. Maternity units were encouraged to formulate and update protocols relating to preeclampsia and eclampsia management. In spite of the early senior clinician involvement in many of the cases, substandard care was still apparent in 10 out of 17 direct deaths, which equated to 59%. However, this represented a significant reduction from 80% in the previous two triennia. The most frequent mode of death from hypertensive disorders of pregnancy was the development of acute respiratory distress syndrome (ARDS), a rare complication of preeclampsia usually attributable to fluid overload.[10]

The use of $MgSO_4$ for secondary prevention of eclampsia was very much in its infancy during this triennium. At this time, diazepam and phenytoin were in routine use for eclampsia with very limited clinical use of $MgSO_4$. In 1998, at the time of publication of the confidential enquiry report for 1994–1996, the pilot trial by the Magpie Trial Collaboration Group had just commenced.[10]

Another focus of recommendations for this triennium surrounded education for both patients and medical professionals. In relation to patients, the report highlighted the significance of routine antenatal education and advising women on the symptoms relating to preeclampsia and the importance of women with these symptoms during their pregnancy to attend for formal assessment. As for health professionals, it was recommended that medical and midwifery staff participated in continued education on preeclampsia. The emphasis was on the importance of accurate diagnosis, assessment and prompt referral for patients with preeclampsia from medical professionals working in community and regional centers to specialist centers (Box 17.2).[10]

Box 17.2: Key learning points from the early 1990s

- Hypertensive disease in pregnancy was the second highest cause of maternal mortality
- Senior clinician input in the management of preeclamptic and eclamptic patients
- Strict fluid balance in patients with preeclampsia and eclampsia
- Antenatal patient education on the signs and symptoms of hypertensive disease in pregnancy and the importance of seeking medical assessment
- Early suggestions for magnesium sulfate ($MgSO_4$) use for secondary prevention of eclampsia

---

The Late 1990s (1997–1999)

Hypertensive disease in pregnancy again remained the second largest contributor to direct maternal deaths in this triennium; however, the overall rate had fallen from 9.1 per million maternities to 7.1 per million maternities. As with the previous triennium, thromboembolic disease was again the leading cause of direct maternal deaths. The overall MMR was 11.4 per 100,000 maternities, which represented a slight decrease in overall MMRs compared to 1994–1996. In this triennium, 15 maternal deaths were attributed to hypertensive disease in pregnancy, five of these from eclamptic seizures occurring in hospital. The greatest single cause of death from preeclampsia or eclampsia was intracranial hemorrhage, suggesting failure of adequate antihypertensive treatment.[11]

Specific recommendations arising in this triennial report stressed the importance of checking blood pressure and urine for protein as a minimum in the diagnostic workup for pregnant women with headache or new epigastric pain. Additionally, caution was recommended with the use of automated blood pressure devices, owing to their tendency to underestimate blood pressure in preeclampsia. In relation to specialist intensive care for women with preeclampsia, it was suggested that such services should be utilized and mobilized early in women with severe preeclampsia. In women with severe preeclampsia who require admission to an intensive care unit, caution should be given to avoid rapid discharge of such patients.[11]

The importance of strict fluid balance in women with severe preeclampsia was again highlighted and it was recommended that fluid intake should be restricted to 85 mL/hour. This recommendation was part of a wider guideline for the management of severe preeclampsia within the report. In addition to this, it was suggested that clear written management protocols for severe preeclampsia should direct both initial and ongoing treatment of these patients while in hospital (Box 17.3).[11]

Box 17.3: Key learning points from the late 1990s

- Hypertensive disease in pregnancy remained the second highest cause of maternal mortality
- Intracranial hemorrhage was the most common cause of death from preeclampsia and eclampsia
- Headache and new onset epigastric pain require a blood pressure and urine protein check as a minimum assessment
- Fluid restriction to 85 mL/hour in women with preeclampsia and eclampsia
- Clear written management plans for patients with hypertensive disease in pregnancy
- Avoid early discharge from intensive care units

The Early 2000s (2000–2002)

As with the preceding two triennia, hypertensive disorders in pregnancy were the second most common cause of direct maternal mortality, with 14 deaths attributed to hypertensive disease in pregnancy.[4,12] Again, thromboembolic disease was the leading cause of direct maternal mortality. However, the number of maternal deaths from this cause continued to decline. The overall MMR was 13.1 per 100,000 maternities corresponding to a slight increase from 1997 to 1999 which was not statistically significant. There were a total of 391 maternal deaths, 106 of these were direct, 155 indirect, 36 coincidental and 94 late. In keeping with trends from the previous two triennia, MMRs from preeclampsia and eclampsia remained the same.[12]

The foremost fault in clinical care in this triennium was insufficient treatment of hypertension resulting in intracranial hemorrhage. The recommendations focused on management protocols which aimed to avoid life-threatening levels of systolic hypertension ($\geq$ 160 mm Hg), in order to avoid and reduce the risk of intracerebral hemorrhage. Additional features highlighted in reports from previous triennia again flowed through into this report including late involvement of consultant obstetricians, substandard care in relation to recognition of new severe headache or epigastric pain, both within hospitals and the community (Box 17.4).[12]

Box 17.4: Key learning points arising from early 2000s

- Importance of treating life-threatening systolic hypertension to avoid the risk of intracranial hemorrhage
- Early involvement of consultant obstetricians in cases complicated by preeclampsia and eclampsia
- Recognizing the significance of new onset severe headache or epigastric pain

---

The Mid 2000s (2003–2005)

This triennium saw 18 direct maternal deaths attributed to hypertensive disease in pregnancy, ranking equal second place with genital tract sepsis as the leading causes of direct deaths. As with the preceding three triennial reports, the leading cause of direct maternal death was thromboembolism. The overall MMR for the triennia was 14 per 100,000 maternities indicating a slight but not statistically significant rise compared to the previous report. This was attributed to better case ascertainment.[4]

Of the 18 deaths, 10 died from intracranial hemorrhage, two from cerebral infarction, two from multiorgan failure, one from massive liver infarction and three from other causes. The vast majority of these women died from intracranial hemorrhage, a reflection of poor control of systolic blood pressure, as the most frequent basis of substandard care. Intracranial hemorrhage again featured as a common cause of death as highlighted in the preceding triennial reports.[4]

This was the first triennial report which included the "top 10", priority areas.[4] The treatment of systolic hypertension was highlighted as an area of top priority as insufficient treatment of systolic hypertension in women with preeclampsia was the single most important contributing factor in substandard care in the triennium. It was suggested that pregnant women with a systolic blood pressure of 160 mm Hg or more require antihypertensive treatment, with consideration to commencement of such therapy at lower blood pressures if there is clinical concern about rapid deterioration or development of severe hypertension.[4]

Further recommendations for this triennium included avoiding the use of syntometrine (oxytocin + ergometrine) for the active management of the third stage of labor in women with hypertension or when the blood pressure has not been checked in labor, as ergometrine is contraindicated in hypertensive disease. In addition, care should be taken when preeclamptic women require an anesthetic, particularly in relation to avoiding the pressor effects associated with intubation.[4] This was highlighted in two cases. In the first case, an eclamptic woman on $MgSO_4$ required an emergency Cesarean section secondary to fetal bradycardia, having had eclamptic seizures at home in early labor. Following intubation for general anesthetic, she had a seizure as a result of an increase in blood pressure to 209/120 mm Hg. Despite antihypertensive therapy, she was found to have an intracranial hemorrhage postpartum. The second case involved a fit and healthy woman with an unremarkable antenatal course who underwent induction of labor as she was postdates. Her induction was postponed due to service demands and she subsequently developed fulminating preeclampsia and fetal distress necessitating Cesarean delivery under general anesthesia. Sadly, she was unable to be woken from the anesthetic, and imaging revealed a massive intracranial hemorrhage (Box 17.5).[4] These cases highlight the difficult balance between obstetric and anesthetic concerns, and the difficulties faced with unstable critically unwell hypertensive pregnant women.

> **Box 17.5:** Key learning points arising from mid 2000s
>
> - Intracranial hemorrhage again was the most common cause of death from preeclampsia and eclampsia
> - Treatment of systolic hypertension at levels of 160 mm Hg or lower if clinical concern as a top priority
> - Avoid syntometrine for active management of third stage in women with elevated blood pressure in labor

The Late 2000s (2006–2008)

The Saving Mothers Report (2006–2008)

This was the most recent confidential enquiry report conducted by CMACE. In the future, the National Perinatal Epidemiology Unit (NPEU) will be responsible for conducting the confidential enquiries. The overall MMR for this triennium was 11.39 per 100,000 maternities representing a statistically significant decline in maternal mortality when compared to the last triennium. Genital tract sepsis was the leading cause of direct maternal mortality in this triennium, with hypertensive disease in pregnancy remaining the second highest cause of direct maternal mortality. Deaths from thromboembolic disease, the foremost reason for direct maternal mortality in the UK for over 20 years ranked third. The reduction in the overall maternal mortality was attributed to the reduction in direct deaths as a result of thromboembolism;

however, there was no reduction in the number of deaths from preeclampsia or eclampsia. Figure 17.2 shows the principal causes of maternal deaths in this triennium, noting that preeclampsia and eclampsia are the fifth most common cause of overall maternal mortality in the UK in these triennia. Cardiac disease was the leading cause of both indirect and overall maternal mortality in this triennium.[1]

Of the 22 women who died as a result of hypertensive disease in pregnancy, 14 died from cerebral causes (nine from intracranial hemorrhage and five from anoxia secondary to cardiac arrest following an eclamptic seizure); three from liver complications (two from necrosis and one from subcapsular hemorrhage); two women died from multiorgan failure, two from complications of acute fatty liver of pregnancy and one from intra-abdominal hemorrhage of unknown cause. It is interesting to note that the majority of maternal deaths were a result of intracranial hemorrhage, again reflecting issues of inadequate management of systolic hypertension. Unfortunately substandard care was a factor in 20 of the 22 deaths, with 14 of these deaths classified as having major issues in relation to substandard care. Substandard care occurred in both the hospital and the community; four cases were attributed to errors made by general practitioners (GP), mainly due to failure of appropriate referral to specialist care.[1] Examples of how these women were incorrectly managed by their GP include one woman with preeclampsia being commenced on antihypertensive medication, instead of specialist referral; a second woman with extensive proteinuria being referred for urological investigation and a third woman with jaundice, who then developed hemolysis, elevated liver enzymes, low platelets (HELLP) syndrome being referred by her GP to the community midwife. Underlying factors contributing to errors in care by GPs are related to the increasing separation of GPs from antenatal care with resultant deskilling in this area. In addition to mistakes in care in the community, both GPs and emergency departments need to address the significance and urgency of epigastric pain in pregnant women. The following case summarizes the important nature of epigastric pain.[1] A woman

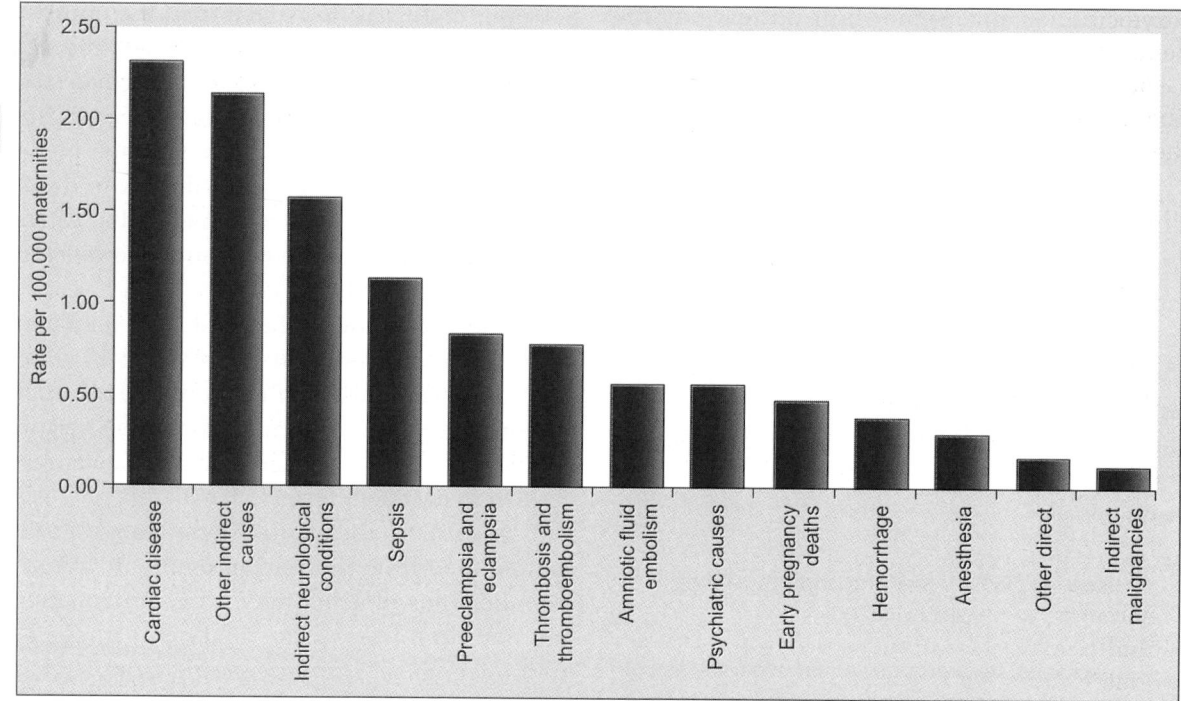

Fig. 17.2: Causes of maternal mortality in the UK between 2006 and 2008 per 100,000 maternities
Source: Modified from Lewis G. (2011). Centre for Maternal and Child Enquiries (CMACE). Saving Mothers' Lives. Reviewing maternal deaths to make motherhood safer: 2006–2008. The Eighth Report on Confidential Enquiries into Maternal Deaths in the United Kingdom. [online] Available from www.cdph.ca.gov/data/statistics/Documents/MO-CAPAMR-CMACE-2006-08-BJOG-2011.pdf. [Accessed May, 2013].

presented to an emergency department in early third trimester with epigastric pain. Her blood pressure was greater than 150/90 mm Hg and she had proteinuria +++. She was diagnosed as having "gastritis" and discharged home, where she collapsed and died shortly afterward. Autopsy showed a cerebral hemorrhage and the typical histological features of preeclampsia.

For the second triennia running, management of systolic hypertension in preeclampsia featured in the "top 10 recommendations". Again, this was the "single most serious failing in the clinical care provided to mothers with preeclampsia". It is important to recognize that systolic hypertension predisposes to the increased risk of cerebral hemorrhage, and high systolic blood pressures should be considered as a medical emergency. The advice regarding the level of systolic blood pressure and clinical situation in which to initiate treatment did not differ from that of the previous triennia and this has led to similar recommendations being made in the National Institute for Health and Clinical Excellence (NICE) guideline on hypertension in pregnancy.[1,6] This is an example of how the confidential enquiry process and organizations, such as NICE, are integrated in informing and improving clinical practice. The NICE hypertension in pregnancy guideline recommends a target blood pressure of 150 mm Hg for antihypertensive therapy to be commenced, with the first agent of choice being oral labetalol for moderate preeclampsia.[16] In severe preeclampsia, treatment may be either oral or intravenous with labetalol, nifedipine or hydralazine or a combination of these medications.[1,16]

The management of the third stage of labor was again a common theme with this and the previous triennia.[1] In this triennium, three women who died from cerebral hemorrhage developed very high blood pressures after giving birth and all were administered syntometrine for active management of third stage. The confidential enquiry report concluded that syntometrine should not be used as a routine drug for the management of the third stage of labor, advising that syntocinon (oxytocin) was as effective to avoid postpartum hemorrhage (PPH) without the adverse side effects associated with syntometrine. The NICE guideline has also supported the recommendation of the use of intramuscular oxytocin as the routine medication for the active management of third stage (Box 17.6).[1]

> **Box 17.6:** Key learning points arising from late 2000s
>
> - Importance of the treatment of systolic hypertension as per NICE guidelines
> - Avoid use of syntometrine for active management in third stage in women with elevated blood pressure in labor

■ INTERNATIONAL PERSPECTIVES

Maternal mortality and morbidity is an imperative global health challenge. Reducing maternal mortality and improving maternal health worldwide was set as a millennium development goal 5 (MDG 5) by the United Nations. The target of MDG 5 is to reduce the MMR by three quarters by 2015 as well as attain universal access to reproductive health.[17] This goal was set in 1990, and although many developing countries have made significant strides to achieve this goal, and with only 2 more years to go, the target is unlikely to be met.[14,17] There are many reasons why achieving this goal has been difficult including the lack of reliable and accurate data, especially in relation to developing countries, where maternal mortality is not only high, but systems of reporting maternal deaths are often lacking, and fail to take into consideration maternal deaths that occur in the home setting.[14] Approximately 358,000 maternal deaths occurred worldwide in 2008 representing a 34% reduction from 1990. In spite of this decline in maternal mortality, the divide between developed and developing nations is obvious with 99% of these maternal deaths occurring in developing countries.[14] Of these deaths, 87% arose in sub-Saharan Africa and South Asia, accounting for 313,000 of the 358,000 maternal deaths worldwide in 2008. The true tragedy behind all these statistics is both the loss of a young woman with all her life ahead of her but also the hard fact that many of the deaths are preventable.[3] Postpartum hemorrhage remains the most significant cause of death

from childbirth in developing countries but it is important not to lose focus on the prevention and management of hypertensive disease in pregnancy, with the many valuable lessons learnt from the UK confidential enquiries.[14]

South African Perspective

South Africa established a confidential enquiry into maternal deaths in October 1997. For the triennium of 2005–2007, about 4,077 maternal deaths were reported, representing an increase from the previous triennia, but this was likely to have represented improved reporting and reflecting the increased number of maternal deaths due to nonpregnancy-related infections such as human immunodeficiency virus (HIV). There is a wide variation in the MMR in South Africa due to varying reporting systems and infrastructure in different provinces. Examples of MMR in different parts of South Africa vary from anywhere between 150 per 100,000 live births to 578 per 100,000 live births. The majority of maternal deaths occur outside health institutions and are therefore not reported or included in the confidential enquiry.[9]

The top five causes of maternal deaths in South Africa include: (1) nonpregnancy-related infection (43.7%); (2) complications of hypertension (15.7%); (3) obstetric hemorrhage [12.4% including both antepartum hemorrhage (APH) and PPH]; (4) pregnancy-related sepsis (9%); and (5) pre-existing maternal disease (6%). These five causes have not changed since the previous triennia. There were a total of 1,819 direct maternal deaths from 2005 to 2007 with 622 of these deaths attributed to hypertension, making hypertension the leading cause of direct maternal deaths in South Africa, remaining unchanged from 1999 to 2007. In the 2005–2007 triennial report, maternal deaths as a result of hypertensive disease were noted to reduce by 13.7%. This was felt to be due to adherence of national guidelines on the management of hypertension (Table 17.2).

As with the more recent reports from the UK confidential enquiries, the South African confidential enquiry has also adopted "10 key recommendations" as part of their report. Unlike the "top 10 recommendations" of the UK confidential enquiry report, which often specify diseases or aspects of disease management to target, those

Table 17.2: A comparison of direct cause maternal mortality in South Africa over three triennia (comparison by percentage of overall mortality rates)

Causes	1999–2001		2002–2004		2005–2007	
	Number (N)	Rate (%)	Number (N)	Rate (%)	Number (N)	Rate (%)
Hypertension	507	20.7	628	19.1	622	15.7
PPH	240	9.8	313	9.5	383	9.7
Pregnancy-related sepsis	210	8.6	274	8.3	223	5.6
Abortion	120	4.9	114	3.5	136	3.4
Acute collapse	134	5.5	107	3.2	128	3.2
APH	100	4.1	129	3.9	108	2.7
Anesthetic related	76	3.1	91	2.8	107	2.7
Ectopic pregnancy	27	1.1	47	1.4	55	1.4
Embolism	48	2	64	1.9	57	1.4

Abbreviations: PPH, postpartum hemorrhage; APH, antepartum hemorrhage)
Source: Modified from NCCEMD (2008). Saving Mothers 2005–2007. Fourth Report on Confidential Enquiry into Maternal Deaths in South Africa. Expanded Executive Summary. [online] Available from www.doh.gov.za/docs/reports/2007/savingmothers.pdf. [Accessed May, 2013].

in the South African report are more general with a focus on policy, protocol, professional development and training.[9]

New Zealand Perspective

New Zealand has a Perinatal and Maternal Mortality Review Committee (PMMRC), which is responsible for the production of a report on perinatal and maternal mortality since 2005. This review committee also works in collaboration with the AMOSS to report on rare conditions associated with maternal morbidity.[18] Prior to this, the review of maternal mortality was conducted by the Maternal Mortality Review Committee, but this ceased in 1995.[7]

The MMR in New Zealand in 2007 was 16.8 per 100,000 maternities compared with 23 per 100,000 maternities in 2006. In 2007, there were 11 maternal deaths from 65,602 maternities; of these deaths five were direct, five indirect and one unclassifiable. Of the direct deaths, two were attributed to preeclampsia, making this the most common cause of direct maternal death in 2007.[18] Recommendations arising from this report relating to hypertension in pregnancy included adopting evidence-based management of hypertension in pregnancy, as advised by the Society of Obstetric Medicine of Australia and New Zealand.[18] Further

specific details surrounding each maternal death in New Zealand are not contained in the report.[18]

Australian Perspective

Australia has one of the lowest rates of maternal mortality worldwide. However, there is much inequality amongst the indigenous Aboriginal and Torres Strait Island population.[19] Between 1997 and 1999, the overall MMR was 8.2 per 100,000 confinements representing a decreasing trend in the MMR over the preceding 24 years. Table 17.3 shows the number of direct, indirect and MMR in Australia between 1973 and 2005. However, the MMR within the Aboriginal and Torres Strait Island population is higher than that of the nonindigenous population.[20] The MMR between 1997 and 1999 in Aboriginal and Torres Strait Islander population was 23.5 per 100,000 confinements compared to 7.2 per 100,000 confinements in the nonindigenous population (Fig. 17.3). This huge disparity reflects the poor health status of the Aboriginal and Torres Strait Island population, and the comparatively higher (three times) MMR than in nonindigenous women has been a common trend over the past three triennial reports.[20] Overall the Aboriginal and Torres Strait Islander populations only contribute 3.1% of total confinements in Australia. Thus, while this population has a higher

Table 17.3: Direct, indirect and maternal mortality rate (per 100,000 confinements) in Australia between 1973 and 2005

Triennium	Direct Deaths	Indirect Deaths	Maternal Mortality Rate
1973–1975	60	32	12.7
1976–1978	52	35	12.8
1979–1981	54	34	12.9
1982–1984	42	25	9.4
1985–1987	32	30	8.5
1988–1990	37	33	9.3
1991–1993	27	22	6.2
1994–1996	46	20	9.1
1997–1999	34	30	8.4
2000–2002	32	52	11.1
2003–2005	29	36	8.4

Source: Modified from Sullivan E, Hall B, King J (2008). Maternal Deaths in Australia 2003–2005. Maternal Death Series Number 3. Cat. No. PER 42. Australian Institute of Health and Welfare. [online] Available from www.aihw.gov. au/WorkArea/DownloadAsset.aspx?id=10737421514. [Accessed May, 2013].

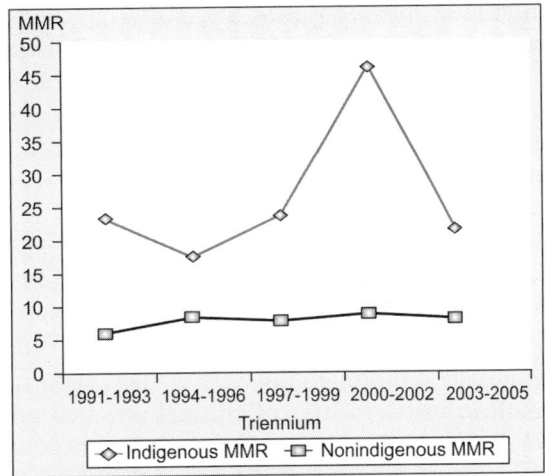

Fig. 17.3: Maternal mortality ratio per 100,000 women giving birth: a comparison between the indigenous and nonindigenous populations in Australia

MMR than the nonindigenous population, the small proportion of confinements dramatically influences the overall MMR in Australia. Additional considerations pertinent to the indigenous communities in Australia include both pre-existing medical comorbidities and living locality of these populations, with many remote from high level medical care, particularly in emergency situations.[20] In addition, this inequality extends to women in rural and remote Australia who inevitably have poor access to maternity services.[21]

Australia has produced triennial reports on maternal deaths, which are currently compiled by the Australian Institute of Health and Welfare (AIHW), and have been in circulation since 1964. The information for the reports is obtained from state and territory maternal death enquiries and the Australian Bureau of Statistics, which then report to the National Advisory Committee on Maternal Deaths.[20]

From 1997 to 1999, there were 90 maternal deaths—34 direct, 28 indirect and 28 incidentals. There was a reduction in direct maternal deaths from 46 in the previous triennium representing a declining trend in direct maternal mortality over the past 15 years. The leading cause of direct maternal death was obstetric hemorrhage with eight maternal deaths; seven of these attributed to PPHs. There were six maternal deaths as a result of hypertensive disease in pregnancy making this the equal third most common cause of direct maternal death along with thromboembolism. Of the hypertensive maternal deaths, two were from cerebral hemorrhage, one from cerebral infarct, one from renal failure, one from ventricular fibrillation and in one death the cause was not established.[20]

Recommendations arising from 1997 to 1999 report included the contraindicated use of ergometrine for third stage management in women with preeclampsia. Women at high risk of hypertensive disease in pregnancy should undergo preconception counseling, while women with a history of preeclampsia, especially if early or recurrent, require counseling about the risks in further pregnancies. As with recommendations arising from the UK confidential enquiry reports, this triennial report advised treatment of severe hypertension, stressing the need for hospitals to have standard protocols for management of hypertension in pregnancy.[20]

The most recent report on maternal deaths in Australia was published in 2008 reflecting the 2003–2005 triennium.[22] In this triennium, there were 65 maternal deaths, accounting for one maternal death for every 11,896 women giving birth, with a MMR of 8.4 per 100,000 women giving birth (confinement). Hypertensive disorders of pregnancy accounted for five maternal deaths making it the second highest cause of direct maternal mortality along with thromboembolism. Amniotic fluid embolism was the leading cause of direct maternal mortality between 2003 and 2005 accounting for eight deaths. This most recent report highlighted the need for improvements to the current system for reporting maternal deaths. It emphasized the deficiency of the current system in obtaining quality information in relation to risk factors, clinical pathways and management in order to provide a thorough analysis of each maternal death in order to inform clinical practice and policy. It also appreciated that the current system of reporting maternal death is multitiered and is not mandatory on a national level. At the present time, maternal deaths are reported at a state and territory level to maternal mortality committees as well as from registered deaths. The AIHWs National Perinatal Statistics Unit then requests this data from each state and territory, where it is then reviewed using the classifications of the confidential enquiries into maternal deaths from the UK as the gold standard.[22]

Information about rare events such as maternal mortality and rare causes of maternal morbidity is collected by the AMOSS as well as state and territory morbidity and mortality review committees.[19] In Australia, data on maternal and perinatal health is required by national, state and territory governments as it is the epidemiological marker of maternal health; however, the review process is handled at a state/territory level with no standardized approach.[7,8,19] It should be noted that in Australia, there is no "nationally agreed method to review or report maternal deaths", nor is there funding at a national level for the collection and production of a report on maternal mortality.[19]

United States of America Perspective

Similar to Australia and many other countries around the world, the United States of America (USA) also lacks a coordinated confidential enquiry process into maternal deaths. It has been recognized that review of maternal deaths facilitates making pregnancy safer, as lessons can be learnt and avoidable factors prevented. In the 1930s, eclampsia was a major cause of maternal

death in the US. However, with the introduction of routine antenatal care, and an emphasis on blood pressure and proteinuria screening for early detection of preeclampsia, this has declined. As with the reports from the UK confidential enquiries, widespread use of $MgSO_4$ saw a reduction in the incidence of eclampsia as well as early induction and delivery in those women with preeclampsia.[23]

In 2010, the MMR in the USA was reported as 12.7 per 100,000 live births. However, variations between the states still exist, from lows of 1.4 deaths per 100,000 live births for Maine, and 4.3 deaths per 100,000 live births for Indiana (lowest MMR for a larger state) reaching as high as 26.0 for Michigan and 41.6 for the District of Columbia.[24]

According to information collected by Amnesty International from the US in 2008–2009, the top five causes of maternal death were: (1) embolism accounting for 20% of maternal deaths; (2) hemorrhage (17% of maternal deaths); (3) preeclampsia and eclampsia 16%; (4) infection 13%; and (5) cardiomyopathy 8%.[24]

There are many factors which contribute to the high MMR in the US including inequality to health care access. Access to healthcare is largely influenced by the need to have private health insurance, which can be out of reach of the more deprived population who tend to belong to the ethnic minority group. As with other countries around the world, it is the ethnic minority group who are at increased risk of death with African-American women four times more likely to die of pregnancy-related complications than white women. In terms of hypertensive disease in pregnancy, African-American and Latina women diagnosed with preeclampsia or eclampsia were 9.9 and 7.9 more likely to die of complications respectively, compared to white women. Furthermore white women in the USA have an increased MMR compared to women in 24 other industrialized countries.[24]

Canadian Perspective

Like Australia, the UK and many other developed countries, Canada has one of the lowest MMRs.[25-27] In 2004, a special report of maternal mortality and severe morbidity was released by the Canadian perinatal surveillance system, modeled on the principles of the UK confidential enquiries.[25-27]

This report focused on both maternal mortality and severe morbidity between 1997 and 2000. During this time, the MMR was 6.1 per 100,000 live births. The leading causes of direct maternal mortality were both pulmonary embolism and pregnancy-induced hypertension, with each accounting for nine maternal deaths and 20.5% of direct maternal deaths. The MMR for hypertensive disease in pregnancy was 0.85 per 100,000 live births. In relation to cause of deaths from hypertensive disease, five women died from intracranial hemorrhage and the other four causes of maternal mortality were not specified. Five of the women who died had received or were receiving medical treatment for their hypertensive disorder prior to their death. It is important to recognize that Canada is a country comprised of many provinces and territories, with diverse reporting methods. Further details surrounding the clinical scenario of these maternal deaths were not included in the report.[25]

CONCLUSION

Valuable lessons have been learnt from the confidential enquiries, with the model from the UK as the gold standard. In the developed world, it is clear that whilst the number of mothers dying from pregnancy-related complications is reducing due to improved access, healthcare and better teamwork, healthcare teams should not be complacent as new challenges such as obesity, older mothers and comorbidities will pose new challenges. It is encouraging to note that in developed countries, a better understanding of the pathophysiology of preeclampsia/eclampsia, appropriate control of blood pressure, fluid management, multidisciplinary teamwork, timely delivery of the fetus and good management guidelines have led to the reduction of deaths from complications of hypertensive disease in pregnancy. However, the numbers dying from hypertensive disorders can still be reduced further as it is treatable and complications are avoidable.

Confidential enquiries into maternal deaths are a valuable tool to review the events that lead to the tragic events. Lessons can always be learnt from such events and practice can be changed in order to benefit the many women who access healthcare when they are pregnant. Unfortunately, in spite of advances in medical and midwifery practice, many women still die as a result of substandard care. It is important that where possible, countries continue to recognize the importance of such an audit so that not only outcomes can be improved, but the goals set by the United Nations (MDG 5) can be also achieved by 2015 and the improvements sustained in the long term (Box 17.7).

Box 17.7: Key learning points from the confidential enquiries

- Hypertensive disease in pregnancy remains an important cause of maternal mortality in both developed and developing countries
- Improving access to routine antenatal care has been pivotal in reducing deaths from hypertension in pregnancy
- Automated blood pressure machines may underestimate blood pressure readings in preeclampsia
- The recognition and treatment of systolic hypertension (> 150 mm Hg systolic) reduces the risk of intracranial hemorrhage
- Women complaining of epigastric pain in pregnancy should have their blood pressure assessed and urine checked for proteinuria before being dismissed as having gastritis
- The use of $MgSO_4$ has reduced the incidence of eclampsia
- Ergometrine is contraindicated in the third stage in women with hypertension
- A multidisciplinary approach to the care of women with severe preeclampsia/eclampsia helps to reduce the morbidity and mortality associated with the disease
- Agreed guidelines for the management of preeclampsia/eclampsia should be available in obstetric units
- Early recognition and transfer to appropriate facilities is vital.

REFERENCES

1. Lewis G. (2011). Centre for Maternal and Child Enquiries (CMACE). Saving Mothers' Lives. Reviewing maternal deaths to make motherhood safer: 2006-2008. The Eighth Report on Confidential Enquiries into Maternal Deaths in the United Kingdom. [online] Available from www.cdph.ca.gov/data/statistics/Documents/MO-CAPAMR-CMACE-2006-08-BJOG-2011.pdf. [Accessed May, 2013].

2. Draycott T, Lewis G, Stephens I. (2011). Executive summary. [online] Available from www.mdeireland. com/pub/SML11_Executive_Summary.pdf. [Accessed May, 2013].

3. World Health Organization. (2004). Beyond the Numbers. Reviewing maternal deaths and complications to make pregnancy safer. [online] Available from whqlibdoc.who.int/publications/2004/9241591838.pdf. [Accessed May, 2013].

4. Lewis G. (2007). Confidential Enquiry into Maternal and Child Health (CEMACH). Saving Mothers' Lives. Reviewing maternal deaths to make motherhood safer: 2003-2005. The Seventh Report of the Confidential Enquiries into Maternal Deaths in the United Kingdom. [online] Available from www.mdeireland.com/pub/SML07_Report.pdf. [Accessed May, 2013].

5. Weindling AM. The confidential enquiry into maternal and child health (CEMACH). Arch Dis Child. 2003;88(12):1034-7.

6. Sullivan E, Pollock W. (2007). Draft options paper for discussion. Maternal Mortality and Morbidity Workshop December 10, 2007. Monitoring of maternal morbidity and mortality in Australia. Part One. Background information and current national and international context. [online] Available from www.preru.unsw.edu.au/preruweb.nsf/resources/ NACMM_2/$file/Microsoft+Word+-+Workshop_ Part+One.pdf. [Accessed May, 2013].

7. Sullivan E, Pollock W. (2007). Draft options paper for discussion. Maternal Mortality and Morbidity Workshop December 10, 2007. Monitoring of Maternal morbidity and mortality in Australia. Part Two. Options for the Future. [online] Available from www.preru.unsw.edu.au/preruweb.nsf/ resources/NACMM_2/$file/Microsoft+Word+- +Workshop_+Part+Two.pdf. [Accessed May 2013].

8. Stewart DE. A broader context for maternal mortality. CMAJ. 2006;174(3):302-3.

9. NCCEMD. (2008). Saving Mothers 2005-2007: Fourth Report on Confidential Enquiries into Maternal Deaths in South Africa. Expanded Executive Summary. [online] Available from www. doh.gov.za/docs/reports/2007/savingmothers.pdf. [Accessed May, 2013].

10. Lewis G, Drife J, Botting B, et al. Why mothers die: report on confidential enquiries into maternal deaths in the United Kingdom, 1994-1996. London, United Kingdom: Department of Health and Her Majesty's Stationary Office, 1998.

11. Lewis G, Drife J (Eds). Why Mothers Die 1997-1999: The Confidential Enquiries into Maternal Death in the United Kingdom, Illustrated Edition. London, United Kingdom: Royal College of Obstetricians and Gynaecologists Press; 2001.

12. Lewis G (Ed). Why Mothers Die 2000-2002: The Sixth Report of the Confidential Enquiries into Maternal Deaths in the United Kingdom, Illustrated Edition. London, United Kingdom: Royal College of Obstetricians and Gynaecologists Press; 2004.

13. Altman D, Carroli G, Duley L, et al. Do women with pre-eclampsia, and their babies, benefit from magnesium sulphate? The Magpie Trial: a randomised placebo-controlled trial. Lancet. 2002;359(9321):1877-90.

14. World Health Organization. (2010). Trends in maternal mortality: 1990 to 2008. Estimates developed by WHO, UNICEF, UNFPA and The World Bank. [online] Available from www.who.int/reproductivehealth/ publications/monitoring/9789241500265/en/. [Accessed May, 2013].

15. Robson S. Pre-eclampsia and eclampsia. In: MacLean AB, Neilson JP (Eds). Maternal Morbidity and Mortality, Illustrated Edition. London, United Kingdom: Royal College of Obstetricians and Gynaecologists Press; 2002.

16. National Institute for Health and Clinical Excellence. (2010). Hypertension in pregnancy: The management of hypertensive disorders during pregnancy. NICE clinical guideline 107. [online] Available from www.nice.org.uk/nicemedia/ live/13098/50418/50418.pdf. [Accessed May, 2013].

17. Rasch V. Maternal death and the Millennium Development Goals. Dan Med Bull. 2007;54(2): 167-9.

18. Perinatal and Maternal Mortality Review Committee. (2009). Perinatal and Maternal Mortality in New Zealand 2007: Third Report to the Minister of Health—July 2008 to June 2009. Wellington: Ministry of Health. [online] Available from www.hqsc.govt. nz/assets/PMMRC/Publications/Third-PMMRC-report-2008-09.pdf. [Accessed May, 2013].

19. Australian Institute of Health and Welfare, Australian Government. (2011). Maternity data in Australia: a review of sources and gaps. AIHW National Perinatal Epidemiology and Statistics Unit. Bulletin 87. [online]. Available from www.aihw.gov.au/ WorkArea/DownloadAsset.aspx?id=10737419978. [Accessed May, 2013].

20. Slaytor EK, Sullivan EA, King JF. (2004). Maternal Deaths in Australia 1997–1999. Australian Institute of Health and Welfare. AIHW Cat. No. PER 24. Maternal Deaths Series Number 1. [online] Available from www.aihw.gov.au/WorkArea/DownloadAsset. aspx?id=10737421517. [Accessed May, 2013].

21. Department of Health and Ageing. (2008). Improving Maternity Services in Australia. A Discussion Paper from the Australian Government. Commonwealth of Australia. [online] Available from www.health.

gov.au/internet/main/publishing.nsf/Content/2
BAF08EE5C0ECDA3CA2575640000CFAC/$File/
Improving_Maternity_Services_In_Australia.pdf.
[Accessed May, 2013].

22. Sullivan E, Hall B, King J. (2008). Maternal Deathsin
Australia 2003-2005. Maternal Death Series Number
3. Cat. No. PER 42. Australian Institute of Health and
Welfare. [online] Available from www.aihw.gov.au/
WorkArea/DownloadAsset.aspx?id=10737421514.
[Accessed May, 2013].

23. Amnesty International. (2010). Deadly Delivery: The
Maternal Health Care Crisis in the USA. [online]
Available from www.amnestyusa.org/research/
reports/deadly-delivery-the-maternal-health-care-
crisis-in-the-usa. [Accessed May, 2013].

24. Xu J, Kochanek KD, Tejada-Vera B, et al. (2009).
Deaths: Preliminary Data for 2007. National Vital
Statistics Reports. [online]. Available from www.
cdc.gov/nchs/data/nvsr/nvsr58/nvsr58_01.pdf.
[Accessed May, 2013].

25. Rusen ID, Liston R. (2004). Special Report on
Maternal Mortality and Severe Morbidity in
Canada. Enhanced Surveillance: The Path to Pre-
vention. [online] Available from publications.
gc.ca/collections/Collection/H39-4-44-2004E.pdf.
[Accessed May, 2013].

26. Lisonkova S, Bartholomew S, Rouleau J, et al.
Temporal trends in maternal mortality in Canada
I: estimates based on vital statistics data. J Obstet
Gynaecol Can. 2011;33(10):1011-9.

27. Lisonkova S, Liu S, Bartholomew S, et al. Temporal
trends in maternal mortality in Canada II: estimates
based on hospitalization data. J Obstet Gynaecol
Can. 2011;33(10):1020-30.

Index

Note: Page numbers in **bold** and *italic* refer to tables and figures respectively.